RECENT ADVANCES
IN DERMATOLOGY

ARTHUR ROOK

MD FRCP

Consultant Dermatologist, Addenbrooke's Hospital, Cambridge
Civil Consultant in Dermatology to the Royal Air Force

RECENT ADVANCES IN DERMATOLOGY

EDITED BY

ARTHUR ROOK

NUMBER FOUR

CHURCHILL LIVINGSTONE

Edinburgh London and New York

1977

CHURCHILL LIVINGSTONE
Medical Division of Longman Group Limited

Distributed in the United States of America by
Longman Inc., 19 West 44th Street, New York,
N.Y. 10036, and by associated companies,
branches and representatives throughout
the world

First published 1977

ISBN 0 443 01318 7
Library of Congress Cataloging in Publication Data
Rook, Arthur J.
    Recent advances in dermatology. No. 4.
    Includes bibliographies and index.
    1. Skin—Diseases—Addresses, essays, lectures.
    I. Title. [DNLM: 1. Dermatology—Period.
    W1 RE105UJ]
RL75.R63 1977   616.5   76–41899

Printed in Great Britain

PREFACE

In this fourth edition of *Recent Advances in Dermatology* I have continued the policy on which the third edition was based. Reviewers of that edition have in general endorsed my conviction that, despite the multiplicity of monographs, reports of symposia and review articles covering most specialised aspects of dermatology, there is a need for practical reviews on the laboratory and clinical aspects of common diseases. With one exception the topics selected are different from those included in the third edition, so that the two volumes may be regarded as complementary. Topical therapy has been covered again because in our patients' interests the voluminous literature requires frequent expert and critical reassessment. The chapters on Opportunism and Skin Infections and on Sexually Transmitted Diseases survey increasingly important aspects of the relationship between host and potential pathogens. The third edition considered bacterial, fungal and viral infections from a different viewpoint.

Authors have been asked to review the literature of the past ten years—in the case of topical therapy, only the last four—but to do so selectively, to provide a critical, useful and readable chapter rather than a comprehensive but dreary catalogue of all the relevant publications of the decade. Some authors have very properly chosen to include some references to older work, when by doing so the new work can be better seen in context, and more clearly understood.

Cambridge, 1976   ARTHUR ROOK

CONTRIBUTORS

BERNARD ACKERMAN MD
Skin and Cancer Unit, New York University Medical Center, New York, N.Y., U.S.A.

JOHN ALMEYDA MB BS MRCP
Consultant Dermatologist, Enfield Group Hospitals

BRIAN BAGNALL PhD
Animal Health Division, Smith, Kline & French Laboratories Limited, Mundells, Welwyn Garden City, Hertfordshire

R. D. CATTERALL FRCP (Edin)
Director, James Pringle House, The Middlesex Hospital, London; Consultant Physician in Sexually Transmitted Diseases, St John's Hospital for Diseases of the Skin and the Institute of Dermatology, London

RICHARD C. CONNORS MD
Skin and Cancer Unit, New York University Medical Center, New York, N.Y., U.S.A.

JOHN H. EPSTEIN MD
Department of Dermatology, University of California Medical Center, San Francisco, California, U.S.A.

KATHERINE GRICE MD(Lond) DCH(Eng)
Consultant Dermatologist, Watford General Hospital and Hemel Hempstead General Hospital

R. R. M. HARMAN MB BS FRCP
Consultant Dermatologist, Royal Infirmary and Southmead Hospital, Bristol

ASHLEY LEVANTINE MB BS MRCP
Consultant Dermatologist, Chichester and Worthing Districts

A. W. McKENZIE MB ChB(Edin) MRCP(Lond)
Consultant Dermatologist, Norwich and Norfolk Hospital

W. C. NOBLE MSc PhD MIBiol MRCPath
Reader in Bacteriology, St John's Hospital for Diseases of the Skin, London

ROBIN D. G. PEACHEY MD FRCP
Consultant Dermatologist, Royal Infirmary, Frenchay Hospital and South-mead Hospital, Bristol

ARTHUR ROOK MD FRCP
Consultant Dermatologist, Addenbrooke's Hospital, Cambridge; Civil Consultant in Dermatology to the Royal Air Force

NEVILLE ROWELL MD FRCP DCH
Consultant Dermatologist, Leeds Regional Health Authority

RICHARD W. SAGEBIEL MD
Department of Pathology, Children's Hospital, San Francisco, California, U.S.A.

J. A. SAVIN MRCP(Lond) MRCP(Edin) DIH
Consultant Dermatologist and Senior Lecturer in Dermatology, Royal Infirmary, Edinburgh

JULIAN VERBOV MD MRCP
Consultant Dermatologist, Liverpool Area Health Authority (Teaching) and Isle of Man Health Services Board; Clinical Lecturer in Dermatology, University of Liverpool

D. S. WILKINSON MD FRCP
Consultant Dermatologist, Buckinghamshire Area Health Authority, High Wycombe District

CONTENTS

1
OPPORTUNISM AND SKIN INFECTIONS

J. A. Savin   W. C. Noble

INTRODUCTION

Traditional distinctions tend to become blurred when dealing with skin infections, and to separate pathogenic from non-pathogenic organisms becomes very difficult. The skin is unique in its galaxy of clinical conditions due to the overgrowth of organisms which are normally resident there—such as trichomycosis axillaris, pityriasis versicolor, and erythrasma. Presumably changes in local resistance are needed for these conditions to occur. Even the word infection is open to debate here. Technically these conditions may not be infections in the usual sense of the word, but as they illustrate so well the response to purely local factors, they will not be excluded from this review.

The term 'opportunistic' should be easy to define precisely. Whether any infection takes place or not, depends on a balance between the attacking qualities of the organism concerned (its virulence), and the resistance to infection of the host. At one end of the scale are those infections in which a highly virulent organism succeeds in breaking the defences of a normally resistant host—a good example of this would be smallpox of the non-vaccinated. At the other end lie those infections with organisms which are usually harmless, but which are able to damage a host whose resistance has been grossly lessened, perhaps by disease or by deliberate immunosuppression. The latter type of situation is easy to accept as opportunistic.

The problem, as with any spectrum, is where to draw the line. Do skin infections with *Staphylococcus aureus*, for example, fall into the opportunistic class? Staphylococcal infections are common enough among those with good general resistance; but many carry the organism on their skin with no clinical sign of infection; some loss of local defence mechanisms is presumably needed for a clinical infection to establish itself. To some extent all infections may be in this sense opportunistic. The skin is again unique in that local alterations, for example in humidity, temperature, sebum content or mechanical integrity, can easily be recognised as playing a major part in allowing some of the common skin diseases to develop. Much of the work on the role of local factors has been with organisms, such as *Staphylococcus aureus*, which some will regard as opportunistic while others do not.

Definitions of opportunism also feel the strain when it comes to patients with common, relatively harmless infections, such as with the wart virus, which may proliferate in conditions of low resistance. Studies, such as those of Morison (1974), showing the high incidence of warts in patients with lack of cellular rather than of humoral immunity, have been of great value in increasing our understanding of the way in which these infections are limited in the normal person.

One further problem in terminology comes with the contrast between an infection, clinically recognisable as such, and colonisation of an area of skin with pathogens, recognisable by in vitro culture but not by the usual physical signs of infection. One important example of this is the regular colonisation of some common dermatoses, such as psoriasis and atopic eczema, with *Staphylococcus aureus*. These dermatoses seem to provide a more favourable environment for growth than normal skin. In this sense this proliferation of organisms is opportunistic.

We have preferred to widen rather than to restrict the opportunistic concept, believing that to allow the discussion to embrace some common skin conditions will be of more value than simply dealing with unusual organisms, admittedly important, but seldom seen in skin clinics. However, widening the definition of opportunism, and hence the scope of the chapter, carries its own disadvantages: the subject matter becomes so great that all areas cannot be discussed in depth, nor can the references quoted be a complete list. Patchiness and omissions must inevitably follow this plan, and only a limited number of selected topics can be dealt with here.

Resistance to infection is a complicated process depending on both non-specific and specific factors. In the non-specific group are included the mechanical integrity of the skin and mucous membranes; contain non-specific bactericidal secretions, for example lysozyme; and finally phagocytosis and the inflammatory response to infection. These mechanisms are reinforced by specific immune responses both humoral and cellular.

Recent advances in this field, therefore, can be split into two major parts. First, there are gains in our knowledge of the qualities of the organisms themselves which allow them to be pathogenic: their attack mechanisms, how they spread, how the different species interact, and the way in which improved identification and classification have helped our understanding of their epidemiology. Secondly, and here the gain has been immense, there is new knowledge about defence mechanisms. Immunology has gone ahead faster than any other branch of medicine over the last few years. We have chosen not to expand this chapter by including a detailed exposition of immunological principles: these can be found elsewhere. However, some knowledge of this is required for an understanding of opportunism. There can be no more beautiful demonstration of immunological principles than the range of defects seen in candidosis.

CANDIDOSIS

Candida albicans is a classic opportunistic pathogen. Candidosis ranges from a brief, trivial, surface infection of the otherwise fit, to an overwhelming and often fatal systemic infection. The seriousness of the infection is roughly proportional to the degree to which the host's defences are compromised. The organism has two growth phases: yeast cells (blastospores) and mycelium. It is a fair working rule that the organism exists as a commensal in the yeast phase only, but that the mycelial phase, with its very clearly defined ultra-structural organelles (Cawson and Rajasingham, 1972), is always to be found in clinical candidal infections. Antigenically the two phases are now known to be both qualitatively and quantitatively different (Evans et al, 1973). So far routine tests for serum antibodies have used only cytoplasmic antigen extracted from the blastospore phase, and this may have given rise to false positive reactions in patients carrying the organism as a commensal. The use of a specific mycelial antigen might help here but the main defence against candida is not through circulating antibodies; indeed it is a deficiency of cellular immunity which is commonly found in chronic mucocutaneous candidosis.

Candidosis is best viewed as an extremely sensitive biological detector of weakness in the body defence system; and, while it is convenient to divide immunological defences into humoral and cellular events, they really form an interlocking series of reactions reinforced by non-specific defence mechanisms such as phagocytosis.

Transient Infections

Even in the common transient local infections, predisposing factors can often be found; for example, candidosis of the groin of healthy male soldiers (Lynch, Minkin and Smith, 1969) was associated with a higher bodyweight than controls, and also a higher incidence of diabetes in the family, and a more frequent intake of systemic steroids in the preceding three months. The birth control pill may also have an effect: in one study women taking the pill were found to harbour *Candida* in the vulva twice as often as controls (Oriel et al, 1972), though this has not been a universal finding (Spellacy et al, 1971). In a separate study (Oriel and Waterworth, 1975), both tetracycline and minocycline rapidly increased the isolation of vaginal yeast even though minocycline has an anticandidal action as well as an antibacterial one. The clinical picture of erosio interdigitale blastomycetica can only be produced experimentally with local occlusion and high humidity (Rebora, Marples and Kligman, 1973).

Candidal vulvo-vaginitis is common in pregnancy. The emphasis has swung away from a purely local cause for this, such as an alteration of pH due to high glycogen content of the vaginal epithelium leading to an increased fermentation by lactobacilli, towards those immunological changes in pregnancy which may act to prevent rejection of the fetus with its range of foreign antigens. Cellular immunity in pregnancy is reduced (Finn et al, 1972), perhaps by an inhibitory serum factor (St Hill, Finn and Denye, 1973).

Newborn infants with candidosis tend to have lower levels of leucocyte myeloperoxidase than uninfected children (Renz et al, 1974), and these workers feel that at least some of the activity of clotrimazole in their study may have been due to stimulating myeloperoxidase activity. Reports of the way in which topical steroids can predispose to candidosis, for example in lichen planus (Cawson, 1968), paved the way for the obvious side effect of oropharyngeal candidosis affecting asthmatics using beclomethasone dipropionate inhalations (Milne and Crompton, 1974).

Systemic Candidosis

Systemic candidosis must be separated from mucocutaneous candidosis. It is seen against a background of severe illness. A characteristic eruption has been described (Bodey and Luna, 1974) which is quite distinct from that of chronic mucocutaneous candidosis. It consists of a variable number of well-circumscribed, firm, raised, red nodules ranging from 0.5 to 1.0 cm in diameter, and was seen in 10 of their 77 patients with systemic candidosis. Biopsy of these nodules showed yeast bodies and pseudohyphae in the dermis and in the blood vessels.

The neutrophil may be a major participant in the defence against systemic candidosis which is seen mainly in those with haematological malignancies. Leukopenia seems to predispose to it. Phagocytosis of *Candida* is not always accompanied by efficient killing of the organism. In one study (Lehrer and Cline, 1969), phagocytosis of *Candida* was successfully achieved by leucocytes from a patient with myeloperoxidase deficiency, and from three patients with chronic granulomatous disease, whose neutrophils fail to generate hydrogen peroxide, but despite this the intracellular *Candida* organisms were not killed.

Chronic Mucocutaneous Candidosis

Mucocutaneous candidosis is a rare condition with many causes. An increasing accuracy in pinpointing the exact deficiency in the host is now being knit together with an improved clinical and genetic classification. This must lead to a better chance of rational treatment for an affected individual, based upon an understanding of the mechanisms operating in his particular case. The problem is a complex one, and deficiencies may not be confined to a single area. For example, a child with a lifelong history of both recurrent pyogenic infection and mucocutaneous candidosis, showed a diminished neutrophil chemotactic responsiveness to account for the former, and a defect in cell-mediated immunity for the latter (Clark et al, 1973).

Investigations of chronic mucocutaneous candidosis have shown a spectrum of immunodeficiency and current classifications may not yet be complete. The comprehensive classification by Higgs and Wells (1973), has been chosen here as the most convenient framework for discussion. The outline of this classification is, for convenience, shown in Table 1.1.

They divided their cases into two main groups. In the first, the infection was associated with one of the defined immunodeficiency syndromes which are dominated by severe infections of various types. Examples include the Swiss type of agammaglobulinaemia, hereditary thymic dysplasia, and the DiGeorge syndrome. Patients in this group thrive poorly and die in early childhood although this is usually from viral or bacterial pneumonia rather than from candidosis. The use of antifungal agents and attempts at grafting fetal tissues, such as bone marrow cells, have met with little success. Fatal graft versus host reactions tend to occur, though this risk seems to be substantially reduced if only HL-A compatible tissue is transplanted.

Table 1.1 Classification of chronic mucocutaneous candidosis (based on Higgs and Wells, 1973)

Group I	Associated with primary immunodeficiencies e.g. Swiss-type agammaglobulinaemia, or hereditary thymic dysplasia
Group II	Candidosis is the main clinical feature
	1. Familial chronic mucocutaneous candidosis
	2. Diffuse chronic mucocutaneous candidosis with or without granulomata
	3. Candida endocrinopathy syndrome
	4. Acquired, e.g. in thymoma

Their second main group, with its four subdivisions, consists of patients who may develop chronic mucocutaneous candidosis early in childhood, but who usually survive at least to early adult life, and whose candidosis of mouth, skin and nails, is responsible for the main clinical features.

Their first subdivision consisted of individuals with the recessively inherited form of mucocutaneous candidosis which they had previously defined (Wells et al, 1972). These patients tend to have responded poorly to prolonged applications of local antifungal agents. Tests of cell-mediated immunity were abnormal in many, but the pattern was variable and did not correlate precisely with the clinical state. One important finding was the high incidence of latent iron deficiency. Iron is important for mitosis and iron deficiency per se seems to associate with reduced cell-mediated immunity both in adults (Jonson et al, 1972) and in malnourished children (Bhaskaram and Reddy, 1975). Wells and Higgs noted the reversal of negative to positive delayed skin tests to Candida in several of their patients after iron therapy, but clinical improvement was not confined to those who showed this change. They felt that iron therapy might have improved the quality of the oral epithelium indirectly, and that the unusual difficulty found in raising the serum iron levels could indicate a fundamental defect in iron metabolism.

It is hard to know how to reconcile this with the known anticandidal effect of transferrin. The systemic candidosis of some patients with leukaemia has been associated with high serum iron levels and an accompanying saturation of iron-binding capacities (Caroline, Rosner and Kozinn, 1969). In vitro, iron-binding proteins such as transferrin inhibit bacterial growth by binding iron so efficiently that none is available to the microorganisms. Some organisms, in reply, also produce iron-binding substances, siderophores, and it has been suspected (*Lancet*, 1974) that the ability of an organism to compete with its host for iron is a feature of pathogenicity.

In mucocutaneous candidosis, the predominant effect may rest upon depressed cell-mediated immunity; other factors may include low levels of myeloperoxidase, and possibly upon changes in the growth of other organisms in the mouth, caused by the low iron levels, which would normally have suppressed growth of the yeast. Other mechanisms may be involved such as the decreased serum complement activity noted in one family with chronic mucocutaneous candidosis (Drew, 1973).

Their next subdivision was termed 'diffuse chronic mucocutaneous candidosis' and included some with granulomas. Though susceptible to bacterial chest and skin infections they usually survive childhood. A detailed analysis of the immunological investigations of 26 patients of this type was published by Valdimarsson et al (1973). Four main immunological patterns emerged. Five patients failed to produce macrophage migration inhibition factors (MIF) in vitro, although the lymphocytes were normally activated to DNA synthesis after challenge with *Candida* antigen. This finding supported the original suggestion of MIF deficiency made first by Chilgren et al in 1969.

If lymphocytes do not release MIF, macrophages will tend not to appear at the site of antigenic stimulus where a mutually stimulating action between lymphocytes and macrophages may be needed for a normal expression of delayed hypersensitivity, and the effective elimination of organisms. Treatment with leucocytes from an HL-A compatible sibling has been highly successful in one case (Valdimarsson et al, 1973); the grafted cells remained competent in the recipient, and the clinical benefit persisted for the 17 months of observation afterwards.

Two patients with adequate MIF, but defective macrophages, were detected; interestingly both showed granuloma formation, a feature not seen in those with defective MIF formation. Nine patients with absent delayed hypersensitivity also failed to produce MIF but their lymphocytes were not activated by *Candida* in vitro. This was thought to have been due to a factor in their serum specifically inhibiting *Candida*-induced lymphocyte transformation. In the 10 other patients no abnormalities of humoral or cellular immunity could be found.

'Immunological rehabilitation' will depend upon the exact range of defects encountered in a particular patient. Attention must also be directed to associated immunoglobulin abnormalities in view of the report of impaired IgG precipitating antibodies to *Candida*, and lowered salivary IgA antibodies to *Candida*, in some cases (Lehner, Wilton and Ivanyi, 1972).

Transfer factor (TF) is a non-antigenic substance isolated from leucocytes which is capable of transferring immunological reactivity. Its use avoids the risk of graft versus host reactions, and sensitisation to HL-A and other antigens. Successful treatment with transfer factor has been recorded (Pabst and Swanson, 1972; Valdimarsson et al, 1972b; Mackie et al, 1975), sometimes aided by the use of amphotericin B (Feigin et al, 1974). This treatment seems likely to help only those patients with reduced lymphocyte transformation to *Candida*, rather than those with inadequate production of MIF as their primary fault. For the latter, a transfusion of HL-A compatible leucocytes is a possibility: in one patient (Valdimarsson et al, 1972a), already referred to above, a remarkable response persisted for a 17 month period of observation, implying that the grafted cells were remaining functionally competent in the recipient.

The *Candida*-endocrinopathy syndrome is inherited as an autosomal recessive trait. Its known associations have increased to include Hashimoto's disease, pernicious anaemia, chronic active hepatitis and alopecia areata (Stankler and Bewsher, 1972). The incidence of organ-specific antibodies (Blizzard, Chee and Davis, 1967), suggests an autoimmune mechanism. One recent 26-year-old patient has been reported to have developed multiple squamous cell carcinomata of the oral cavity (Richman et al, 1975). This early onset might suggest a defective immunological surveillance, but also *Candida albicans* seems able to induce epithelial hyperplasia (Cawson, 1973).

The final group of cases was of cutaneous candidosis occurring for the first time later in life, usually over the age of 50; in some ways these echo the endocrine-candidosis group, with a thymic tumour underlying a tendency to autoimmune diseases such as myasthenia gravis (Montes et al, 1968; Schoch, 1971), as well as defective cellular immunity.

DERMATOPHYTE INFECTIONS

In general, the balance between the dermatophyte and its host is less evenly poised than is the case with *Candida*. Unlike *Candida*, chronic dermatophyte skin infections are common in many apparently healthy people. This could imply that local factors such as mechanical trauma (Abdallah, 1971), blistering (Rosenthal and Baer, 1966), moisture (Allen and Taplin, 1973), and the anatomy of the toe spaces, are of more importance than are alterations in immunity.

Nevertheless there has been a steady stream of reports of extravagant fungal infections in those with abnormal immunity: for example, a *Microsporum equinum* infection of the scalp of an adult taking prednisolone for breast carcinoma (O'Grady, English and Warin, 1972), mycetoma formation by *Trichophyton rubrum* in a patient on prednisone for asthma (Burgoon et al, 1974), subcutaneous abscesses in a patient on steroids for pemphigoid (Thorne and Fusaro, 1971), and a chronic *Epidermophyton floccosum* infection in a lymphoma patient with immune deficiency (Levene, 1973). Mixed dermatophyte and *Candida* infections have been seen in patients with thymic tumours (Baer et al, 1964; Savin, unpublished observations). Bagnall and Grünberg (1972) quote the very striking example of an epidemic of generalised *Trichophyton mentagrophytes* infections in capuchin monkeys: only those grossly debilitated by worm parasites were affected.

The whole subject of the immunocompetence of those with chronic fungal infections has recently come under review. While it is local factors which are of the greatest importance in acquiring an infection, it has been stated that 80 per cent of men chronically infected with dermatophytes have failed to reject this infection for immunological reasons (Jones, Reinhardt and Rinaldi, 1974). They suggest the mechanism may either be a relatively specific lack of cell-mediated immunity to trichophytin, or a curious response in which a brisk type I humoral immunity antagonises cell-mediated immunity. The propensity of atopics to develop immediate humoral immunity seems to be linked with their special liability to dermatophytosis (Jones, Reinhardt and Rinaldi, 1973), and supporting this is the association of asthma or hay fever, rather than atopic dermatitis itself, with chronic fungal infections.

There are of course differences between the types of fungus. Hanifin, Ray and Lobitz (1974) investigated one group of patients with *T. rubrum* infections, and another with *T. mentagrophytes* infections, for immediate and delayed cutaneous reactivity to trichophytin. The *T. rubrum* cases were likely to show either no reactivity at all, or only the immediate type; while the mentagrophytes cases usually had delayed hypersensitivity, with or without the immediate type. Curiously, Knight (1973) noted that a positive delayed reaction to trichophytin did not affect the ease with which he could infect human volunteers with *T. mentagrophytes*; in this his findings differed from those of Jones et al (1974) who found a close association between cell-mediated immunity to trichophytin and resistance to fungal infection.

Several other factors may be important in determining whether a patient develops a chronic fungal infection. For example, a significant number of elevated glucose-tolerance curves was found in one study of 29 patients with recurrent *T. rubrum* infections (Jolly and Carpenter, 1969), There may be interactions between the normal skin flora and the fungus: *T. mentagrophytes*, for instance, can, by its penicillin production, increase the proportion of penicillin resistant bacteria in the area (Bibel and Lebrun, 1975). The role of serum fungal inhibitory factors is not yet understood (Carlisle et al, 1974).

Racial differences must also be considered in assessing results. Blank, Mann and Reale (1974) have found differences between caucasoids and negroids in Philadelphia with respect to their experience of dermatophyte infections. Of children attending the clinics, 91.5 per cent were negroid, and perhaps these differences were due to socioeconomic status. But the observations of Allen and Taplin (1973) in Vietnam, that US servicemen, both caucasoid and negroid, became infected with zoophilic *T. mentagrophytes*, whilst the Vietnamese military and civilian population were infected with *T. rubrum*, might imply genuine racial differences.

IMMUNOSUPPRESSION

By immunosuppression is meant a state in which established immunity and the response to new antigens are impaired (Bagshawe, 1972). The term covers changes in cell-mediated as well as antibody-mediated immunity. Whilst immunosuppression may occur naturally in diseases of the lympho-reticular system, it may also be induced for therapeutic reasons and the dermatologist can expect to be shown patients suffering from common infective conditions in an unusual form or from previously rare infections. The subject of immunosuppression and skin infection has been reviewed by Savin and Noble (1975) and for full references the reader is referred to this article.

Skin disease must be seen in perspective in relation to other disease. Eickhoff et al (1972) in a study of 216 patients with renal transplants found that skin infection (22 per cent) was less common than lung (42 per cent) or urinary tract (35 per cent) infection. Turcotte (1972) found six cases of herpes simplex, four of cellulitis and three of herpes zoster amongst 93 transplant patients at risk for a total of 1000 months.

Viral Infections

Perhaps the most interesting development here has been the suggestion that Hodgkin's disease itself is an infective condition, with a long incubation period, transmitted by person-to-person contact (Vianna et al, 1972). Their study of an extended 'epidemic' at a high school in New York State suggested that contacts sometimes developed other types of lymphoma also. The relationship between Hodgkin's disease, infectious mononucleosis and the EB virus, has been discussed in detail (*Lancet*, 1972). However, it would be premature to judge this difficult issue before further evidence is available. It has, of course, been long known that various forms of malignancy, including lymphomata, may be induced by immunosuppression (Allison, 1970). Transfer factor prepared from patients with Hodgkin's disease in remission may prove to be a useful line of treatment (Ng et al, 1975).

Serum copper estimations seem to be a valuable way of assessing the activity of Hodgkin's disease, the level tending to rise as the disease becomes more active. Herpes zoster infections are undoubtedly particularly common in patients with Hodgkin's disease: it has now been shown that serum copper levels fall steadily for as long as 200 days before the episode of shingles (Thorling and Thorling, 1974).

Infections with other viruses in immunosuppression are now very well documented. Extensive herpes simplex may lead to the death of renal transplant patients (Montgomerie et al, 1969) and is also seen in patients with lymphomata (Lynfield, Farhangi and Runnels, 1969). Viral warts can be very frequent in Hodgkin's disease and Perry and Harman (1974) feel that the appearance of luxuriant warts should suggest the possibility of immune deficiency. Brodersen, Genner and Brodthagen (1974) in a study of tuberculin sensitivity, found that children with warts had a mean zone of induration of 10 mm compared with about 15 mm in controls. They point out that it is not possible to decide whether the reduced sensitivity results from the wart infection or whether the warts are a marker for defective cellular immunity. Extensive molluscum contagiosum has been recorded in two patients treated with methotrexate and prednisone (Rosenburg and Yusk, 1970). Varicella may also be associated with mortality in cancer patients (Armstrong et al, 1970) and is more common in those on active therapy than those in remission (Feldman, Hughes and Daniel, 1975). Cytomegalovirus, giant orf and severe progressive vaccinia, have all been described in immunologically compromised patients.

Fungal Infections

Infection with some unusual fungi has been reported, including *Fusarium solani* in acute leukaemia (Cho et al, 1973) and *Phoma* species in induced immunosuppression (Young, Kwon-Chung and Freeman, 1973). More common fungi such as *Pityrosporum, Candida* and *Histoplasma* have all been implicated in secondary disease of patients with some form of immunosuppression.

Bacterial Infections

Infections with the acid-fast bacilli have attracted some attention. *Mycobacterium tuberculosis* was troublesome in patients with neoplastic disease (Kaplan, Armstrong and Rosen, 1974): the severity of tuberculosis being directly related to the vigour of the antineoplastic therapy. *M. marinum* and *M. cheloni* have also been in evidence (Sage and Derrington, 1973; Aaronson and Park, 1974; Graybill et al, 1974). Fraser et al (1975) believe the administration of prednisone and azathioprine to have prevented the granulomatous cell-mediated response and to have resulted in a cellulitic inflammatory reaction to *M. kansasii*.

Non-staphylococcal toxic epidermal necrolysis (scalded skin syndrome) has been reported as associated with deficient cell-mediated immunity in leukaemia, during renal failure, in lymphoma patients, in a patient receiving prednisolone and azathioprine and in drug abuse. In experimental systems, the staphylococcal form of toxic epidermal necrolysis (TEN) can be potentiated by prednisolone and azathioprine (Wiley et al, 1974). *Pseudomonas aeruginosa* may cause blood stream infection with secondary skin lesions during cancer chemotherapy and *Escherichia coli* may also be associated with skin lesions.

Most immunosuppressive agents lack selectivity, and interfere, to some degree with both cellular and humoral immunity. If a generalisation is possible, it is that most of the case reports are of viral, fungal or Gram-negative bacillary infection, suggesting that the main effect is on cell-mediated immunity. It is not easy to separate the complications of immunosuppression from those of bone marrow suppression.

SUPERINFECTION OF EXISTING SKIN DISEASE

It has long been known that skin affected by several dermatoses provides a favourable area for the multiplication of bacteria, including pathogens such as *Staphylococcus aureus*, with or without clinical signs of infection. The dissemination of scales infected in this way has been responsible for several notable epidemics (e.g. Payne, 1967); and the superinfection of the skin disease may do considerable harm to the patients themselves as in the epidemic of acute glomerulonephritis associated with infected scabies (Svartman et al, 1972).

The normal commensal skin flora has recently been divided (Selwyn, 1975) into those strains ('inhibitors') which can in vitro inhibit the growth of other organisms by the production of antibiotic substances, and those which cannot. 'Inhibitor' organisms of this sort were detected in specimens from about one quarter of a normal population. The presence of inhibitor organisms was found to be associated with a significantly low rate of colonisation of skin lesions with potential pathogens in Selwyn's study of patients with skin disease. This protective effect was particularly striking for pathogens acquired after admission into hospital. It applied only to Gram-positive pathogens; indeed the incidence of Gram-negative organisms was slightly higher in the presence of 'inhibitors', perhaps by a mechanism similar to the production of Gram-negative folliculitis in antibiotic treated acne (Fulton et al, 1968), or the curious acneform eruption which can be caused by tetracycline due to the unopposed growth of *P. orbiculare* (Bean, 1971). Further studies of the interactions between the normal skin flora and potential pathogens are clearly due and may be of great value.

Patients with atopic eczema seem to show an especially heavy and frequent colonisation with pathogens, which often cause episodes of clinical infection. A study of 20 children with persisting infantile eczema, over a period of one year (Smith, Alder and Warin, 1975), has shown that if staphylococci are involved, the organisms found in a series of infections in a single patient were likely to be of the same strain in each attack, arising from persistently colonised sites on the patient's own skin. Streptococci were isolated less often than staphylococci, and the few patients with more than one episode of strepto-coccal sepsis yielded different serological types on each occasion. Streptococcal infections seemed to be derived from the infected throats of contacts, rather than by a reactivation of strains colonising the eczema.

Scaling, exudation, and fissuring, all favour the growth of pathogens in atopic eczema, but the idea of an underlying defect in immunological defences in atopy is gaining support. The existence of eczema vaccinatum and herpe-ticum has long suggested this, the most likely explanation being a defect in cell-mediated immunity (Turk, 1970). In addition, a transient IgA deficiency in infancy has formed the basis of an attractive hypothesis about the patho-genesis of atopic eczema (Gerrard, 1973). Other infections have recently been shown to associate with atopy, particularly chronic dermatophytosis (Jones, Reinhardt and Rinaldi, 1973), and molluscum contagiosum (Blattner, 1967). Studies of cell-mediated immunity in atopic dermatitis have yielded confusing results. Anderson and Hjorth (1975) found a slight but significant reduction in the percentage and absolute number of thymus-dependent lymphocytes in a group of patients with atopic eczema, supporting the findings of Luckasen et al (1974) but not those of Schopf and Bohringer (1974). Grove, Reid and Forbes (1975) found some evidence of immuno-deficiency, as judged by a failure to mount delayed hypersensitivity reactions to intradermal antigens, but could detect no abnormality in T- and B-lymphocytes in peripheral blood. Anderson and Hjorth suggest that lympho-cyte function may be impaired by a high IgE level. The final position has yet to be resolved.

Psoriasis contrasts with eczema in its colonisation. Nystrom et al (1971) showed that psoriatic lesions harbour rather fewer *Staphylococcus aureus* organisms than do other chronic dermatoses. Indeed Noble and Savin (1968), using contact plates, found that, while some plaques of psoriasis carried high counts of *Staphylococcus*, there was no statistically significant difference from nearby unaffected skin. Lynfield, Ostroff and Abraham (1972), using a similar contact plate method, confirmed that there was no significant difference between the flora of the psoriatic plaque and adjacent normal skin. This may only be due to a spill-over of organisms on to the surrounding skin, as com-paring a psoriatic plaque with normal skin on a symmetrical site on the opposite side of the body, demonstrated heavier carriage on the psoriasis. They also found, by serial stripping, that staphylococci were most numerous on the surface, but were still demonstrable in the deeper layers, for example after as many as 20 tape strippings. They were able to devise a simple method, using iodine and alcohol, to sterilise plaques and reduce the hazard of the spread of infected scales to other patients in a surgical ward. The quantitative scrubbing method used by Marples, Heaton and Kligman (1973) on psoriatic plaques is more difficult to assess, as the surface scaling of psoriasis is so different from that of normal skin. They found colonisation with staphylococci more frequently, and more heavily, on psoriatic patches than on normal skin. Occlusion with a plastic film led to an explosive increase in staphylococci, and heavily colonised plaques became recognisably redder and more oedematous than before, though not showing the usual signs of infection. These plaques sometimes failed to respond to topical steroid therapy until they had been treated by a topical antibiotic.

No discussion of staphylococci in psoriasis would be complete without mentioning the finding of coagulase positive staphylococci in blood cultures from six out of seven patients with generalised pustular psoriasis (McFadyen and Lyell, 1971). Systemic antibiotic therapy directed against these organisms seemed to terminate episodes of pustulation. The authors speculated that the admittedly sterile pustules in this condition may represent an ide reaction to the circulating organisms. This work has never been substantiated however and Matta (1974) in a careful study, which included a thorough cleaning of the skin, found no staphylococci or other organisms in 17 of 18 blood cultures from eight patients with generalised pustular psoriasis.

HUMIDITY

Naturally Occurring Disease

The effect of humidity on the formation of skin lesions has received some attention recently. The most dramatic studies of natural infection have been those of Allen and Taplin (1973) who found that after four months of exposure to high humidity in Vietnam, 73 per cent of serviceman had fungus lesions of the body or groin. Sulzberger and Akers (1969) described how 70 per cent of lost combat man-days were through skin disease during the rainy season, while in the dry season this fell to 18 per cent. Taplin and his colleagues (1973) relate the prevalence of pyoderma in South America to altitude and to temperature in areas that they describe as 'all humid', though no figures are given. Singh (1973a), from India, showed how the incidence of pyoderma is highest in months when both the temperature and the humidity are high, rather than when either alone is at a maximum. Taplin, Zaias and Rebell (1965) had previously noted how microbial skin lesions became worse in those introduced to a humid tropical environment. The effect of high humidity is to increase enormously the number of organisms on the surface. In the Transvaal, twice as many patients with tinea versicolor present during the summer as during the winter (Finlay, 1974).

Experimental Work

The experiments of O'Brien (1950) demonstrated that increasing local humidity could induce miliaria-like lesions, though the role of organisms in this disease has been the subject of some debate. Although there is no relation between the absolute number of cocci and diptheroids, or Gram-negative rods, and the production of miliaria, the magnitude of the increase may relate to the severity of the induced miliaria.

Humidity has been found to be of great importance in bacterial infections. Savin (1967) found that the *Pseudomonas* lesions associated with a contaminated steroid cream were especially severe in patients who had been treated with polythene occlusion. To produce a vesiculo-pustular rash of the toe webs by experimental applications of *Pseudomonas aeruginosa* requires excessive hydration and the use of water-soaked cotton pads (Hojyo-Tomoka, Marples and Kligman, 1973). *Pseudomonas cepacia*, which causes onion skins to rot, will also infect feet that are water sodden (Taplin, Bassett and Mertz, 1971). Singh (1974) showed that the response was greater when the skin surface was broken during experimental *Pseudomonas* infection. Ammonette and Rosenberg (1973) reported a series of patients whose infection of the toe-web was primarily due to *Proteus* sp. and *Pseudomonas aeruginosa*: all 12 of their patients had tight interdigital spaces in which contact and friction between toes was inevitable, and 10 of the 12 had been using an antibacterial soap. Their remark, that no fungi were isolated, is interesting in the light of the suggestion by Leyden and Kligman (1975) that fungi may be only the precipitating cause of tinea pedis, and that bacterial takeover occurs. They feel that drying the feet with aluminium compounds may be helpful; this is analogous to the drying induced by aluminium compounds in axillary deodorants. An excessive sweating of the feet certainly seems to be responsible for the proliferation of organisms, thought to be streptomycetes and corynebacteria (Young, 1974), found in patients with pitted keratolysis.

Another relevant study is that of Wright and Alexander (1974). The bacterial flora of the external auditory meatus, originally Gram-positive, changes after diving or prolonged exposure to water from the city drinking supply. All their subjects developed otitis externa and the flora gradually became predominantly Gram-negative. Invasion followed tissue maceration; however, when sterile water was used infection and otitis externa did not occur.

McBride, Duncan and Knox (1975) examined the effect of general humidity on the body flora. High temperature and humidity increased the incidence of Gram-negative bacilli, including *Pseudomonas*, on the skin. However, there were great and unexplained individual differences in response. The flora reverted to normal very rapidly on return to a normal environment. They had earlier (Duncan, McBride and Knox, 1969) described how an increase in both temperature and humidity was needed experimentally to bring about changes in the bacterial skin flora.

Knight (1972) reviewed experimental fungus infections in man and concluded that high skin humidity was one of the most important factors. The site of infection was important too in that moist areas, such as the groin, were less likely to heal quickly at the end of the experiment. He found (Knight, 1973) that an experimental fungal lesion could be induced by applying 10^4

spores in 0.05 ml of sterile water to the upper arm and occluding the site for 72 h. If the occlusive dressing became loose, lesions did not occur. Others have used essentially similar methods (Singh, 1973b; Desai, 1974). Local variations have been found in the response: Taplin (personal communication) noted that *T. rubrum* lesions lasted especially long in the humid climate of Miami, and that they could be exacerbated by personal stress as well as climatic conditions.

Rebora, Marples and Kligman (1973a, b) found that a pustular dermatitis could be induced experimentally with *Candida albicans* by applying the yeast to the skin under occlusion. The severity of the lesions was dose related. Applied to the finger-webs under occlusion, *C. albicans* produced typical erosio interdigitalis blastomyetica, a lesion which is well known to occur mainly in those whose hands are kept wet at work. Those affected by candidiasis of the groin were 10 per cent heavier than controls in one study (Lynch, Minkin and Smith, 1969): this might have been related to a higher local humidity in deeper groin folds.

It is probably a gross over-simplification to assume that, in any experimental situation, only one factor has been altered. For example, since most of the studies on increased humidity have relied on local occlusion, it is inevitable that the local temperature has also been raised. The site is also important in experimental infections. Duncan, McBride and Knox (1970) found that it was easier to infect the lower leg or thigh than the arm or back using staphylococci under occlusion, and speculated that circulatory factors might be responsible for this.

Occlusion may alter the sweating of an area for some time after it has been removed and so a return to normal is not truly seen. All of these factors must be taken into account in interpreting experimental skin infections, and in addition host susceptibility may be changed by exposure to the experimental infection itself.

THE NEWBORN SKIN

Newborn skin is widely regarded as an excellent culture medium for staphylococci (Hurst, 1960). In utero the child is protected by the defence mechanisms of its mother until it develops its own systems. Cellular immunity starts when stem cells from the liver or spleen enter the thymus at about the eighth week of gestation, and is complete by the sixteenth week. Immunoglobulin synthesis begins with the production of IgM at about $10\frac{1}{2}$ weeks, IgG at 12 weeks and IgA at 30 weeks (Lawton and Cooper, 1973).

Granulocytes are first seen in the liver at eight weeks, but neonatal granulocytes may still have a low bactericidal capacity towards staphylococci in the first 12 h of life (Coen, Grush and Kauder, 1969). Macrophage function is also poor in neonatal rats but this has not been demonstrated in humans. The complement system, which plays an important role in enhancing the phagocytosis of organisms to which the body has never been exposed, starts to develop at 12 weeks and at term levels of its components have reached slightly more than half of the adult level. Low birth weight infants have diminished opsonic activity against all test particles, particularly Gram-negative organisms (Miller, 1969). Newborn infants who develop candidosis tend to have lower levels of leucocyte myeloperoxidase than normal children (Renz et al, 1974).

Fetal infections, in utero, occur through the placenta and the bloodstream following maternal infection, rather than directly on to the fetal skin (Plotkin, 1975). However, at parturition, organisms come into direct contact with the child's skin: either as part of the 'amniotic infection syndrome' associated with premature rupture of the membranes, or from the birth canal, or from the environment. Amniotic fluid itself does not seem to inhibit the growth of lactobacilli, staphylococci or diphtheroids found in the vagina. Indeed it seems to be a good culture medium (Sarkany and Gaylarde, 1968).

The colonisation of a newborn child's skin is of great interest. Evans, Akpata and Baki (1971) comparing cultures from the vaginal vault at term with the developing skin flora of the newborn child, felt that, while *Staphylococcus epidermidis* in about half of the children studied was derived from the cervical canal of the mother, otherwise the skin organisms correlated poorly with the vaginal flora, and seemed to come from postpartum sources in the nursery. Seasonal factors seemed to be of great importance (Evans et al, 1973a), with a reduced staphylococcal colonisation in autumn and winter. *Escherichia coli* and *Pseudomonas* showed peaks in the summer. Additional humidity greatly increased the *E. coli* and *Pseudomonas* levels in the nares, and outbreaks of infection secondary to contaminated humidifiers have been recorded (Moffet and Allan, 1967). The massive study by McAllister et al (1974) showed that colonisation has reached its height in all areas by the sixth day of life, and again emphasised the preponderance of Gram-negative organisms during the hexachlorophane era.

The combination of possible immuno-incompetence and exposure to pathogens makes frank skin infection a likely alternative to colonisation with skin commensals. Fetal malnutrition, particularly, is associated with significant depression of T-lymphocytes and reduced cellular immunity, and with this goes an increased liability to infections (Chandra, 1975). Premature infants show an increased incidence of nasal *Pseudomonas* and umbilical staphylococci (Evans, Akpata and Baki, 1970), although this may be secondary to extra handling by the staff.

Unfortunately the use of antibiotics in the newborn is made difficult by the range of possible infecting organisms, and by deficiencies in ability to metabolise drugs; for example glucuronyl-transferase deficiency leads to toxic blood levels of chloramphenicol. The subject has been well reviewed by Davies (1975). It is for this reason that regimes of skin and umbilical care with purely local antiseptics and antibiotics are so well established. Umbilical sterility is especially important in neonates whose blood sugar levels are monitored through the umbilical vessels.

Hexachlorophane proved to be of great value in reducing colonisation by, and clinical infections with, *Staphylococcus aureus*; however, its use has now been discouraged since it has been associated with a specific degenerative central nervous system lesion (Shuman, Leech and Alvord, 1974). The barrier function of the skin is poorly developed in premature infants below 38 weeks of gestational age (Nachman and Esterly, 1971); and they may also have a limited ability to metabolise and excrete the substance (Kopelman, 1973). So, despite the extra liability of these children to infections, the use of hexachlorophane is strongly contraindicated; there may, however, be more acceptable alternatives (McHattie et al, 1974).

One of the problems associated with the use of hexachlorophane had been the high colonisation rate by Gram-negative organisms. This has also been recorded in adults (Evans et al, 1973b). In the nursery other contributory factors will have operated, particularly the high level of hand carriage of Gram-negatives by staff using hexachlorophane hand cleaners (Bruun and Solberg, 1973), and the colonisation of humidifiers, and even wick-type air-fresheners by *Pseudomonas* (Vanhegan and Mitchell, 1975). The balance was disturbed very shortly after the use of hexachlorophane in neonatal nurseries was stopped, and several sharp epidemics of skin infections with *Staphylococcus aureus* were recorded (*British Medical Journal*, 1974; McAllister et al, 1974; Hyams et al, 1975). In the study of Hyams et al, the staphylococcal colonisation rate rose from 2.2 to 67 per cent. Previous figures, during the hexachlorophane era, had showed that Gram-negative organisms had colonised the nares, umbilicus and groins to the almost total exclusion of *Staphylococcus aureus*. The implantation of the reputedly non-pathogenic *Staphylococcus aureus* 502A, as a way of preventing colonisation by more sinister strains, seems to have fallen out of favour since the many reports of frank infections with strain 502A itself (Blair and Tull, 1969).

INFECTIONS IN DIABETES MELLITUS

Bacterial infections are still an important trigger of diabetic coma, and remain a major cause of death (Biegelman and Warner, 1973). However, this does not answer the problem of whether skin infections are especially common or especially severe in diabetics. Indeed, Somerville and Lancaster-Smith (1973) in their study of the skin flora in diabetics, could not confirm the earlier finding (Smith, O'Connor and Willis, 1966) of an increased nasal carriage rate in diabetics. In one study of nearly 4000 people, a standard inquiry of recent skin infections revealed no difference between diabetics and non-diabetics (Welborn et al, 1966). Despite the rather inadequate clinical proof of an association with bacterial infection, laboratory workers have continued to investigate possible pathological mechanisms: this conflict has been recently reviewed (Savin, 1974).

Using plasma with added glucose, Robson and Heggers (1969) noted that Gram-positive organisms grew well in high sugar levels while Gram-negative organisms did not. Leucocyte function tests on cells from diabetics who were poorly controlled, but not ketotic (Bagdade, Root and Bulger, 1974), showed depressed phagocytosis and poor killing of a test organism. The deficient chemotaxis of polymorphs from diabetics can be returned to normal after incubation with insulin and glucose (Mowat and Baum, 1971). The findings with lymphocytes from diabetics are less unanimous, and the earlier suggestion of a poor response to phytohaemagglutinin (Brody and Merlie, 1970) has not been confirmed (Ragab, Hazlett and Cowan, 1972).

In contrast to staphylococcal infections, the association between diabetes and erythrasma (Montes et al, 1969) was confirmed in the study of Somerville and Lancaster-Smith (1973). They also showed that the carriage of fluorescent diptheroids on clinically normal skin was more common in diabetes than in other populations. Apart from this, their 98 adult diabetics, under good diabetic control, had a skin flora similar to non-diabetics of the same age. However, conditions on the skin of diabetics may be more favourable to bacterial activity than normal skin. Newly diagnosed, and untreated diabetics have high skin levels of free fatty acids, perhaps due to enhanced bacterial lipolysis (Gloor, Marckardt and Friedrich, 1975). The same workers also found high levels of free cholesterol, a feature which they had already noted in patients with impetigo, and which they feel could be an important predisposing factor to susceptibility to bacterial infections.

The difficulty in defining diabetes itself has been another stumbling block in interpreting the literature on this subject. For example, Calandra and Lisi (1974) found that 52.5 per cent of their series of patients with herpes zoster had diabetes using their criteria: however, using these criteria 24.3 per cent of their clinically healthy subjects fitted within the definition of diabetes. This, of course, is very much higher than the usually quoted figures. This whole area of research needs meticulous methodology and it will be of great interest to follow future developments.

ADVANCES IN MICROBIOLOGICAL KNOWLEDGE

Advances in microbial taxonomy are slow; but however tiresome they may be for those who must struggle to learn new names they may reveal new facets of infection, especially opportunist infection. Unfortunately there are few changes in our recent knowledge of the skin flora which can be set alongside those of Baird-Parker's classification of the *Micrococcaceae* (Baird-Parker, 1963, 1974) which showed that only one group (out of 15 groups of coagulase-negative cocci) was responsible for the colonisation of Spitz–Holter hydrocephalus valves and the Starr–Edwards heart prosthesis. That this same group (Baird-Parker S II or Biotype I) should in addition be the most common in lesions of acne is also interesting. The more recent schemes devised by Schleifer and Kloos (Kloos, Tornabene and Schleifer, 1974; Kloos and Schleifer, 1975; Schleifer and Kloos, 1975) may provide greater refinement and have already demonstrated apparent geographical differences in coccal carriage.

Amongst the diphtheroids, redefinition of the anaerobic species by Marples and McGinley (1974) and by phage typing (Jong, Ko and Pulverer, 1975) must eventually lead to a greater understanding of the role of *Corynebacterium* (*Propionibacterium*) *acnes* not only in acne but in systemic infection (Duborgel, 1974).

The work of Pitcher (1975, 1976) on the aerobic diphtheroid flora of the skin seems certain to lead to a deeper knowledge of trichomycosis, erythrasma and body odour. His studies on the composition of the cell wall of aerobic skin diphtheroids shows that only about 60 per cent are members of the genus *Corynebacterium*, the remainder form a heterogeneous mass involving perhaps six other genera, some of which may be important in disease. It seems likely that some organisms whose natural home is in the soil, or in dairy products, will prove to be capable of causing infection under some circumstances.

Perhaps the most striking new pathogen has been the alga *Prototheca* now known as an agent of human disease. Both cutaneous and systemic infection were comprehensively reviewed by Sudman (1974).

The toxic enzymes of bacteria are providing much interest to microbial chemists and others. This work must be seen as contributing to our knowledge of skin infection, the more scientific workers who can be drawn into dermatology the faster will advances be made into understanding this facet of dermatology (Noble, 1976). Four areas may be singled out as growing points in our knowledge. One of the most advanced is staphylococcal toxic epidermal necrolysis (STEN). This disease has recruited microbial chemists and geneticists to the ranks of skin researchers. It is now known that STEN is caused by a toxin complex of molecular weight about 20 000 produced mainly by *Staphylococcus aureus* strains of phage group II (the type 71 complex), though other phage groups are sometimes involved. The genetic information controlling abundant production of the toxin is carried on a plasmid, though chromosomal information may result in minimum quantities being formed. The toxin acts on the stratum granolosum, and although its gross effect cannot be distinguished from the drug-induced form in eliciting the Nikolsky sign, the ultrastructural picture is quite different. This subject has recently been reviewed by Wuepper, Dimond and Knutson (1975) and Noble (1976).

The second area in which advances are being made is that of *Mycobacterium ulcerans* infections, frequently termed Buruli ulcers. This disease has excited the attention of immunologists and epidemiologists. The bare facts are that, although found throughout the tropical world, *M. ulcerans* infections are most frequent in the Buruli county of Uganda where most of the research effort has been concentrated. Human to human transmission apparently does not occur, and it seems probable that the organism is acquired from vegetation associated with swamps, perhaps via an insect vector. The toxin produces an extensively undermined ulcer with necrosis of the subcutaneous fat. Surgical excision and skin grafting are still the treatment of choice. Although cases may clear eventually, this may not occur for a long period, by which time extensive tissue damage may have led to contractures of the limbs (Barker, 1974; Noble, 1976).

Erysipelothrix has been less extensive investigated although there has been an increased interest in this organism recently, especially in Germany (Heggers, Buddington and McAllister, 1974; Leimbeck and Bohm, 1975; Krasemann and Muller, 1975).

The fourth organism to arouse attention is *Pseudomonas aeruginosa*. Experimental investigations have failed to reveal how *Ps. aeruginosa* is able to infect skin even when given the assistance of a steroid and occlusion (Savin, 1967). Lesions in mice can be obtained which may be necrotic or simply pustular with an absence of erythema or apparent systemic effects (P. M. White, personal communication). In dogs it has not proved possible to induce a permanent pyoderma (Wooley et al, 1974). Experimental burns are susceptible to colonisation however (Carney, Dyster and Jones, 1973; Stieritz and Holder, 1975). Enzymes under study in relation to skin disease include those affecting vascular permeability (Kusama, 1974), protease enzymes (Muszynski, 1973), the slime layer (Mates and Zand, 1974) and the exotoxin which affects cellular and mitochondrial respiration (Pavlovskis, 1972). A promising line of treatment is the use of vaccines (Jones and Lowbury, 1972) either to whole cells or to specific fragments such as the slime layer.

Our knowledge of interactions between organisms at the skin surface is slowly increasing. Selwyn (1975) has described the carriage of antibiotic-producing strains of cocci in skin lesions, and shown how possession of a producer strain may help to prevent secondary infection in diseases such as eczema and to a lesser extent psoriasis. Dermatophyte fungi are also good producers of antibiotics, and N. Youssef (personal communication) has found strains to produce penicillin when grown on stratum corneum in vitro. A reinvestigation of the interchange of substances at the skin surface is clearly overdue. Murphy (1975) has demonstrated how slight is our knowledge of the chemicals permitting or preventing growth of organisms.

Other microbial interactions may be relevant to the skin, but we do not yet know how far organisms are able to alter the environment in their own favour. Schwab (1975) has reviewed the suppression of immune responses by microorganisms. The most interesting organism from the skin aspect is *Corynebacterium parvum* which is being extensively studied as a therapeutic anticancer agent (Scott, 1974), acting as a powerful stimulant of the reticuloendothelial system, and also having an effect on antitumour cellular immunity (Kirschner, Glaser and Herberman, 1975). *C. parvum* may prove to be indistinguishable from the *C. acnes* complex, and could be a member of the normal flora in some, perhaps many, individuals.

Antibiotics may alter the milieu sufficiently to affect the bacterial flora. For example, patients receiving antibiotics for acne acquire Gram-negative bacilli in the nares more frequently than those not receiving antibiotics and resistant organisms may emerge (Fulton et al, 1968; Aly et al, 1970; Bayston, 1974). Clinically this may be accompanied by a Gram-negative folliculitis (Leyden, 1973; Plewig and Braun-Falco, 1974). However, we should be cautious in interpreting all effects of antibiotics as directly antimicrobial since Lacey (1969) showed that applying neomycin to skin allowed neomycin-resistant *Staph. aureus* to persist longer on the skin, perhaps due to its effect in binding the skin fatty acids.

Finally, studies on the interaction between organisms at high population levels are only at a preliminary stage. Aly and his colleagues (1975), correlating in vivo and in vitro characteristics, found that persons with a high count of normal flora (micrococcaceae and diphtheroids) were more likely to resist innocula of *Staph. aureus* and *Candida albicans* than those with low skin counts. There may also be unsuspected reactions between pathogens; for example Wallin and Gnarpe (1975) have reported the suppression of *N. gonorrhoeae* by *C. albicans* and suggest that this may be a cause of false negative gonococcal culture results.

REFERENCES

INTRODUCTION

Morison, W. L. (1974) Survey of viral warts, herpes zoster and herpes simplex in patients with secondary immune deficiencies and neoplasms. *British Journal of Dermatology*, **91,** Suppl. 10, 18–19.

CANDIDOSIS

Bhaskaram, C. & Reddy, V. (1975) Cell-mediated immunity in iron and vitamin deficient children. *British Medical Journal*, **3,** 522.

Blizzard, R. M., Chee, D. & Davis, W. (1967) The incidence of adrenal and other antibodies in the sera of patients with idiopathic adrenal insufficiency (Addison's disease). *Clinical and Experimental Immunology*, **2,** 19–30.

Bodey, G. P. & Luna, M. (1974) Skin lesions associated with disseminated candidosis. *Journal of the American Medical Association*, **229,** 1466–1468.

Caroline, L., Rosner, F. & Kozinn, P. J. (1969) Elevated serum iron, low unbound transferrin and candidosis in acute leukaemia. *Blood*, **34,** 441–451.

Cawson, R. A. (1968) Treatment of oral lichen planus with betamethasone. *British Medical Journal*, **1,** 86–89.

Cawson, R. A. (1973) Induction of epithelial hyperplasia by *Candida albicans*. *British Journal of Dermatology*, **89,** 497–503.

Cawson, R. A. & Rajasingham, K. C. (1972) Ultrastructural features of the invasive phase of *Candida albicans*. *British Journal of Dermatology*, **87,** 435–443.

Chilgren, R. A., Meuwissen, H. J., Quie, P. G., Good, R. A. & Hong, R. (1969) The cellular immune defect in chronic mucocutaneous candidosis. *Lancet*, **1,** 1286–1288.

Clark, R. A., Root, R. K., Kimball, H. R. & Kirkpatrick, C. H. (1973) Defective neutrophil chemotoxis and cellular immunity in a child with recurrent infections. *Annals of Internal Medicine*, **78,** 515–519.

Drew, J. H. (1973) Chronic mucocutaneous candidosis with abnormal function of serum complement. *Medical Journal of Australia*, **2**, 77–80.

Evans, E. G. V., Richardson, M. D., Odds, F. C. & Holland, K. T. (1973) Relevance of antigenicity of *Candida albicans* growth phase to diagnosis of systemic candidiasis. *British Medical Journal*, **4**, 86–87.

Feigin, R. D., Shackleford, P. G., Eisen, S., Spitler, L. E., Pickering, L. K. & Anderson, D. C. (1974) Treatment of mucocutaneous candidosis with transfer factor. *Pediatrics*, **53**, 63–70.

Finn, R., Hill, C. A. St, Govan, A. J., Ralfs, I. G., Guerney, F. J. & Denye, V. (1972) Immunological responses in pregnancy and survival of fetal homograft. *British Medical Journal*, **3**, 150–152.

Higgs, J. M. & Wells, R. S. (1973) Chronic mucocutaneous candidiasis: new approaches to treatment. *British Journal of Dermatology*, **89**, 179–190.

Hill, C. A. St, Finn, R. & Denye, V. (1973) Depression of cellular immunity in pregnancy due to a serum factor. *British Medical Journal*, **3**, 513–514.

Jonson, D. H. M., Jacobs, A., Walker, D. M. & Dolby, A. E. (1972) Defect of cell-mediated immunity in patients with iron deficiency anaemia. *Lancet*, **2**, 1058–1059.

Lancet (1974) Iron and resistance to infection. *Lancet*, **2**, 323–326.

Lehner, T., Wilton, J. M. A. & Ivanyi, L. (1972) Immunodeficiencies in chronic mucocutaneous candidiasis. *Immunology*, **22**, 775–787.

Lehrer, R. I. & Cline, M. J. (1969) Interaction of *Candida albicans* with human leucocytes and serum. *Journal of Bacteriology*, **98**, 996–1004.

Lynch, E. B., Minkin, W. & Smith, E. B. (1969) Ecology of *Candida albicans* in candidiasis of the groins. *Archives of Dermatology*, **99**, 154–160.

Mackie, R. M., Cochran, R., de Souza, M. & Paratt, D. (1975) The treatment of chronic mucocutaneous candidosis with transfer factor. *Scottish Medical Journal*, **20**, 278.

Milne, L. J. R. & Crompton, G. K. (1974) Beclomethazone dipropionate and orophargageal candidosis. *British Medical Journal*, **3**, 797–798.

Montes, L. F., Carter, R. E., Moreland, N. & Ceballos, R. (1968) Generalised cutaneous candidosis associated with diffuse mycopathy and thymoma. *Journal of the American Medical Association*, **204**, 351–354.

Oriel, J. D., Partridge, B. M., Denny, M. J. & Coleman, J. C. (1972) Genital yeast infections. *British Medical Journal*, **4**, 761–764.

Oriel, J. D. & Waterworth, P. M. (1975) Effect of minocycline and tetracycline on the vaginal yeast flora. *Journal of Clinical Pathology*, **28**, 403–406.

Pabst, H. F. & Swanson, R. (1972) Successful treatment of candidiasis with transfer factor. *British Medical Journal*, **2**, 442–443.

Rebora, A. E., Marples, R. R. & Kligman, A. M. (1973) Experimental infection with *Candida albicans*. *Archives of Dermatology*, **108**, 69–73.

Renz, M., Cohen, M., Farquhar, J. W. & Harkness, R. A. (1974) Elevation of myeloperoxidase activity in infants with oral candidiasis treated with clotrimazole. *Postgraduate Medical Journal*, **50**, Suppl. I, 30–34.

Richman, R. A., Rosenthal, I. M., Solomon, L. M. & Karachorlu, K. V. (1975) Candidosis and multiple endocrinopathy, with oral squamous cell carcinoma complications. *Archives of Dermatology*, **111**, 625–627.

Schoch, E. P. (1971) Thymic conversion of *Candida albicans* from commensalism to pathogenism. *Archives of Dermatology*, **103**, 311–319.

Spellacy, W. N., Zaias, N., Buhi, W. C. & Birk, S. A. (1971) Vaginal yeast growths and contraceptive practices. *Obstetrics and Gynaecology*, **38**, 343–349.

Stankler, L. & Bewsher, P. D. (1972) Chronic mucocutaneous candidiasis, endocrine deficiency and alopecia areata. *British Journal of Dermatology*, **86**, 238–245.

Valdimarsson, H., Moss, P. D., Holt, P. J. L. & Hobbs, J. R. (1972a) Treatment of chronic mucocutaneous candidiasis with leucocytes from HL-A compatible sibling. *Lancet*, **1**, 469–472.

Valdimarsson, H., Woods, L. B. S., Hobbs, J. R. & Holt, P. J. L. (1972b) Immunological features in a case of chronic granulomatous candidiasis and its treatment with transfer factor. *Clinical and Experimental Immunology*, **11**, 151–163.

Valdimarsson, H., Vamamura, M. H., Wells, R. S., Hobbs, J. R. & Holt, P. J. L. (1973) Immune abnormalities associated with chronic mucocutaneous candidiasis. *Cellular Immunology*, **6**, 348–361.

Wells, R. S., Higgs, J. M., MacDonald, A., Valdimarsson, H. & Holt, P. J. L. (1972) Familial chronic mucocutaneous candidiasis. *Journal of Medical Genetics*, **9**, 302–310.

DERMATOPHYTE INFECTIONS

Abdallah, M. A. (1971) The role played by mechanical trauma in dermatophyte infection. *Mykosen*, **14**, 595–597.

Allen, A. M. & Taplin, D. (1973) Epidemic *Trichophyton mentagrophytes* infections in servicemen. *Journal of the American Medical Association*, **226**, 864–867.

Baer, R. L., Bart, R. S., Stritzer, R. & Michaelides, P. (1964) Exfoliative Erythrodermie und Thymom, gleichzeitiges Vorkommen einer ungewöhnlichen generalisierten Dermatose, 'universeller' cutaner Candidiasis und eines Thymoms: Bericht eines Falles. *Hautartz*, **15**, 413–418.

Bagnall, B. G. & Grünberg, W. (1972) Generalised *Trichophyton mentagrophytes* ringworm in capuchin monkeys (*Cebus nigrivitatus*). *British Journal of Dermatology*, **87**, 565–570.

Bibel, D. J. & Lebrun, J. R. (1975) Effect of experimental dermatophyte infection on cutaneous flora. *Journal of Investigative Dermatology*, **64**, 119–123.

Blank, F., Mann, S. J. & Reale, R. A. (1974) Distribution of dermatophytes according to age, ethnic group, and sex. *Sabouraudia*, **12**, 352–361.

Burgoon, C. F. Blank, F., Johnson, W. C. & Grappe, S. F. (1974) Mycetoma formation in *Trichophyton rubrum* infection. *British Journal of Dermatology*, **90**, 155–162.

Carlisle, D. H., Inouve, J. C., King, R. D. & Jones, H. E. (1974) Significance of serum fungal inhibitory factor in dermatophytosis. *Journal of Investigative Dermatology*, **63**, 239–241.

Hanifin, J. M., Ray, L. F. & Lobitz, W. C. (1974) Immunologic reactivity in dermatophytosis. *British Journal of Dermatology*, **90**, 1–8.

Jolly, H. W. & Carpenter, C. L. (1969) Oral glucose tolerance studies in recurrent *Trichophyton rubrum* infections. *Archives of Dermatology*, **100**, 26–28.

Jones, H. E., Reinhardt, J. H. & Rinaldi, M. G. (1973) A clinical, mycological and immunological survey for dermatophycosis. *Archives of Dermatology*, **108**, 61–65.

Jones, H. E., Reinhardt, J. H. & Rinaldi, M. G. (1974) Immunologic susceptibility to chronic dermatophytosis. *Archives of Dermatology*, **110**, 213–220.

Knight, A. G. (1973) Human models for in vivo and in vitro assessment of topical antifungal compounds. *British Journal of Dermatology*, **89**, 509–514.

Levene, G. M. (1973) Chronic fungal infection (*E. floccosum*), erythroderma, immune deficiency and lymphoma. *Proceedings of the Royal Society of Medicine*, **66**, 745–746.

O'Grady, K. J., English, M. P. & Warin, R. P. (1972) *Microsporum equinum* infection of the scalp in an adult. *British Journal of Dermatology*, **87**, 175–179.

Rosenthal, S. A. & Baer, R. L. (1966) Experiments of biology of fungus infections of the feet. *Journal of Investigative Dermatology*, **47**, 568–576.

Thorne, E. & Fusaro, R. (1971) Subcutaneous *Trichophyton rubrum* abscesses. *Dermatologica*, **42**, 167–170.

IMMUNOSUPPRESSION

Aaronson, C. M. & Park, C. H. (1974) Sporotrichoid infection due to *Mycobacterium marinum*, lesions exacerbated by corticosteroid infiltration. *Southern Medical Journal*, **67**, 117–118.

Allison, A. C. (1970) Tumour development following immunosuppression. *Proceedings of the Royal Society of Medicine*, **63**, 1077–1080.

Armstrong, R. W., Gurwith, M. J., Waddell, D. & Merigan, T. C. (1970) Cutaneous interferon production in patients with Hodgkin's disease and other cancers infected with varicella or vaccinia. *New England Journal of Medicine*, **283**, 1182–1187.

Bagshawe, K. D. (1972) Immunosuppression. *British Journal of Hospital Medicine*, **6**, 677–684.

Brodersen, I., Genner, J. & Brodthagen, H. (1974) Tuberculin sensitivity in BCG vaccinated children with common warts. *Acta dermato-venereologica*, **54**, 291–292.

Cho, C. T., Vats, T. S., Lowman, J. T., Brandsberg, J. W. & Tosh, F. E. (1973) *Fusarium solani* infection during treatment for acute leukaemia. *Journal of Pediatrics*, **83**, 1028–1031.

Eickhoff, T. C., Olin, D. B., Anderson, R. J. & Schafer, L. A. (1972) Current problems and approaches to diagnosis of infection in renal transplant recipients. *Transplantation Proceedings*, **4**, 693–697.

Feldman, S., Hughes, W. T. & Daniel, C. B. (1975) Varicella in children with cancer. Seventy-seven cases. *Pediatrics*, **56**, 388–397.

Fraser, D. W., Buxton, A. E., Jaji, A., Barker, C. F., Rudnick, M. & Weinstein, A. J. (1975) Disseminated *Mycobacterium kansasii* infection presenting as cellulitis in a recipient of a renal homograft. *American Review of Respiratory Diseases*, **112**, 125–129.

Graybill, J. R., Silva, J., Fraser, D. W., Lordon, R. & Rogers, Edna (1974) Disseminated mycobacteriosis due to *Mycobacterium abscessus* in two recipients of renal homografts. *American Review of Respiratory Diseases*, **109**, 4–10.

Kaplan, M. H., Armstrong, D. & Rosen, P. (1974) Tuberculosis complicating neoplastic disease: a review of 201 cases. *Cancer (Philadelphia)*, **33**, 850–858.

Lancet (1972) Clustering in Hodgkin's disease. *Lancet*, **2**, 907–908.

Lynfield, Y. L., Farhangi, M. & Runnels, J. L. (1969) Generalised herpes simplex complicating lymphoma. *Journal of the American Medical Association*, **207**, 944–945.

Montgomerie, J. Z., Becroft, D. M. O., Croxson, M. C., Doak, P. B. & North, J. D. K. (1969) Herpes simplex virus infection after renal transplantation. *Lancet*, **2**, 867–871.

Ng, R. P., Alexopoulos, C. G., Moran, C. J. & Bellingham, A. J. (1975) Transfer factor in Hodgkin's disease. *Lancet*, **2**, 901–903.

Perry, T. L. & Harman, L. (1974) Warts in diseases with immune defeats. *Cutis*, **13**, 359–362.

Rosenburg, E. W. & Yusk, J. W. (1970) Molluscum contagiosum. Eruption following treatment with prednisone and methotrexate. *Archives of Dermatology*, **101**, 439–441.

Sage, R. E. & Derrington, A. W. (1973) Opportunistic cutaneous *Mycobacterium marinum* infection mimicking *Mycobacterium ulcerans* in lymphosarcoma. *Medical Journal of Australia*, **2**, 434–437.

Savin, J. A. & Noble, W. C. (1975) Immunosuppression and skin infection. *British Journal of Dermatology*, **93**, 115–120.

Thorling, E. B. & Thorling, K. (1974) Serum copper in Hodgkin's disease before and after herpes zoster. *Lancet*, **2**, 1396–1397.

Turcotte, J. G. (1972) Infection and renal transplantation. *Surgical Clinics of North America*, **52**, 1501–1512.

Vianna, N. J., Greenwald, P., Brady, J., Polan, A. K., Dwork, A., Mauro, J. & Davies, J. P. N. (1972) Hodgkin's disease: cases with the features of a community outbreak. *Annals of Internal Medicine*, **77**, 169–180.

Wiley, B. B., Allman, S., Rogolsky, M., Nordon, C. W. & Glasgow, L. A. (1974) Staphylococcal scalded skin syndrome: potentiation by immunosuppression in mice; toxin-mediated exfoliation in a healthy adult. *Infection and Immunity*, **9**, 636–640.

Young, N. A., Kwon-Chung, K. J. & Freeman, J. (1973) Subcutaneous abscess caused by *Phoma* sp. resembling *Pyrenochaete romeroi*. Unique fungal infection occurring in immunosuppressed recipient of renal allograft. *American Journal of Clinical Pathology*, **59**, 810–816.

SUPERINFECTION

Anderson, E. & Hjorth, N. (1975) B-lymphocytes, T-lymphocytes and phytohaemaggutinins responsiveness in atopic dermatitis. *Acta dermato-venereologica*, **55**, 345–349.

Bean, S. F. (1971) Acneiform eruption from tetracycline. *British Journal of Dermatology*, **85**, 585–586.

Blattner, R. J. (1967) Molluscum contagiosum: eruptive infection in atopic dermatitis. *Journal of Paediatrics*, **70**, 997–999.

Fulton, J. E., McGinley, K., Leyden, J. & Marples, R. (1968) Gram-negative folliculitis in acne. *Archives of Dermatology*, **98**, 349–353.

Gerrard, J. W. (1973) Transient IgA deficiency and pathogenesis of infantile atopic eczema. *Lancet*, **2**, 448.

Grove, D. I., Reid, J. G. & Forbes, I. J. (1975) Humoral and cellular immunity in atopic eczema. *British Journal of Dermatology*, **92**, 611–618.

Jones, H. E., Reinhardt, J. H. & Rinaldi, M. G. (1973) A clinical, mycological and immunological survey for dermatophycosis. *Archives of Dermatology*, **108**, 61–65.

Jones, H. E., Reinhardt, J. H. & Rinaldi, M. G. (1974) Immunologic susceptibility to chronic dermatophytosis. *Archives of Dermatology*, **110**, 213–220.

Luckasen, J. R., Sabad, A., Goltz, R. W. & Kersey, J. H. (1974) T- and B-lymphocytes in atopic eczema. *Archives of Dermatology*, **110**, 375–377.

Lynfield, Y. L., Ostroff, G. & Abraham, J. (1972) Bacteria, skin sterilisation and wound healing in psoriasis. *New York State Journal of Medicine*, **72**, 1247–1250.

Marples, R. R., Heaton, C. L. & Kligman, A. M. (1973) *Staphylococcus aureus* in psoriasis. *Archives of Dermatology*, **107**, 568–570.

Matta, M. (1974) Blood and pustule culture in pustular psoriasis. *British Journal of Dermatology*, **90**, 309–312.

McFadyen, T. & Lyell, A. (1971) Successful treatment of generalised pustular psoriasis (von Zumbusch) by systemic antibiotics controlled by blood culture. *British Journal of Dermatology*, **85**, 274–276.

Noble, W. C. & Savin, J. A. (1968) Carriage of *Staphylococcus aureus* in psoriasis. *British Medical Journal*, **1**, 417–419.

Nystrom, B., Molin, L. & Rajka, G. (1971) Isolation ward treatment for dermatoses. *Acta dermato-venereologica*, **51**, 301–304.

Payne, R. W. (1967) Severe outbreak of surgical sepsis due to *Staphylococcus aureus* of unusual type and origin. *British Medical Journal*, **4**, 17–20.

Schopf, E. & Bohringer, H. (1974) Zellvermittelte Immunität bei Neurodermitis atopica. *Hautarzt*, **25**, 420–426.

Selwyn, S. (1975) Natural antibiosis among skin bacteria as a primary defence against infection. *British Journal of Dermatology*, **93**, 487–493.

Smith, R. J., Alder, V. G. & Warin, R. P. (1975) Pyogenic cocci in infantile eczema throughout one year. *British Medical Journal*, **3**, 199–201.

Svartman, M., Potter, E. V., Tinklea, J. F., Poon-King, T. & Earle, D. P. (1972) Epidemic scabies and acute glomerulo-nephritis in Trinidad. *Lancet*, **1**, 249–251.

Turk, J. L. (1970) Contribution of modern immunological concepts to an understanding of diseases of the skin. *British Medical Journal*, **3**, 363–368.

HUMIDITY

Allen, A. M. & Taplin, D. (1973) Epidemic *Trichophyton mentagrophytes* infection in servicemen. *Journal of the American Medical Association*, **226**, 864–867.

Ammonette, R. A. & Rosenburg, E. W. (1973) Infection of the toewebs by Gram-negative bacteria. *Archives of Dermatology*, **107**, 71–73.

Desai, S. C. (1974) Experimental trichophyton infections in humans and some observations on the biology of *T. rubrum* infections. *British Journal of Dermatology*, **91**, 713–714.

Duncan, W. C., McBride, M. E. & Knox, J. M. (1969) Bacterial flora: the role of environmental factors. *Journal of Investigative Dermatology*, **52**, 479–484.

Duncan, W. C., McBride, M. E. & Knox, J. M. (1970) Experimental production of infections in humans. *Journal of Investigative Dermatology*, **54**, 319–323.

Finlay, G. H. (1974) Fungous diseases of the skin in the Transvaal. *Transactions of the St John's Hospital Dermatological Society*, **60**, 63–72.

Hojyo-Tomoka, M. T., Marples, R. R. & Kligman, A. M. (1973) *Pseudomonas* infection in superhydrated skin. *Archives of Dermatology*, **107**, 723–727.

Knight, A. G. (1972) A review of experimental human fungus infections. *Journal of Investigative Dermatology*, **59**, 354–358.

Knight, A. G. (1973) Human models for in vitro and in vivo assessment of topical antifungal compounds. *British Journal of Dermatology*, **89**, 509–514.

Leyden, J. J. & Kligman, A. M. (1975) Aluminium chloride in the treatment of symptomatic athlete's foot. *Archives of Dermatology*, **111**, 1004–1010.

Lynch, P. J., Minkin, W. & Smith, E. B. (1969) Ecology of *Candida albicans* in candidiasis of the groin. *Archives of Dermatology*, **99**, 154–160.

McBride, M. E., Duncan, W. C. & Knox, J. M. (1975) Physiological and environmental control of Gram-negative bacteria on skin. *British Journal of Dermatology*, **93**, 191–199.

O'Brien, J. P. (1950) The aetiology of poral closure II. The role of staphylococcal infection in miliaria rubra and bullous impetigo. *Journal of Investigative Dermatology*, **15**, 102–133.

Rebora, A., Marples, R. R. & Kligman, A. M. (1973a) Erosio interdigitalis blastomycetica. *Archives of Dermatology*, **108**, 66–68.

Rebora, A., Marples, R. R. & Kligman, A. M. (1973b) Experimental infection with *Candida albicans*. *Archives of Dermatology*, **108**, 69–73.

Savin, J. A. (1967) *Pseudomonas aeruginosa* infections in a skin ward. *Transactions of the St John's Hospital Dermatological Society*, **53**, 75–79.

Singh, G. (1973a). Heat, humidity and pyodermas. *Dermatologica*, **147**, 343–347.

Singh, G. (1973b) Experimental *Trichophyton* infection of intact human skin. *British Journal of Dermatology*, **89**, 595–599.

Singh, G. (1974) *Pseudomonas* infections of skin, an experimental study. *International Journal of Dermatology*, **13**, 90–93.

Sulzberger, M. B. & Akers, W. A. (1969) Impact of skin diseases on military operations. *Archives of Dermatology*, **100**, 702.

Taplin, D., Zaias, N. & Rebell, G. (1965) Environmental influences on the microbiology of the skin. *Archives of Environmental Health*, **11**, 546–550.

Taplin, D., Bassett, D. C. J. & Mertz, P. M. (1971) Foot lesions associated with *Pseudomonas cepacia*. *Lancet*, **2**, 568–571.

Taplin, D., Lansdell, L., Allen, A. M., Rodriguez, R. & Corks, A. (1973) Prevalence of streptococcal pyoderma in relation to climate and hygiene. *Lancet*, **1**, 501–503.

Wright, D. N. & Alexander, J. M. (1974) Effect of water on the bacterial flora of swimmers' ears. *Archives of Otolaryngology*, **99**, 15–18.

Young, C. N. (1974) Pitted keratolysis—a preliminary report. *Transactions of the St John's Hospital Dermatological Society*, **60**, 77–85.

NEWBORN SKIN

Blair, E. B. & Tull, A. H. (1969) Multiple infections among newborns resulting from colonisation with *Staphylococcus aureus* 502A. *American Journal of Clinical Pathology*, **52**, 42–49.

British Medical Journal (1974) Staphylococcal skin sepsis in a hospital. *British Medical Journal*, **2**, 287.

Bruun, J. N. & Solberg, C. O. (1973) Hand carriage of Gram-negative bacilli and *Staphylococcus aureus*. *British Medical Journal*, **2**, 580–582.

Chandra, R. K. (1975) Fetal malnutrition and post-natal immunocompetence. *American Journal of Diseases of Children*, **129**, 450–454.

Coen, R., Grush, O. & Kauder, E. (1969) Studies of bactericidal activity and metabolism in full-term neonates. *Journal of Pediatrics*, **75**, 400–406.

Davies, P. A. (1975) Antimicrobial therapy in the neonatal period. *British Journal of Hospital Medicine*, **14**, 517–526.

Evans, H. E., Akpata, S. O. & Baki, A. (1970) Factors influencing the establishment of the neonatal bacterial flora. 1. The role of host factors. *Archives of Environmental Health*, **21**, 514–519.

Evans, H. E., Akpata, S. O. & Baki, A. (1971) Relationship of the birth canal to the bacterial flora of the neonatal respiratory tract and skin. *Obstetrics and Gynaecology*, **37**, 94–97.

Evans, H. E., Akpata, S. O., Baki, A. & Glass, L. (1973a). Flora in newborn infants: annual variation in prevalence of *Staphylococcus aureus*, *Escherichia coli* and streptococci. *Archives of Environmental Health*, **26**, 275–276.

Evans, Z. A., Rendtorff, R. C., Robinson, H. & Rosenberg, E. W. (1973b) Ecologic influence of hexachlorophene on skin bacteria. *Journal of Investigative Dermatology*, **60**, 207–214.

Hurst, V. (1960) Transmission of hospital staphylococci among newborn infants. II. Colonisation of the skin and mucous membranes of the infants. *Pediatrics*, **25**, 204–214.

Hyams, P. J., Counts, G. W., Monkus, E., Feldman, R., Kicklighter, J. L. & Gonzalez, C. (1975) Staphylococcal bacteremia and hexachlorophene bathing. Epidemic in a newborn nursery. *American Journal of Diseases of Children*, **129**, 595–599.

Kopelman, A. E. (1973) Cutaneous absorption of hexachlorophane in low birth weight infants. *Journal of Pediatrics*, **82**, 972–975.

Lawton, A. R. & Cooper, M. D. (1973) Development of immunity: phylogeny and ontogeny. In *Immunologic Disorders in Infants and Children*, ed. Steihm, E. R. & Fulginiti, V. A., p. 28. Philadelphia: W. B. Saunders.

McAllister, T. A., Givan, J., Black, A., Turner, M. J., Kerr, M. M. & Hutchison, J. H. (1974) The natural history of bacterial colonisation of the newborn in a maternity hospital. *Scottish Medical Journal*, **19**, 119–124.

McHattie, J. C., Crossan, M., Talvkdar, C., Elder, R. & Murdock, A. I. (1974) A comparison of hexachlorophene and lactate on growth of skin flora in healthy term newborn infants. *Canadian Medical Association Journal*, **110**, 1248–1250.

Miller, M. E. (1969) Phagocytosis in the newborn: humoral and cellular factors. *Journal of Pediatrics*, **74**, 255–259.

Moffet, H. L. & Allan, D. (1967) Colonisation of infants exposed to bacterially contaminated mists. *American Journal of Diseases of Children*, **114**, 21–25.

Nachman, R. L. & Esterly, N. B. (1971) Increased skin permeability to hexachlorophane of skin with increasing gestational age. *Journal of Pediatrics*, **79**, 628–632.

Plotkin, S. A. (1975) Routes of fetal infection and mechanisms of fetal damage. *American Journal of Diseases of Childhood*, **129**, 444–449.

Renz, M., Cohen, M., Farquhar, J. W. & Harkness, R. A. (1974) Elevation of myeloperoxidase activity in infants with oral candidosis treated with clotrimazole. *Postgraduate Medical Journal*, **50**, Suppl. I, 30–34.

Sarkany, I. & Gaylarde, C. G. (1968) The effect of amniotic fluid on bacterial growth. *British Journal of Dermatology*, **80**, 241–243.

Shuman, R. M., Leech, R. W. & Alvord, E. C. (1974) Neurotoxicity of hexachlorophene in the human. I. A clinicopathologic study of 248 children. *Pediatrics*, **54**, 689–695.

Vanhegan, R. I. & Mitchell, R. G. (1975) *Pseudomonas* infection associated with colonisation of wick-type air freshness. *British Medical Journal*, **3**, 785.

INFECTIONS IN DIABETES MELLITUS

Bagdade, J. D., Root, R. K. & Bulger, R. J. (1974) Impaired leucocyte function in patients with poorly controlled diabetes. *Diabetes*, **23**, 9–15.

Biegelman, P. M. & Warner, N. E. (1973) Thirty-two fatal cases of severe diabetic keto-acidosis including a case of mucomycosis. *Diabetes*, **22**, 847–850.

Brody, J. I. & Merlie, K. (1970) Metabolic features of lymphocytes from patients with diabetes mellitus, similarities to lymphocytes in chronic lymphoblastic leukaemia. *British Journal of Haematology*, **19**, 193–201.

Calandra, P. & Lisi, P. (1974) Skin and diabetes. II. Incidence of diabetes in a group of patients with herpes zoster. *Italian General Review of Dermatology*, **11**, 207–213.

Gloor, M., Marckardt, V. & Friedrich, H. C. (1975) Biochemical and physiological parti-cularities on the skin surface of diabetics. *Archives of Dermatological Research*, **253**, 185–194.

Montes, L. F., Dobson, H., Dodge, B. G. & Knowles, J. R. (1969) Erythrasma and diabetes mellitus. *Archives of Dermatology*, **99**, 674–680.

Mowat, A. G. & Baum, J. (1971) Chemotaxis of polymorphonuclear leucocytes from patients with diabetes mellitus. *New England Journal of Medicine*, **284**, 621–627.

Ragab, A. H., Hazlett, B. & Cowan, P. H. (1972) Response of peripheral blood lymphocytes from patients with diabetes mellitus, to phytohaemagglutinin and *Candida albicans* antigen. *Diabetes*, **21**, 906–907.

Robson, M. C. & Heggers, J. P. (1969) Effect of hyperglycaemia on survival of bacteria. *Surgical Forum*, **20**, 56–57.

Savin, J. A. (1974) Bacterial infections in diabetes mellitus. *British Journal of Dermatology*, **91**, 481–487.

Smith, J. A., O'Connor, J. J. & Willis, A. T. (1966) Nasal carriage of *Staphylococcus aureus* in diabetes mellitus. *Lancet*, **2**, 776–777.

Somerville, D. A. & Lancaster-Smith, M. (1973) The aerobic cutaneous microflora of diabetic subjects. *British Journal of Dermatology*, **89**, 395–400.

Welborn, J. A., Curnow, D. H., Wearne, J. T., Cullen, K. J., McCall, M. G. & Stenhouse, N. S. (1968) Diabetes detected by blood sugar measurement after a glucose load: report from the Busselton survey. *Medical Journal of Australia*, **2**, 778–783.

ADVANCES IN MICROBIOLOGICAL KNOWLEDGE

Aly, R., Maibach, H. I., Rahman, R., Shinefield, H. R. & Mandel, A. D. (1975) Correlation of human in vivo and in vitro cutaneous antimicrobial factors. *Journal of Infectious Diseases*, **131**, 579–583.

Aly, R., Maibach, H. I., Strauss, W. G. & Shinefield, H. R. (1970) Effects of a systemic antibiotic on nasal bacterial ecology in man. *Applied Microbiology*, **20**, 240–244.

Baird-Parker, A. C. (1963) A classification of micrococci and staphylococci based on physiological and biochemical tests. *Journal of General Microbiology*, **30**, 409–428.

Baird-Parker, A. C. (1974) The basis for the present classification of staphylococci and micrococci. *Annals of the New York Academy of Sciences*, **236**, 7–14.

Barker, D. J. P. (1974) Mycobacterial skin ulcers. *British Journal of Dermatology*, **91**, 473–474.

Bayston, R. (1974) Effects of cloxacillin on the flora of the skin and anterior nares. *Archives of Diseases in Childhood*, **49**, 826–827.

Carney, S. A., Dyster, R. E. & Jones, R. J. (1973) The invasion of burned skin by *Pseudomonas aeruginosa*. *British Journal of Dermatology*, **88**, 539–545.

Duborgel, S. (1974) Etude de Corynebacteries Anaerobes Isolées à partir de 9000 hemocultures. *Annales de biologie clinique*, **32**, 487–491.

Fulton, J. E., McGinley, K., Leyden, J. & Marples, R. (1968) Gram-negative folliculitis in acne vulgaris. *Archives of Dermatology*, **98**, 349–353.

Heggers, J. P., Buddington, R. S. & McAllister, H. A. (1974) Erysipelothrix endocarditis diagnosis by fluorescence microscopy. Report of a case. *American Journal of Clinical Pathology*, **62**, 893–806.

Jong, E. C., Ko, H. L. & Pulverer, G. (1975) Studies on bacteriophages of *Propionibacterium acnes*. *Medical Microbiology and Immunology*, **161**, 263–271.

Jones, R. J. & Lowbury, E. J. L. (1972) Early protection of vaccines against *Pseudomonas aeruginosa* colonising burns. *British Journal of Experimental Pathology*, **53**, 659–664.

Kirschner, H., Glaser, M. & Herberman, R. B. (1975) Suppression of cell-mediated tumour immunity by *Corynebacterium parvum*. *Nature*, **257**, 396–398.

Kloos, W. E. & Schleifer, K. H. (1975) Isolation and characterisation of staphylococci from human skin. II. Descriptions of four new species: *Staphylococcus warneri*, *Staphylococcus capitis*, *Staphylococcus hominis* and *Staphylococcus simulans*. *International Journal of Systematic Bacteriology*, **25**, 62–79.

Kloos, W. E., Tornabene, T. G. & Schleifer, K. H. (1974) Isolation and characterisation of micrococci from human skin, including two new species: *Micrococcus lylae* and *Micrococcus kristinae*. *International Journal of Systematic Bacteriology*, **24**, 79–101.

Krasemann, Christina & Muller, H. E. (1975) The virulence of *Erysipelothrix rhusiopathiae* strains and their neuraminidase production. *Zentralblatt für Bakteriologie und Hygiene*, *I. Abteil, Originale A*, **231**, 206–213.

Kusama, H. (1974) Presence of co-factor for the vascular permeability factor of *Pseudomonas aeruginosa*. *Infection and Immunity*, **10**, 1185–1188.

Lacey, R. W. (1969) Loss of the antibacterial action of the skin after topical neomycin. *British Journal of Dermatology*, **81**, 435–439.

Leimbeck, R. & Bohm, K. H. (1975) Investigations on toxic fractions of swine erysipelas bacteria (*Erysipelothrix rhusiopathiae*). *Zentralblatt für Bakteriologie und Hygiene. I. Abteil, Originale A*, **230**, 367–368.

Leyden, J. J., Marples, R. R., Mills, O. H. & Kligman, A. M. (1973) Gram-negative folliculitis—a complication of antibiotic therapy in acne vulgaris. *British Journal of Dermatology*, **88**, 533–538.

Marples, R. R. & McGinley, K. J. (1974) *Corynebacterium acnes* and other anaerobic diphtheroids from human skin. *Journal of Medical Microbiology*, **7**, 349–356.

Mates, A. & Zand, P. (1974) Specificity of the protective response induced by the slime layer of *Pseudomonas aeruginosa*. *Journal of Hygiene (Cambridge)*, **73**, 75–84.

Murphy, Catherine T. (1975) Nutrient materials and the growth of bacteria on human skin. *Transactions of the St John's Hospital Dermatological Society*, **61**, 51–57.

Muszynski, Z. (1973) Enzymatic and toxigenic activity of culture filtrates of high and low virulent strains of *Pseudomonas aeruginosa* on mice. *Pathology and Microbiology*, **39**, 135–147.

Noble, W. C. (1976) The increasing interest in microbial skin disease. *International Journal of Dermatology* (in press).

Pavlovskis, O. R. (1972) *Pseudomonas aeruginosa* exotoxin: effect on cellular and mitochondrial respiration. *Journal of Infectious Diseases*, **126**, 48–53.

Pitcher, D. G. (1975) Cell wall composition of aerobic cutaneous 'diphtheroid' organisms. *Journal of Medical Microbiology*, **8**, Piii.

Pitcher, D. G. (1976) The taxonomy of cutaneous diphtheroid organisms. Ph.D. thesis London University.

Plewig, G. & Braun-Falco, O. (1974). Gram-negative follikulitis. *Hautarzt*, **25**, 541–546.

Savin, J. A. (1967) *Pseudomonas aeruginosa* infections in a skin ward. *Transactions of the St John's Hospital Dermatological Society*, **53**, 75–79.

Schleifer, K. H. & Kloos, W. E. (1975) Isolation and characterisation of staphylococci from human skin. I. Amended description of *Staphylococcus epidermidis* and *Staphylococcus saprophyticus* and descriptions of three new species: *Staphylococcus cohnii*, *Staphylococcus haemolyticus* and *Staphylococcus xylosus*. *International Journal of Systematic Bacteriology*, **25**, 50–61.

Schwab, J. H. (1975) Suppression of the immune response by microorganisms. *Bacteriological Reviews*, **39**, 121–143.

Scott, M. T. (1974) *Corynebacterium parvum* as a therapeutic anticancer agent. *Seminars in Oncology*, **1**, 367–378.

Selwyn, S. (1975) Natural antibiosis among skin bacteria as a primary defence against infection. *British Journal of Dermatology*, **93**, 487–493.

Stieritz, D. D. & Holder, I. A. (1975) Experimental studies of the pathogenesis of infections due to *Pseudomonas aeruginosa*: description of the burned mouse model. *Journal of Infectious Diseases*, **131**, 688–691.

Sudman, M. S. (1974) Protothecosis. A critical review. *American Journal of Clinical Pathology*, **61**, 10–19.

Wallin, J. & Gnarpe, H. (1975) Possible inhibitions of *N. gonorrhoeae* by *C. albicans*. A clinical study. *British Journal of Venereal Diseases*, **51**, 174–175.

Wooley, R. E., Blue, J. L., Scott, T. A. & Belcher, M. K. (1974) Attempt to induce *Pseudomonas* pyoderma in the dog. *American Journal of Veterinary Research*, **35**, 807–810.

Wuepper, K. D., Dimond, R. L. & Knutson, D. D. (1975) Studies on the mechanism of epidermal injury by a staphylococcal epidermolytic toxin. *Journal of Investigative Dermatology*, **65**, 191–200.

2
THE SEXUALLY TRANSMITTED DISEASES

R. D. Catterall

The increase in the incidence of the majority of the sexually transmitted diseases first became apparent in the late 1950s and has continued throughout the last decade. The high prevalence of the diseases throughout the world has caused anxiety among public health authorities in many countries and the World Health Organisation designated 1975 as sexually transmitted diseases year. The subject received considerable attention at the 28th World Health Assembly in May of that year. A document entitled 'Social and Health Aspects of Sexually Transmitted Diseases: Need for a Better Approach' (World Health Organisation, 1975a) was prepared by a group of experts and sent to all member governments. It recommended a complete review of their services against the diseases and indicated ways in which improvements might be made.

The enlargement of the European Economic Community in 1972 and the moves towards mutual recognition of university degrees and specialist training programmes, leading eventually to the free migration of doctors in all the nine countries of the community, highlighted the different systems in use in the United Kingdom and the other eight countries. In Britain venereology and dermatology have been separate specialties for over 50 years and the training programmes for trainee specialists are quite different (Catterall and Nicol, 1975), whereas in Europe in the majority of instances dermatology and venereology are practised by the same specialist and the training programmes for dermatovenereologists, although heavily weighted towards dermatology, contain some essential training in venereology. These differences lead to difficulties in agreement about the mutual recognition of specialist training, and free migration of dermatovenereologists, dermatologists and venereo-logists within the European Economic Community with mutual recognition of qualifications and training is not yet possible. Nevertheless, the discussions which have taken place at the Monospecialist Committee of Dermato-venereology have led to useful exchanges of information and a better under-standing of the services in the different countries.

The true incidence of the various sexually transmitted diseases is difficult to ascertain because of the different methods of obtaining figures and the great under-reporting which exists in most countries. Nevertheless, it has been estimated by the World Health Organisation that each year about 250 million people are infected with gonorrhoea throughout the world and about 50 million people with syphilis (World Health Organisation, 1975b). The incidence of all the other sexually transmitted diseases is unknown. In England, the figures refer only to patients attending National Health Service clinics which serve a total population of just over 46 million people. In 1974 the commonest condition diagnosed was non-specific genital infection with 84 213 cases compared with 58 139 cases of gonorrhoea. There were 35 457 cases of candidosis, 19 011 cases of trichomoniasis and 18 733 cases of genital warts. Genital herpes accounted for 5245 cases and there were 3641 cases of syphilis. Pediculosis pubis was diagnosed 4936 times and scabies 2742 times. Treponemal disease, other than syphilis, was found in 1066 patients, but the tropical venereal diseases, such as chancroid and lymphogranuloma venereum, were only diagnosed 46 and 43 times respectively. Over 80 per cent of cases of early syphilis seen at the larger clinics occurred in homosexual men (Department of Health and Social Security, 1974).

Cases of genital herpes, warts and several other genitourinary conditions are also increasing in incidence and the work carried out in the majority of clinics has expanded considerably during the past decade. Only about 20 per cent of the patients attending the clinics are now found to have classical venereal diseases such as syphilis and gonorrhoea. The majority are found to have other sexually transmitted conditions or related diseases and because of this trend the name of the specialty has been called into question by many physicians. Some think that the old-term venereal diseases should now be abandoned and the diseases called the sexually transmitted diseases. Many believe that it would be in the patients' interests, that it would make referrals by general practitioners easier and that it would help recruitment to the specialty, if the name was changed to genitourinary medicine and the specialists practising it were called genitourinary physicians. This proposed change of name has been approved by the Royal College of Physicians and the Department of Health and Social Security and several departments in university teaching hospitals have already adopted the new name. As a result, the final break with dermatology has come about in the United Kingdom and, as its new name implied, the specialty is now concentrating its major attention on the medical diseases of the genitourinary tract.

The last decade has also seen important developments and improvements in the service for sexually transmitted diseases in the United Kingdom. Several new clinics have been built and there are now 220 specialist clinics in the United Kingdom. All the university teaching hospitals have a clinic and undergraduate medical students receive clinical and laboratory teaching. A postgraduate course in sexually transmitted diseases of one university term of three months duration is now organised twice a year in London by the British Postgraduate Medical Federation and a diploma in venereology is awarded to successful candidates, following an examination, by the Society of Apothecaries of London. Research is only carried out at a limited number of centres but the quality of much of it has improved greatly. The Medical Society for the Study of Venereal Diseases remains the most active society in the world devoted exclusively to the subject and it publishes the *British Journal of Venereal Diseases* six times yearly. As yet there is no academic chair in the subject in the United Kingdom, but agreement has been reached with the Middlesex Hospital Medical School and London University for the creation of a chair in genitourinary medicine provided funds to finance it can be found from independent sources (Catterall, 1976).

Non-specific Genital Infection

Non-specific genital infection (NSGI) is now the commonest sexually transmitted disease diagnosed in the United Kingdom and in 1974 84 213 cases were recorded in the clinics. It is most usually detected as non-specific urethritis (NSU) in men and it is now much more prevalent than gonorrhoea, there being 70 988 cases of NSU in men in 1974 as compared with 38 466 cases of gonorrhoea in men in the same year. It has also been recognised that several other organs in the genitourinary tract may be infected such as the cervix, prostate, bladder, fallopian tubes and rectum. The association of the condition with diseases of the eye, such as inclusion conjunctivitis, punctate keratitis and uveitis, and the recognition of the relapsing nature of its most serious complication, Reiter's disease, has stimulated a considerable amount of research into its cause in recent years (King, 1972). The attempts to identify the cause or causes of the condition have tended to be at the expense of epidemiological, clinical and social aspects of the disease and much work remains to be done.

The search for the causes have taken several forms. The two principal agents which have been studied in detail are members of the genus *Chlamydia*, especially those of subgroup A, and the mycoplasmas, particularly the so-called T-strains. Various other organisms, such as staphylococci, diphtheroids and corynebacteria, have been studied but at present the available evidence does not suggest that they are responsible for many cases. Some observers have suggested that non-specific genital infection may be an autoimmune disease or due to allergy. There is little or no experimental evidence to support either of these contentions.

Inclusion bodies in urethral epithelial cells from the urethra of patients with non-specific urethritis have been observed for over 60 years and they have also been known to be present in cells from the conjunctiva in patients with inclusion conjunctivitis. In 1957 T'ang and others succeeded in culturing the causative agent of trachoma in the yolk sacs of fertile hen eggs. Shortly afterwards, Jones, Collier and Smith (1959) isolated a similar agent from patients with inclusion conjunctivitis and patients with non-specific urethritis. It is now believed that the agent responsible for inclusion conjunctivitis and 'non-specific' genital infections cannot be distinguished from the agent causing trachoma and the two conditions are believed to be due to a single organism. The agent concerned is a member of the group of organisms known as *Chlamydia* and its correct name is currently *Chlamydia trachomatis*. It is neither a virus nor a bacterium. Although restricted to obligate intracellular growth, it has a characteristic development cycle and multiplies by binary fission. It contains both DNA and RNA, has a cell wall, ribosomes and enzyme systems and its growth is inhibited by sulphonamides and antibiotics of the tetracycline group.

Isolation of the agent in yolk sac has been shown to be a relatively insensitive method of diagnosis and has been replaced by culture in irradiated McCoy cells (Dunlop et al, 1969). These techniques have been well described by Gordon and his colleagues (Gordon et al, 1969) and the techniques have been improved and simplified by Darougar, Cubitt and Jones (1974). The development of a microimmunofluorescent technique by Wang, Grayston and Gale (1973) has provided a useful technique for immunological classification and the identification of serotypes of the different strains of the organism.

Chlamydia have been isolated from cases of untreated non-specific urethritis in men, of cervicitis in women and of proctitis in both sexes. They have also been isolated from the genital tracts of both sexual partners in a number of instances. Dunlop and his colleagues (1972) have shown that *Chlamydia* of subgroup A can be isolated from 44.5 per cent of cases of non-specific urethritis in men and these results have been confirmed elsewhere. Richmond, Hilton and Clarke (1972) have isolated *Chlamydia* from 81 per cent of men with postgonococcal non-specific urethritis. Urethroscopy sometimes showed appearances of the urethra resembling the follicles found in the conjunctiva in cases of inclusion conjunctivitis and similar follicles have been demonstrated on the cervix of women with non-specific cervicitis.

Chlamydia are definitely pathogenic in the eye. The evidence now suggests that *Chlamydia* of subgroup A are associated with a significant proportion of non-specific genital infections and may well be one of the causes of the condition. However, it has yet to be proved that they are not opportunist organisms establishing themselves on already damaged tissue or that they are normal inhabitants of the genital tract which become easier to detect when there is infection from another cause.

The possible relationship between organisms of the genus *Mycoplasma* and non-specific genital infection is even more uncertain. These organisms can be grown on culture in many cases of urethral and genital infection, although the results have varied in different studies. The same organisms have, however, been found slightly less frequently in patients with no evidence of past or present genitourinary infection. More recently attention has been directed to a special variety of mycoplasma described by Shepard (1956) in which the colonies were considerably smaller than those of *Mycoplasma hominis* and which, because of the tiny size of the colonies, were called 'T-strains'. These strains have been isolated in over 70 per cent of cases of non-specific urethritis but they have also been found, usually less frequently, in the genitourinary tracts of apparently healthy people (Shepard, 1970). The role of mycoplasmas in non-specific genital infection remains a matter of speculation. Whether they cause the condition, are commensals or are non-pathogenic organisms, which become pathogenic under certain conditions, is unknown and has so far defied all attempts to clarify the situation. However, it is the general view of those who have studied the condition that they are unlikely to be the cause of many cases of non-specific genital infection.

The most important complications of the disease in men include follicular conjunctivitis, punctate keratitis, anterior uveitis, epididymitis, vesiculitis, cystitis, prostatitis, Reiter's disease and possibly ankylosing spondylitis. Postgonococcal non-specific urethritis occurs in about 10 to 20 per cent of men and it is widely believed that the agent causing non-specific urethritis is acquired at the same time as the gonococcus, but manifests itself later because of its longer incubation period. The most distressing personal consequence of the disease is frequently the psychological reaction which it provokes in the patient, particularly in relapsing cases. Anxiety, depression and a lowering of morale are very common and some patients become totally obsessed by their genitalia and their symptoms have important consequences on their work, leisure, family life and happiness.

Non-specific genital infection in women is difficult to diagnose and the criteria for diagnosis are unsatisfactory. The diagnosis is usually based on the knowledge of infection in the male sexual partner, symptoms such as vaginal discharge, dysuria or frequency and clinical evidence of genital infection in the form of cervicitis, urethritis or vaginitis. There is an excess of leucocytes on microscopical examination of stained slides of the secretions and cultures are sterile or grow only commensal organisms.

Complications in women include salpingitis, bartholinitis and Reiter's disease, as well as conjunctivitis, punctate keratitis and anterior uveitis. Babies born to mothers with non-specific genital infection may develop inclusion conjunctivitis during the first few days of life and *Chlamydia* of subgroup A can frequently be isolated from the infants' conjunctiva, the cervix of the mother, and in some instances, the urethra of the father.

It is now widely believed that non-specific proctitis occurs as a sexually transmitted disease in homosexual men and also in some women.

Treatment

As the causes of non-specific genital infection are unknown treatment must be empirical. If no treatment is given or the patient is given a placebo, in the majority of cases the symptoms and signs will diminish and may eventually disappear in the course of the next few weeks. Relapse is frequent but the incidence of complications is unknown. Withholding treatment causes considerable discomfort to the patient and produces increasing anxiety, as well as subjecting others to the risk of infection.

Controlled clinical trials and clinical experience indicate that antibiotics of the tetracycline group are superior to other antibiotics and chemotherapeutic agents. Tetracycline and oxytetracycline have been the most popular remedies and doses have varied from 250 to 500 mg 6-hourly for periods ranging from 5 to 21 days or longer (John, 1971). It has been suggested that patients with chlamydial infections require longer treatment than those in whom the agent cannot be demonstrated. Nevertheless cure rates vary greatly in different studies and range from 55 to 85 per cent. In general, recurrences increase with time and are related to the thoroughness and frequency of follow-up tests. Repeated relapses occur in about 10 to 15 per cent of men despite all treatment and may persist for periods varying from six months to three years, after which the disease often tends to disappear spontaneously. Some of these patients may have impaired cell-mediated immunity. There is no evidence of any general protective immunity following infection but localised tissue concentrations of plasma cells and immunoglobulins in the cervix and urethra have been demonstrated in biopsy specimens from infected patients, suggesting that there may be some local immune response (Chipperfield and Evans, 1972).

Reiter's disease

The most serious complication of non-specific genital infection is Reiter's disease. In the United Kingdom this interesting condition appears to have a sexually transmitted origin in the vast majority of cases although in some areas of Europe and Asia it is reported in association with bacillary dysentery and non-specific diarrhoea. In some cases the patient may have gonorrhoea. It is unlikely that either gonorrhoea or dysentery are the cause of the Reiter's disease, but it is possible that the damage to the urethral and intestinal mucosae by these organisms may act as a predisposing factor. The true incidence of the disease is unknown but it has been suggested that between 1 and 2 per cent of patients with non-specific genital infection will subsequently develop Reiter's disease. The condition is recognised and diagnosed predominantly in men but it does occur in women, although it is particularly difficult to be certain of the diagnosis in them. In 1974, 492 cases were diagnosed in the clinics in England, 447 in men and 25 in women (Department of Health and Social Security, 1974).

Recently important research work by Brewerton and his colleagues (1973) has established that the majority of the patients who develop Reiter's syndrome possess the histocompatibility antigen HLA-27 (W27), whereas the majority of those with non-specific genital infection who do not have this antigen do not develop the condition. Furthermore a close correlation between the occurrence of sacro-iliitis and uveitis with the presence of HLA-27 has been demonstrated. It seems probable that the possession of HLA-27 histocompatibility antigen predisposes patients to the development of arthritis and other clinical manifestations after certain types of infection.

Lawrence (1974) studied the relatives of a series of patients with Reiter's disease, the majority of whom were examined both clinically and radio-logically. Psoriasis was found to be nine times more common in male relatives of patients with Reiter's disease than in the general population and was almost as frequent as in psoriatic families. Ankylosing spondylitis was eight and bilateral sacroiliac involvement was three times as frequent in the relatives of those with the disease as in the control group. He concluded that there was a genetic association with both psoriasis and ankylosing spondylitis.

The possible role of *Chlamydia* as an aetiological agent in the development of Reiter's disease has been reviewed by Dunlop et al (1967). So far the results are unconvincing but improved methods of culturing the agent and new immunological tests may help to clarify the position in the future. The situation with regard to *Mycoplasma* as a causative agent has been well reviewed by McCormack and colleagues (1973) and they concluded that the available evidence did not suggest that the organism was a likely initiating factor.

So the cause of Reiter's disease remains unknown, but it is becoming increasingly clear that a significant number of patients have multiple relapses leading to eventual residual damage to joints, painful deformities of the feet, sacro-iliitis and stiffness of the spine and recurrent attacks of uveitis. The less common manifestations of the disease such as thrombophlebitis of the deep veins of the legs, conduction defects in the heart, aortic valvular disease, neuralgic amyotrophy, encephalopathy, optic neuritis, amyloidosis and changes indistinguishable from ankylosing spondylitis are now more widely recognised.

Numerous drug regimes have been advocated for the treatment of Reiter's disease but there have been very few controlled clinical trials. The usual therapy consists of bed rest, tetracycline and analgesics, such as aspirin derivatives, phenylbutazone or indomethacin. Steroids are usually only given to patients with rapidly progressive florid disease. Gold therapy has been advocated in protracted and severe cases. Cytotoxic and immunosuppressive drugs have been used by some workers, particularly folic acid antagonists. The greatest experience has been with methotrexate (Farber, Forshner and O'Quinn, 1967) and aminopterin, but the number of reported cases is small and it is not yet established that these preparations produce sufficient benefit to justify the obvious dangers of their use. Treatment of anterior uveitis with atropine and prednisolone drops is usually supervised by an ophthalmologist. As Reiter's disease is usually associated with genital infection correct manage-ment should include investigation of the sexual partners.

Gonorrhoea

It is now generally recognised that measures taken to try to control this disease throughout the world have failed and the condition is completely out of control in most countries. The rate per 100 000 of population of reported cases in the United States rose from 129.8 in 1957 to 410.5 in 1974 (American Social Health Association, 1975). In England there were 58 139 cases in 1974 and the rate per 100 000 of population was 95.6 in 1968 and 134.2 in 1974. However, it should be pointed out that standards of diagnosis and reporting vary greatly from country to country and in most areas there is gross under-reporting of cases, so the true incidence of the disease is unknown.

Some of the reasons for failure of control are the decreasing sensitivity of the gonococcus to antibiotics, the short incubation period making it difficult to interrupt the chain of infection, the highly infectious nature of the disease, the lack of protective immunity, variable standards of diagnosis, treatment and management by physicians and lack of proper health education, especially for young people.

Morton (1971) has drawn attention to the social factors which have influenced the situation throughout the past 20 years. He believes that prosperity has brought more leisure and given to many the time and impetus to demand greater freedom, especially sexually. At the same time restraints on behaviour resulting from influences by the family, religion, social custom, neighbours and public opinion have declined. Juhlin (1968) studied a group of patients with gonorrhoea and a control group in Uppsala, Sweden. He concluded that the increase in gonorrhoea was probably due to the availability and widespread use of contraceptive pills and the growth of sexual freedom.

The most important development in the clinical aspects of gonorrhoea in recent years has been the recognition that symptomless infection was more frequent in men than had previously been suspected, especially in the urethra, rectum and pharynx and tonsils. Equally important has been the increased incidence of complications of the infection in both sexes.

Both Handsfield et al (1974) and Perera and Lim (1975) have drawn attention to the fact that an increasing number of men have no symptoms of gonorrhoea yet gonococci can be found in tests taken from the urethral wall. Other investigators have described similar findings and it is probable that asymptomatic men now constitute about 10 per cent of all patients with the disease. It has long been recognised that over 50 per cent of women with gonococcal infections have no symptoms but the importance of symptomless anorectal infections in patients of both sexes has been stressed in recent years. For example, Olsen (1971) showed that inclusion of rectal smears and cultures in the routine examination of women for gonorrhoea would increase the yield by between 2 and 6 per cent and Bhattacharyya and Jephcott (1974) recommended that rectal examination and sampling were an essential part of the investigation of all named female contacts of men with the disease.

In the past oropharyngeal gonorrhoea has been regarded as uncommon. However, an increasing number of cases are being recognised, especially in the United States of America, Sweden and Denmark. The majority of authors stress that symptoms are usually slight or absent and the clinical appearance has no special characteristics. They recommend that all those patients who have had orogenital sexual contact, especially homosexual men, should have throat samples taken (Stolz and Schuller, 1974).

The rising incidence of gonococcal salpingitis has been the subject of several reports in recent years. Rees and Annels (1969) found salpingitis in 61 (10.6 per cent) of 606 consecutive cases of gonorrhoea, whereas Weström (1975) stated that in Sweden 20 per cent of infected patients developed pelvic inflammatory disease and of 415 women with salpingitis 88 (21.2 per cent became sterile as a result of the infection. The frequency of ectopic pregnancy, chronic dyspareunia, sterility and relapsing chronic pelvic inflammatory disease in young girls and women is related by many other Scandinavian authors to the high incidence of gonorrhoea in these age groups.

In recent years an increasing number of cases of gonococcal septicaemia have been recognised. Holmes, Counts and Beaty (1971) described a series of patients with disseminated gonococcal infection, two of whom had meningitis, two endocarditis and one fatal pericarditis. Seventy-nine per cent of the patients were women and the dissemination seemed to occur during menstruation or pregnancy. Danielsson (1971) in Sweden stated that the majority of his patients presented with bouts of fever, arthralgia, arthritis and skin rashes, which usually gave the clue to the diagnosis and Barr and Danielsson (1971) described the gonococcal skin lesions in detail. They are usually few in number and tend to affect the distal parts of the limbs. They are discrete and begin as pinpoint erythematous macules, becoming papular, vesiculopustular and haemorrhagic. The fully developed lesion is raised, slightly umbilicated and the centre contains grey necrotic material surrounded by an irregular haemorrhagic border or an erythematous halo. Healing occurs in three to four days, leaving some residual brownish discolouration but permanent scarring is rare.

Gonococci can usually be found in the genital tract although genital symptoms are rare. Blood cultures may be positive but the gonococcus is difficult to grow in the blood as it is from joint fluid or the skin lesions. Better results are usually obtained by fluorescent techniques from the material from the skin. The condition usually responds satisfactorily to penicillin which should be given in large doses for several days.

An interesting condition of gonococcal perihepatitis has also been diagnosed more commonly in recent years. It is more frequent in women with pelvic inflammatory diseases but has also been found in men (Kimball and Knee, 1970). The condition presents with sudden pain in the right upper abdomen, worse on deep breathing and coughing. There is fever, nausea and occasionally vomiting. There is great tenderness on palpation of the right side of the upper abdomen and the condition suggests acute cholecystitis, pyelonephritis, pleurisy, subphrenic abscess, renal calculus or even a perforated peptic ulcer. The ESR is raised and a chest x-ray may show a small pleural effusion on the right side. Genital tests may show evidence of urethritis, cervicitis or salpingitis and, if antibiotics have not been given, gonococci may be found. A late complication may be adhesions between the surface of the liver, the diaphragm and the anterior abdominal wall.

The gonococcus has been a greatly neglected organism by microbiologists and research workers. However, there are now indications that greater interest is being taken in the bacterium and the volume and quality of research work has increased in recent years. In clinical practice rapid presumptive diagnoses are made by microscopical examination of Gram-stained smears and confirmed by cultural diagnosis, either by direct inoculation in the clinic of highly nutrient culture media, such as McLeod's heated blood agar, selective media, such as Thayer–Martin medium or Columbia agar or by the inoculation of a transport medium, such as that described by Stuart. Confirmation of identity by the oxidase reaction, Gram staining of selected colonies and fermentation reactions are widely used and in skilled and dedicated hands produce excellent results. Sensitivity testing of strains of gonococci is commonly undertaken, but unfortunately no standard technique is employed and the results are usually not comparable. There is still no serological test for the disease and the gonococcal complement fixation test has been abandoned in most centres because of its lack of sensitivity and specificity.

Fluorescent antibody testing for gonococci was originally introduced by Deacon in 1959 and the techniques have been greatly modified and developed in recent years. The test depends upon the principle that antibody to gonococci when conjugated with fluorescein isothiocyanate produces a highly specific stain for gonococci, which can be easily visualised under a suitable microscope. Non-specific fluorescence and both false positive and false negative results have proved to be a major difficulty but considerable progress has been made to reduce these to acceptable levels. The test can be carried out by the 'direct' technique on smears of material taken directly from the patient or by the 'indirect' method, in which culture plates are inoculated and incubated for 18 or 30 h before the strains are stained and examined on microscope slides. The success of the test depends upon the specificity of the antiserum employed and considerable progress has been made so that the delayed fluorescent antibody test is not only used in diagnosis of infection but is also used to replace fermentation reactions to establish the exact identity of the *Neisseria* concerned.

Cultural methods have been greatly improved by the introduction of selective media, which suppress the growth of other organisms and allow the gonococcus to grow more freely. This has resulted in improved isolation rates, especially in samples from the pharynx and rectum. Modifications of the Thayer–Martin medium, containing vancomycin, colistin and nystatin have proved the most popular but there is still considerable debate as to whether the addition of trimethoprim is beneficial as it would prevent overgrowth of the plate with *Proteus* species and other contaminants. Some workers believe that the use of selective media inhibits the growth of too many strains and Reyn (1969) has suggested the use of a combination of a selective and non-selective medium for each strain.

Attempts to develop a transport and growth medium, using modified Thayer–Martin medium with the addition of trimethoprim, in a special bottle containing carbon dioxide, in order to save time in establishing the diagnosis, were promising under laboratory conditions but proved to be disappointing under ordinary clinical conditions.

Serum immunoglobulin levels in uncomplicated gonorrhoea in men mostly fall within the normal range, but in some cases, and in those with complications, levels of IgM, IgG and IgA may be raised. Local immunoglobulin production in the cervix in women with gonococcal cervicitis has been demonstrated by Chipperfield and Evans (1972) in biopsy specimens and in some cases it seems probable that the gonococcus may be eliminated from the endocervix by this method. Various attempts have been made to develop a sensitive and specific serological test using such techniques as precipitin formation, haemagglutination, flocculation, fluorescence and radioimmunoassay. Tests using purified gonococcal pili as antigen have given encouraging initial results but disadvantages and unexpected difficulties have emerged.

In 1971 Swanson, Kraus and Gotschlich demonstrated conclusively that gonococci of Kellog's types I and II, namely those virulent for the human host, showed pili under the electron microscope. Later Ward and Watt (1972) showed zones of adherence between gonococci and epithelial cells and Swanson (1973) suggested that the pili were probably concerned with attachment to the tissue cells. It has now been demonstrated that the attachment of gonococci to epithelial cells causes the cells to throw out pseudopodial processes and eventually ingest the cell. Electron microscope studies suggest that the gonococci survive in the cells for several hours.

Attempts to produce a vaccine have so far been unsuccessful and the natural history of the disease, which indicates that there is little or no evidence of the development of protective immunity in those infected with the organism, does not encourage the hope that a vaccine would be protective against further reinfection. Nevertheless, research into the gonococcus and its effects in the host has gathered considerable momentum and great progress has been made. However, there are still many areas of total ignorance and much further work is required.

Penicillin remains the most popular preparation used in the treatment of gonorrhoea in both sexes. Cure rates are related to both the dosage and the number of relatively resistent strains of organisms in the region. Over the past 25 years there have been a series of cycles in which the failure rates of treatment have risen and this has been followed by higher dosage schedules with temporary improvements in the cure rates. In South-East Asia and the west coast of the United States of America single dose treatment with aqueous procaine penicillin has now reached levels of 4.8 or 6.4 mega units. In 1969 Olsen and Lomholt published a report from Greenland where the morbidity rate for gonorrhoea was 10 000 per 100 000 of the population. In 1963 about 80 per cent of local strains showed reduced sensitivity to penicillin and treatment failure rates were of the order of 27 per cent. To try to overcome this serious situation they instituted a treatment regime of 5 mega units of benzyl penicillin G in 8 ml of 0.5 per cent lignocaine, preceded by 1 g of probenecid orally. The cure rate was 99 per cent. Before the trial started 80 per cent of strains showed reduced sensitivity to penicillin and at the end of a two-year period only 19 per cent of strains were in this group.

Other treatment schedules that are in current use and have been subjected to clinical trials are ampicillin, 2 g, preceded by 1 g of probenecid and followed by a further dose of 2 g of ampicillin 12 h later; co-trimoxazole four tablets every 12 h for three days; kanamycin 2 g intramuscularly in a single dose; spectinomycin hydrochloride 2 g intramuscularly once only; and tetra-cycline 500 mg 6-hourly for three days. Many other antibiotics are effective against the disease.

Gonorrhoea is now one of the commonest and most important communicable diseases in the world. If it is to be brought under control undergraduate and postgraduate education throughout the world must be improved, clinical services for diagnosis and treatment extended, research encouraged and expanded and contact tracing made more effective. With rapid air travel international contact tracing has become of great importance and greater efforts are needed in all countries to make this possible.

Candidosis

Infestation of the genital tract with the fungus *Candida albicans* has been increasing during the past decade and it is now the commonest infectious agent isolated from women attending clinics for sexually transmitted diseases. It has been observed to be sexually transmitted in certain cases since 1920 and about 10 per cent of the male sexual partners of women with vaginal candidosis were found by Diddle et al (1969) to have candidal balanoposthitis. Certain factors appear to cause the organism to produce a symptomatic clinical condition where previously it has been a commensal. They include pregnancy, glycosuria, the administration of broad spectrum antibiotics, steroids, immunosuppressive drugs, and more recently it has been shown that gestogenic contraceptive pills can also exacerbate vaginal candidosis (Catterall, 1971). Species of *Candida* can frequently be recovered from the stools, the oral cavity, the nails, the external ears and the intertrigenous areas and Pedersen (1969) isolated the organism from the rectum in 69 per cent of pregnant women.

Urethritis in men due to *Candida albicans* is relatively uncommon and usually only occurs in an already damaged urethra (Rohatiner, 1966). Balanitis and balanoposthitis are the commonest manifestations in men and Catterall (1966) reported four patients with soreness and ulceration of the penis commencing 6 to 24 h after intercourse with their wives, all of whom were infested with the fungus. He postulated that this was a hypersensitivity phenomenon as *Candida* could not be found in the men and their clinical condition responded immediately to 1 per cent hydrocortisone cream.

In addition to vulval irritation, vaginal discharge and sometimes dysuria, Barr (1972) points out that women frequently complain of dyspareunia and notice burning and itching immediately after intercourse. The most difficult problem is to assess the significance of asymptomatic candidosis in women. The mycelium seen on Gram-stained smears is usually due to *Candida albicans* but there are many advantages to culturing it on Sabouraud's maltose-peptone agar and carrying out the germ tube test. Oriel et al (1972) found yeasts in culture from 138 (26 per cent) of 533 women and *Candida albicans* accounted for 112 (81 per cent), *Torulopsis glabrata* for 22 (16 per cent) and other yeasts for only 4 (3 per cent).

Unfortunately treatment is still with local applications of antifungal agents and the results are likely to remain unsatisfactory until a safe, efficient, systemic preparation is available. A large variety of new and old antifungal agents are available such as clortrimazole (Canesten), candicin (Candeptin), amphotericin (Fungilin), nifurate (Magmilor), natamycin (Pimafucin) and hydragraphen (Penotrane). It is extremely difficult to assess their relative merits and nystatin, which is available as vaginal pessaries, oral tablets and ointment or cream, is probably as effective as any and has few or no side effects. Relapse is frequent. In such cases a long course of treatment over several months using a decreasing number of pessaries a week, the application of nystatin cream to the vulva and perineum, oral nystatin to clear the intestine and investigation of the sex partners is indicated. Search should also be made for any predisposing factors (Nicol, 1971).

Trichomoniasis

The parasite *Trichomonas vaginalis* is widely accepted as being the commonest cause of vaginal discharge in women and it has been stated that one woman in every five is infested at some time during the sexually active period of her life. The percentage of their male sexual partners found to harbour the parasite varies from 13 to 60 per cent and the great majority of them are symptomless carriers. Of men presenting with non-gonococcal urethritis between 5 and 10 per cent are found to be infested (Dunlop and Wisdom, 1965). The sexual transmission of the disease now seems firmly established (Catterall and Nicol, 1969) but means of transmission other than sexual may sometimes occur (Valent and Cătár, 1967). Berggren (1969) found the incidence of trichomoniasis in Swedish women to be 7.4 per cent, but in patients with cervical carcinoma in situ and invasive carcinoma the rate was four times greater and he and other authors have discussed the role of the parasite in the development of cervical cancer.

The association of trichomoniasis with other sexually transmissible diseases has been increasingly recognised and in Russia Lopatin and Kolesnikova (1971) found that 34.5 per cent of women with gonorrhoea also had concomitant trichomoniasis. Block (1968) drew attention once again to the observation that trichomoniasis frequently presents with the symptoms of cystitis. The wide variety of clinical manifestations of the disease have been recently reviewed by Catterall (1972b).

The most widely employed methods of diagnosis are the examination by dark ground microscopy, ordinary light microscopy or phase contrast microscopy of a fresh specimen of secretion, together with the inoculation of cultures usually containing proteolysed liver, human serum and an antibiotic and antifungal agent. There is some difference of opinion about the value of staining techniques but good results have been claimed with Papanicolaou stain, brilliant cresyl blue and, more recently, Boulin's solution of 3 per cent silver nitrate. A variety of techniques has been used to demonstrate specific antibodies in the serum against *T. vaginalis*. Complement fixation tests, immunofluorescent reactions and skin tests have given variable results but recently antibodies in the vaginal secretions of women with the disease have been demonstrated by Ackers et al (1975). Previously Lumsden, Robertson and McNeillage (1966) had described experiments on the isolation, cultivation, preservation at low temperature and infectivity of *T. vaginalis*.

Metronidazole (Flagyl) has been shown to be as effective today as it was in 1960 when it was first introduced into clinical practice. Cure rates of the order of 95 to 98 per cent are often reported at a dosage of 200 mg three times daily for seven days or 400 mg twice daily for five days. Treatment in the first three months of pregnancy is not recommended. Side effects are few and consist of nausea, a bad taste in the mouth, headache, dizziness, skin rashes and drowsiness. The commonest causes of treatment failure are irregular ingestion of the drug, failure of absorption, reinfestation by a sexual partner and inactivation of metronidazole by certain vaginal bacteria. Claims that resistant strains of organisms have been found have not been substantiated.

Various other trichomonacidal agents have been made available. Nimorazole (Naxogen) and nifuratel (Magmilor) have been shown to be effective in treatment and may be useful in cases where metronidazole is not indicated.

Genital Warts

The papilloma virus causing genital warts is sexually transmissible and the incidence of the condition is increasing considerably in England. The treatment takes up a disproportionate amount of the patient's time, not to mention that of the doctor or nurse who gives the treatment and is frequently far from satisfactory. Genital warts are often seen in association with other sexually transmitted diseases and this is particularly so with perianal warts and rectal gonorrhoea. Oriel and Almeida (1970) using an electron microscope and negative staining demonstrated intranuclear virus particles in thin sections of genital warts in 13 of 25 patients.

According to Oriel (1971), who studied a large number of cases, a small number of patients with skin warts elsewhere on the body also have distinctive genital warts, resembling verruca vulgaris, and he considered it was possible that transfer of virus particles had occurred from the skin sites to the genitalia. He also noted that 64 per cent of the sex contacts of patients with condylomata accuminata developed genital warts and that the incubation period could be over two years. A retrospective study by the same author of 500 homosexual patients showed that anal warts were seven times commoner than penile warts and he concluded that there may be other factors besides sexual contact which account for the high incidence of perianal warts. Intrameatal penile warts are a common finding and Halverstadt and Parry (1969) have drawn attention to the frequency of recurrence in this site. Giant condylomata of the penis and more rarely of the anorectal region have been described in recent years.

Very few studies have been carried out on wart virus antibodies and further work is needed to help in the understanding of the natural history of the condition.

Treatment continues to be with podophyllin, trichloracetic acid and cauterisation. Recently Chamberlain, Reynolds and Yoeman (1972) treated a primigravida with the surprising amount of 7.5 ml of 25 per cent podophyllin in compound tincture of benzoin under general anaesthesia. A severe peripheral neuropathy and stillbirth resulted. This example of gross over-dosage has served as a warning that great care should be taken in the use of podophyllin, especially in pregnancy.

Further work is needed on immunological aspects of the condition and especially on treatment methods.

Herpes Genitalis

This condition has become very frequent in venereological practice and is now the commonest cause of genital ulceration in England. The virus causing disease of the genital tract can be distinguished antigenically and biologically and is usually known as herpes virus type 2 to distinguish it from type 1, which is usually isolated from the mouth and face. However, this differentiation does not always occur and type 1 virus is found in genital lesions and type 2 in oral lesions (Smith, Peutherer and Robertson, 1973).

Primary attacks frequently produce severe symptoms in women with fever, generalised malaise and very intense pain in the vulva and vagina, often necessitating complete bed rest. Recently Goldmeir, Pateman and Rodin (1975) have described a series of cases of anorectal herpes with severe pain and retention of urine. Clinical diagnosis is best confirmed by tissue culture on human embryo lung, HeLa cells or the chorioallantoic membrane of eggs.

Various transport media may be used and Rodin et al (1971) have shown that Stuart's transport medium is very satisfactory. The presence of antibodies to herpes virus type 2 in the serum may be helpful but in general their presence is no more than suggestive of the possible diagnosis. Detection of giant multinucleated syncetial cells typical of the condition in cervical cytology specimens is now recognised much more frequently and has drawn attention to the frequency of symptomless infections of the cervix.

Nahmias et al (1969) have described the dangerous complications in newborn infants as a result of infection from the cervix at birth. He puts the risk to the infant as high as 60 per cent and many died of encephalitis, visceral infection and generalised dissemination of the condition. He recommends that caesarian section should be considered in all cases of maternal genital herpes. Other workers have reported an increase in abortion and congenital malformations in cases where the mother was infected early in the pregnancy. In adults encephalitis, meningitis and hepatitis have been described. But the most important association is between genital infection with herpes virus type 2 and the later development of carcinoma of the cervix. Naib et al (1969), Royston and Aurelian (1970) and several others have found significantly higher antibody levels against the virus in patients with carcinoma of the cervix than in matched controls. Further, Aurelian et al (1971) have identified herpes virus type 2 in cervical cancer cells, undergoing degeneration in tissue culture, by electronmicroscopy. Lehner, Wilton and Schillitoe (1975) have considered the evidence that herpes virus type 1 may be associated with the development of squamous cell carcinoma of the lip. At present the evidence in both sites is circumstantial but is strong enough to indicate that patients with herpes of the cervix should be followed closely with regular cervical cytological tests.

Treatment remains disappointing. As it is now well established that the virus invades the sensory nerves and the posterior root ganglia a systemic treatment is essential if cure is to be effected. Idoxuridine alone or dissolved in dimethyl sulphoxide at various strengths applied to the lesions as early as possible has been claimed to shorten the attacks but there is no evidence that it prevents recurrences.

Photodynamic inactivation by sensitisation of the lesions with 0.1 per cent aqueous solution of neutral red or proflavine followed by exposure of the area to either fluorescent or ordinary light has been tried by Felber et al (1971). Relief of symptoms and early healing of lesions was said to occur in some patients, but the method has been criticised because of the theoretical danger that it might encourage the development of malignant changes.

Recently vaccines have been employed by Nasemann (1970) and later by Söltz-Szöts (1971) with interesting results. The vaccine was prepared from herpes virus antigen and herpes in all sites was treated. Söltz-Szöts used influenza A vaccine for patients with herpes zoster and some with recurrent herpes virus infections and thought that the method stimulated the production of interferon. Much work remains to be done but it seems theoretically possible that a satisfactory solution to this very intractable and common problem may eventually result from vaccination.

Syphilis

The incidence of infectious syphilis has been increasing during the past decade with high rates of infection in certain countries, such as the United States of America and Poland, and relatively low rates in others, such as the United Kingdom and Sweden. In most industrial countries the problem is an urban one and the most important high risk group is the promiscuous homosexual male (Fluker, 1972). For example in central and west London 82 per cent of cases of early infectious syphilis occurred in homosexual men. Another important factor in the failure to control the incidence of syphilis has been ignorance of the facts about the disease and lack of clinical experience with patients with the disease among members of the medical profession. Webster (1972) has stressed the fact that undergraduate teaching is frequently inadequate, particularly in the United States. The marked change in the patterns of sexual behaviour and the increasing mobility of large sections of the population are also important factors (Willcox, 1972).

Nevertheless, the gains have been substantial. There has been a sharp fall in deaths from syphilis and cases of cardiovascular and neurosyphilis have become rare. Gummata and the tertiary cutaneous skin and bone lesions are seen infrequently and the incidence of congenital syphilis is now very low. However, latent syphilis, despite some decline in incidence, remains a frequent condition and its differentiation from other treponemal diseases or from the biological false positive phenomenon can present serious diagnostic difficulties.

The essential diagnostic test in primary syphilis is still examination of material from the primary chancre under the dark ground microscope and the identification of *Treponema pallidum*. The fluorescent treponemal antibody test (FTA-ABS) has a high degree of sensitivity and it becomes positive early in the course of the disease. Nevertheless, many patients with early primary chancres have a negative test and a fluorescent technique is available for detecting *T. pallidum* in specimens taken from the lesion itself. Garner and Robson (1968) in Australia obtained excellent results but Kellogg (1970) was less certain about the accuracy of the test.

Secondary syphilis continues to be the great imitator and the diagnosis is frequently missed by the inexperienced. In rare cases the serological tests may be negative, particularly the reagin tests, possibly due to an excess of antibodies in the serum producing the prozone phenomenon, which can be abolished by diluting the serum (Spangler et al, 1964). Uveitis and choroidoretinitis may result in impairment of vision and Schmidt and Goldschmidt (1972) have demonstrated treponemes in the aqueous humour in secondary syphilis. Hepatitis has been regarded as uncommon but several recent reports (Lee, Thornton and Conn, 1971) suggest that it occurs more frequently than is usually supposed. Involvement of the central nervous system is well known but cases of perceptive deafness with the sudden onset of severe impairment of hearing have been described by several authors, including Willcox and Goodwin (1971).

Idsøe, Guthe and Willcox (1972) have demonstrated that patients who are diagnosed as having latent syphilis and are given treatment with penicillin have a good prognosis. A detailed report of 251 patients with neurosyphilis was published by Hooshmand, Escobar and Kopf (1972).

The diagnosis of congenital syphilis in the first few weeks of life may be very difficult. Scotti and Logan (1968) has suggested the use of an FTA-ABS test using fluorescin-labelled IgM conjugate in place of the ordinary fluorescin-labelled antihuman globulin. A positive test shows the presence of IgM antibodies to symphilis produced by the infant as these antibodies do not pass through the placenta from the maternal to the fetal circulation. The limitations of the test have been pointed out by Ackerman (1969). Cremin and Fisher (1970) reviewed the radiological findings in 106 patients with congenital syphilis.

In 1966 Karmody and Schuknecht described 47 patients with deafness due to congenital syphilis. The patients affected early in childhood developed profound bilateral deafness of sudden onset with minimal vestibular dysfunction. Patients affected at a later stage in early or mid-adult life usually presented with vertigo, tinnitus and deafness, frequently indistinguishable from Ménières disease. Morrison (1969) used prednisone to treat 22 patients and 10 showed marked improvement. Kerr, Smyth and Cinnamond (1973) used prednisone and ampicillin and stressed the importance of speech discrimination tests in assessing progress.

There had been several advances in serological tests for syphilis during the past decade. It is convenient to divide these tests into reagin tests and specific tests. The reagin tests measure a non-specific substance called reagin which appears in the serum of patients with syphilis and other treponemal diseases. It is usually measured by complement-fixation tests, such as the Wassermann reaction (WR) or flocculation tests such as the Venereal Disease Research Laboratory test (VDRL), the Kahn, Meinicke, Price or other similar tests.

The specific serological tests use *Treponema pallidum*, or some part of it, as the antigen and, therefore, measure different antibodies in the serum. They include the treponemal immobilisation test (TPI), the fluorescent treponemal antibody test (FTA), the *Treponema pallidum* haemagglutination test (TPHA) and several others.

It is usual to carry out more than one test on each specimen of serum and with the advent of automated tests and improvements in autoanalysers only those tests which can be automated are likely to survive. A common practice is to perform the VDRL test, which is quantified, and the TPHA test on all sera, and, if there are problems in interpretation of the results in conjunction with the clinical history and physical findings, to carry out the FTA-ABS test. With this combination of tests it is usually possible to reach a diagnosis but in a small percentage of cases further help will be needed and the TPI test will usually provide the necessary data.

The FTA-ABS test is the most sensitive and usually becomes positive first in primary syphilis. It has satisfactory specificity but some false positive reactions occur in sera from patients with balanitis and lupus erythematosus. For the follow-up and study of the effects of treatment the titred VDRL test is the most satisfactory and the test should become negative about six to nine months after successful treatment of early infectious syphilis. The TPHA test is a relative newcomer to the serological scene and is very easy to perform. It appears to be somewhere between the FTA-ABS and the VDRL. It remains positive for very many years after apparently successful treatment of early and late syphilis.

False positive reactions occur in the reagin tests for syphilis and may be technical false positive reactions or biological false positive reactions. The former may result from mistakes in labelling specimens, use of faulty reagents in the tests, mistakes in performing the tests and errors in reporting the results. Biological false positive results occur when reagin appears in the patient's serum for reasons other than a treponemal disease. Acute false positive reactions are short-lived and last less than six months and are usually associated with immunisation or vaccination, glandular fever, hepatitis, malaria and certain bacterial and viral infections. Chronic biological false positive reactions usually persist for years or for the rest of life and are frequently one of the serological manifestations of autoimmune disease, especially systemic lupus erythematosus, haemolytic anaemia, Hashimoto's thyroiditis and a variety of other conditions. They are more frequent in young women and are associated with the development of antinuclear, mitochondrial and other autoantibodies, such as rheumatoid factor or cryoglobulins (Catterall, 1972a).

It is important to remember that the finding of a positive test for reagin, confirmed on a second specimen of serum, in the absence of a definite history or adequate clinical evidence of syphilis, should not be immediately diagnosed as latent syphilis, but is a definite indication for the performance of a specific treponemal test to confirm the diagnosis.

Penicillin remains the treatment of choice for syphilis in all its stages. Collart (1970) has shown that the average multiplication time of T. *pallidum* is 30 to 33 h and a minimal concentration of 0.03 i.u. of penicillin per millilitre of serum should be maintained for 7 to 10 days. This is best achieved by daily intramuscular injections of procaine penicillin at a dose of 600 000 units in each injection. Long-acting preparations, such as benzathine penicillin are used with increasing frequency but experience with their use is very limited and no long-term controlled trials have been undertaken. The same limitations apply to the commonly used alternatives to penicillin, namely tetracycline and erythromycin.

The Jarisch–Herxheimer reaction occurs most commonly in patients with secondary syphilis and in patients with neurosyphilis with a raised cell count in the cerebrospinal fluid. Recent work indicates that it is associated with changes in complement, which becomes activated by the classical pathway shortly before the] clinical manifestations of the reaction develop (Fulford et al, 1976). Some physicians claim that it can be prevented or diminished by small doses of steroids before and during the early stages of penicillin treatment (Gudjönsson and Skog, 1968).

Experimental work in syphilis has been mainly directed towards electron microscopical studies of *T. pallidum* (Ovčinnikov and Delektorskij, 1971). These workers have demonstrated trilaminar membranes and a capsule on their outside and have also shown treponemes inside cells, especially macrophages, endothelial cells and monocytes. Collart, Poggi and Dunoyer (1966) have continued their important work on the persistence of treponemes after treatment, the interpretation of which still produces much discussion. Further immunological studies and the presence of other antibodies is syphilitic sera have been studied by Lassus (1969) and lymphocyte migration and transformation test on syphilitic sera have been described by Fulford and Brostoff (1972). Work towards the development of a vaccine against syphilis has been undertaken by Miller (1967, 1972) and Metzyger and Smogór (1969).

Pediculosis Pubis and Scabies (see pp. 69–73)

The frequent association of pediculosis pubis and other sexually transmitted diseases in the same patient has been stressed by Altchek (1970), who states that the finding of one should lead to the search for the others. The increase in the incidence of the condition was underlined by Fisher and Morton (1970) and resistance to various insecticides was discussed by Busvine (1967).

The rising incidence of scabies was demonstrated by Shrank and Alexander (1967) in London and by Pace and Purres (1970) in Canada. Orkin (1971) reviewed the world-wide factors responsible for the increase and stressed population movement and promiscuity.

Cases of acute glomerular nephritis associated with secondarily infected scabies have been published by Hersch (1967) and Allen (1972). An excellent review of the subject was given by Lyall (1967) who points out that scabies should be suspected in all cases of persistent generalised itch and demonstrating *Sarcoptes scabei* establishes the diagnosis beyond doubt.

Treatment, especially with benzyl benzoate, is considered by Maleville and Heid (1972) who recommend that all sexual and domestic contacts should receive epidemiological treatment.

Molluscum Contagiosum

Cobbold and Macdonald (1970) produced strong evidence that molluscum contagiosum was usually a sexually transmitted disease and the same views were held by Lynch and Minkin (1968), who reviewed cases seen in servicemen returning from Korea and Vietnam. Very little work has been done on growing the virus or on treatment and the application of phenol to each individual lesion still seems to be a very popular method of managing the condition.

Chancroid, Lymphogranuloma Venereum and Granuloma Inguinale

These diseases are seen infrequently in temperate climates and individual experience with them is therefore limited. *Haemophilus ducreyi*, the cause of chancroid, is difficult to grow on culture and is usually cultivated on defribrinated rabbit's blood enriched with several other ingredients. A medium using inactivated serum from the patient was described by Borchardt and Hoke (1970). The same authors described a technique for preparing slides for staining using sterile cotton-tipped applicators.

The Ito–Reenstierna intradermal test is rarely performed today because of false positive reactions and the withdrawal of the commercial vaccine. Treatment with sulphonamides, streptomycin or the tetracyclines is usually very satisfactory.

Lymphogranuloma venereum is caused by an agent of the genus *Chlamydia*. The inguinal lymphatic swellings and the constitutional symptoms should suggest the diagnosis, which is usually confirmed by the Frei intradermal test and the complement fixation test. The subject has been well reviewed by Hopsu-Havu and Sonck (1973). Late manifestations include genital lymphatic oedema, anorectal stricture and malignant changes. The most satisfactory treatment is with the tetracyclines but the sulphonamides are also effective early in the course of the disease.

The Donovan bodies causing the rather dramatic granulomatous condition of granuloma inguinale can usually be demonstrated by staining specimens from scrapings of the lesions or from biopsies by Wright's or Giemsa's stain. Lal and Nicholas (1970) found the majority of cases diagnosed to be in men but 52 per cent of their female sexual partners were infected. Malignant changes were described by Davis (1970). Treatment with streptomycin or tetracycline gives successful results in most patients.

Hepatitis B

Since the discovery of Australia antigen (HBAg) and the improved techniques for detecting it, it has become apparent that not all cases were transferred by parenteral means. Reports from several centres (Jeffries et al, 1973;

Fulford et al, 1973) showed an unexpectedly high incidence of the antigen in the serum of patients attending clinics for sexually transmitted diseases and especially in homosexual men. For example, Fulford's study at the Middlesex Hospital showed that antibody was most commonly found among male homosexuals and promiscuous patients of United Kingdom origin, whereas antigen was predominantly found in men of Mediterranean origin. In a totally independent study Heathcote and Sherlock (1973) studied 67 patients admitted to hospital with acute hepatitis. Sexual or domestic contact was thought to be the probable source of infection in 27 patients (40 per cent). Fifteen of the 43 men in the survey were either of homosexual or bisexual orientation (34.9 per cent). More recently Lim and colleagues (1976) have shown that hepatitis B antigen can be found in both semen and saliva and in a detailed study of 200 men they produced evidence that infection was probably related to the practice of orogenital sex and the swallowing of semen.

As a result of these and other studies it is becoming clear that the spread of hepatitis B in industrial countries results from close contact with jaundiced patients or hepatitis antigen carriers. There is growing evidence that the transmission frequently occurs between sexual partners and male homosexuals and bisexuals are especially liable to develop the disease. The practice of swallowing semen is probably an important factor in the passage of the infecting agent and in this sense sexual transmission is one of the most frequent methods of spread of hepatitis B virus.

CONTROL OF THE SEXUALLY TRANSMITTED DISEASES

Control of the incidence of sexually transmitted infections in a community depends upon the provision of a high quality clinical service, freely available to the public in attractive modern clinics, offering a prompt, efficient, scientific diagnostic service and effective treatment and surveillance. This service should be supported by educational programmes for medical students, doctors and nurses as well as other members of the paramedical professions. Education of the public about the simple facts of the sexually transmitted diseases is also vital if attitudes are to be changed and attendance at clinics of those who are at risk is to be encouraged. In addition the tracing of all the contacts of those known to be infected is vital to all methods of control and the system developed in the United Kingdom, based on the use of contact slips, has been shown to be successful in some areas (Morton, 1970; Dunlop, Lamb and King, 1971).

However, the failure to control the incidence of the diseases in most countries has led to attempts to produce vaccines and other methods of stimulating artificial immunity to the common infecting agents. The majority of infections do not result in protective immunity against reinfection later. There are, therefore, many difficulties and serious technical problems to be overcome before effective and safe vaccines are developed. Should, however, suitable methods of immunisation become available as a result of future research work, their eventual use will raise interesting and serious ethical, medical and personal problems. These may be among the most fascinating and important issues concerning the sexually transmitted diseases in the last quarter of the twentieth century.

REFERENCES

Ackerman, B. D. (1969) Congenital syphilis: observations on laboratory diagnosis of intra-uterine infection. *Journal of Pediatrics*, **74**, 457–462.

Ackers, J. P., Lumsden, W. H. R., Catterall, R. D. & Coyle, R. (1975) Antitrichomonal antibody in the vaginal secretions of women infected with *T. vaginalis*. *British Journal of Venereal Diseases*, **51**, 319–323.

Allen, B. R. (1970) Scabies and acute glomerulonephritis. *Lancet*, **1**, 434.

Altchek, A. (1970) Editorial: Epidemic pediculosis and gonorrhea. *Obstetrics and Gynecology*, **35**, 638–641.

American Social Health Association (1975) *Today's VD Control Problem*. New York: American Social Health Association.

Aurelian, L., Strandberg, J. D., Melendez, L. V. & Johnson, L. A. (1971) Herpesvirus type 2 isolated from cervical tumor cells grown in tissue culture. *Science*, **174**, 704–707.

Barr, J. & Danielsson, D. (1971) Septic gonococcal dermatitis. *British Medical Journal*, **1**, 482–485.

Barr, W. (1972) *Clinical Gynaecology*, 1st edn, p. 59. Edinburgh and London: Churchill Livingstone.

Berggren, O. (1969) Association of carcinoma of the uterine cervix and *Trichomonas vaginalis* infestations: frequency of *Trichomonas vaginalis* in preinvasive and invasive cervical carcinoma. *American Journal of Obstetrics and Gynecology*, **105**, 166–168.

Bhattacharyya, M. N. & Jephcott, A. E. (1974) Diagnosis of gonorrhoea in women. *British Journal of Venereal Diseases*, **50**, 109–112.

Block, E. (1968) Förekomsten av Trichomonas vid symtom pa kronisk uretrit hos kvinnor. *Nordisk Medicin*, **80**, 921.

Borchardt, K. A. & Hoke, A. W. (1970) Simplified laboratory technique for diagnosis of chancroid. *Archives of Dermatology*, **102**, 188–192.

Brewerton, D. A., Caffrey, M., Nicholls, A., Walters, D., Oates, J. K. & James, D. C. O. (1973) Reiter's disease and HL-A 27. *Lancet*, **2**, 996–998.

Busvine, J. R. (1967) Inheritance of DDT-resistance in body-lice: a preliminary investigation. *Bulletin of the World Health Organisation*, **36**, 431–434.

Catterall, R. D. (1966) *Candida albicans* and the contraceptive pill. *Lancet*, **2**, 830–831.

Catterall, R. D. (1971) Influence of gestogenic contraceptive pills on vaginal candidosis. *British Journal of Venereal Diseases*, **47**, 45–47.

Catterall, R. D. (1972a) Presidential Address to the M.S.S.V.D.: systemic disease and the biological false positive reaction. *British Journal of Venereal Diseases*, **48**, 1–12.

Catterall, R. D. (1972b) Trichomonal infections of the genital tract. *Medical Clinics of North America*, **56**, 1203–1209.

Catterall, R. D. (1976) In *Proceedings of the Anglo-American Conference on Sexually Transmitted Diseases*, June 1975. New York: Academic Press.

Catterall, R. D. & Nicol, C. S. (1969) Transmission of trichomonas. *British Medical Journal*, **2**, 765.

Catterall, R. D. & Nicol, C. S. (1975) Technical discussion. Geneva: World Health Organisation.

Chamberlain, M. J., Reynolds, A. L. & Yoeman, W. B. (1972) Medical memoranda. Toxic effect of podophyllum application in pregnancy. *British Medical Journal*, **3**, 391–392.

Chipperfield, E. J. & Evans, B. A. (1972) The influence of local infection on immunoglobulin formation in the human endocervix. *Clinical and Experimental Immunology*, **11**, 219–223.

Cobbold, R. J. C. & Macdonald, A. (1970) Molluscum contagiosum as a sexually transmitted disease. *Practitioner*, **204**, 416–419.

Collart, P. (1970) *Revue médicale* (*Paris*), **11**, 1265.

Collart, P., Poggi, G. & Dunoyer, F. R. (1966) Recenti studi sulla sifilide tardiva sperimentale e umana. *Minerva Medica*, **57**, 4478–4486.

Cremin, B. J. & Fisher, R. M. (1970) The lesions of congenital syphilis. Part 1. The early or perinatal lesions. *British Journal of Radiology*, **43**, 333–341.

Danielsson, D. (1971) Gonococcal dermatitis syndrome. *British Medical Journal*, 1, 482.

Darougar, S., Cubitt, S. & Jones, B. R. (1974) Effect of high-speed centrifugation on the sensitivity of irradiated McCoy cell culture for the isolation of *Chlamydia*. *British Journal of Venereal Diseases*, **50**, 308–312.

Davis, C. M. (1970) Granuloma inguinale. *Journal of the American Medical Association*, **211**, 632–636.

Department of Health and Social Security (1974) Annual Report of the Chief Medical Officer of the year 1973, *On the State of the Public Health*. London: HMSO.

Department of Health and Social Security (1975) Annual Report of the Chief Medical Officer for the year 1974, *On the State of the Public Health*. London: HMSO.

Diddle, A. W., Gardner, W. H., Williamson, P. J. & O'Connor, K. A. (1969) Oral contraceptive medications and vulvovaginal candidiasis. *Obstetrics and Gynecology*, **34**, 373–377.

Dunlop, E. M. C., Freedman, A., Garland, J. A., Harper, I. A., Jones, B. R., Race, J. W., du Toit, M. S. & Treharne, J. D. (1967) Infection by bedsoniae and the possibility of spurious isolation. 2. Genital infection, disease of the eye, Reiter's disease. *American Journal of Ophthalmology*, **63**, 1073–1081.

Dunlop, E. M. C. & Wisdom, A. R. (1965) Diagnosis and management of trichomoniasis in men and women. *British Journal of Venereal Diseases*, **41**, 85–89.

Dunlop, E. M. C., Hare, M. J., Darougar, S., Jones, B. R. & Rice, N. S. C. (1969) Detection of *Chlamydia* (*Bedsonia*) in certain infections of man. II. Clinical study of genital tract, eye, rectum, and other sites of recovery of *Chlamydia*. *Journal of Infectious Diseases*, **120**, 463–470.

Dunlop, E. M. C., Lamb, A. M. & King, D. M. (1971) Improved tracing of contacts of heterosexual men with gonorrhoea: relationship of altered female to male ratios. *British Journal of Venereal Diseases*, **47**, 192–195.

Dunlop, E. M. C., Vaughan-Jackson, J. D., Darougar, S. & Jones, B. R. (1972) Chlamydial infection: incidence in 'non-specific' urethritis. *British Journal of Venereal Diseases*, **48**, 425–428.

Farber, G. A., Forshner, J. G. & O'Quinn, S. E. (1967) Reiter's syndrome: treatment with methotrexate. *Journal of the American Medical Association*, **200**, 171–173.

Felber, T. D., Smith, E. B., Knox, J., Wallis, C. & Melnick, J. L. (1971) Photoinactivation may find use against herpesvirus. *Journal of the American Medical Association*, **217**, 270–271.

Fisher, I. & Morton, R. S. (1970) Phthirus pubis infestation. *British Journal of Venereal Diseases*, **46**, 326–329.

Fluker, J. L. (1972) Syphilis. *Practitioner*, **209**, 605–613.

Fulford, K. W. M. & Brostoff, J. (1972) Leucocyte migration and cell-mediated immunity in syphilis. *British Journal of Venereal Diseases*, **48**, 483–488.

Fulford, K. W. M., Dane, D. S., Catterall, R. D., Woof, R. & Denning, J. V. (1973) Australia antigen and antibody among patients attending a clinic for sexually transmitted diseases. *Lancet*, **1**, 1470–1473.

Fulford, K. W. M., Johnson, N., Loveday, C., Storey, J. & Tedder, R. S. (1976) Changes in intravascular complement and antitreponemal antibody titre preceding the Jarisch–Herxheimer reaction in secondary syphilis. *Clinical and Experimental Immunology*, **24**, 483.

Garner, M. F. & Robson, J. H. (1968) An immunofluorescence method for the diagnosis of primary syphilis using an absorption technique. *Journal of Clinical Pathology*, **21**, 576–577.

Goldmeier, D., Bateman, J. R. M. & Rodin, P. (1975) Urinary retention and intestinal obstruction associated with anorectal herpes simplex virus infection. *British Medical Journal*, **2**, 425.

Gordon, F. B., Harper, I. A., Quan, A. L., Treharne, J. D., Dwyer, R. St C. & Garland, J. A. (1969) Detection of *Chlamydia* (*Bedsonia*) in certain infections of man. I. Laboratory procedures: comparison of yolk sac and cell culture for detection and isolation. *Journal of Infectious Diseases*, **120**, 451–462.

Gudjönsson, H. & Skog, E. (1968) The effect of prednisolone on the Jarisch–Herxheimer reaction. *Acta cermato-venereologica*, **48**, 15–18.

Halverstadt, D. B. & Parry, W. L. (1969) Thiotepa in the management of intraurethral condylomata acuminata. *Journal of Urology*, **101**, 729–731.

Handsfield, H. H., Lipman, T. O., Harnisch, J. P., Tronca, E. & Holmes, K. K. (1974) Asymptomatic gonorrhea in men. *New England Journal of Medicine*, **290**, 117–123.

Heathcote, J. & Sherlock, S. (1973) Spread of acute type-B hepatitis in London. *Lancet*, **1**, 1468–1470.

Hersch, C. (1967) Acute glomerulonephritis due to skin disease, with special reference to scabies. *South African Medical Journal*, **41**, 29–34.

Holmes, K. K., Counts, G. W. & Beaty, H. N. (1971) Disseminated gonococcal infection. *Annals of Internal Medicine*, **74**, 979–993.

Hooshmand, H., Escobar, M. R. & Kopf, S. W. (1972) Neurosyphilis. A study of 241 patients. *Journal of the American Medical Association*, **219**, 726–729.

Hopsu-Havu, V. K. & Sonck, C. E. (1973) Infiltrative, ulcerative, and fistular lesions of the penis due to lymphogranuloma venereum. *British Journal of Venereal Diseases*, **49**, 193–202.

Idsøe, O., Guthe, T., & Willcox, R. R. (1972) Penicillin in the treatment of syphilis: the experience of three decades. *Bulletin of the World Health Organisation*, Suppl. **47**, 68 pp.

Jeffries, D. J., James, W. H., Jefferiss, F. J., MacLeod, K. G. & Willcox, R. R. (1973) Australia (hepatitis-associated) antigen in patients attending a venereal disease clinic. *British Medical Journal*, **2**, 455–456.

John, J. (1971) Efficacy of prolonged regimes of oxytetracycline in the treatment of non-gonococcal urethritis. *British Jouranl of Venereal Diseases*, **47**, 266–268.

Jones, B. R., Collier, L. H. & Smith, C. H. (1959) Isolation of virus from inclusion blennorrhoea. *Lancet*, **1**, 902–905.

Juhlin, L. (1968) Factors influencing the spread of gonorrhoea. II. Sexual behaviour at different ages. *Acta dermato-venereologica*, **48**, 82–89.

Karmody, C. S. & Schuknecht, H. F. (1966) Deafness in congenital syphilis. *Archives of Otolaryngology*, **83**, 18–27.

Kellogg, D. S. (1970) The detection of treponema pallidum by a rapid, direct fluorescent antibody darkfield. *Health Laboratory Science*, **7**, 34–41.

Kerr, A. G., Smyth, G. D. L. & Cinnamond, M. J. (1973) Congenital syphilitic deafness. *Journal of Laryngology and Otology*, **87**, 1–12.

Kimball, M. W. & Knee, S. (1970) Gonococcal perihepatitis in a male: the Fitz-Hugh–Curtis syndrome. *New England Journal of Medicine*, **282**, 1082–1085.

King, A. (1972) Non-specific urethritis. *Medical Clinics of North America*, **56**, 1193–1202.

Lal, S. & Nicholas, C. (1970) Epidemiological and clinical features in 165 cases of granuloma inguinale. *British Journal of Venereal Diseases*, **46**, 461–463.

Lassus, A. (1969) Development of rheumatoid factor activity and cyroglobulins: primary and secondary syphilis. *International Archives of Allergy and Applied Immunology*, **36**, 515–522.

Lawrence, J. S. (1974) Family survey of Reiter's disease. *British Journal of Venereal Diseases*, **50**, 140–145.

Lee, R. V., Thornton, G. F. & Conn, H. O. (1971) Liver disease associated with secondary syphilis. *New England Journal of Medicine*, **284**, 1423–1425.

Lehner, T., Wilton, J. M. A. & Shillitoe, E. J. (1975) Immunological basis for latency, recurrences, and putative oncogenicity of herpes simplex virus. *Lancet*, **2**, 60–62.

Lim, K. S., Fulford, K. W. M., Catterall, R. D., Dane, D. S., Taan, V. & Simpson, R. (1976) In *Proceedings of the Anglo-American Conference on Sexually Transmitted Diseases*, June 1975. New York: Academic Press.

Lopatin, A. I. (1970) Trikhomonadnye iazvy polovogo chlena. *Vestnik Dermatologii i Venerologii (Moskva)*, **44**, 78–79.

Lopatin, A. I. & Kolesnikova, N. P. (1971) O gonoreĭno-trikhomonadnykh uretritakh u muzhchin. *Vestnik Dermatologii i Venerologii (Moskva)*, **45**, 53–56.

Lumsden, W. H. R., Robertson, D. H. H. & McNeillage, G. J. C. (1966) Isolation, cultivation, low temperature preservation, and infectivity titration of *Trichomonas vaginalis*. *British Journal of Venereal Diseases*, **42**, 145–154.

Lyell, A. (1967) Diagnosis and treatment of scabies. *British Medical Journal*, **2**, 223–225.

Lynch, P. J. & Minkin, W. (1968) Molluscum contagiosum of the adult: probable venereal transmission. *Archives of Dermatology*, **98**, 141–143.

McCormack, W. M., Braun, P., Lee, Y. H., Klein, J. O. & Kass, E. H. (1973) The genital mycoplasmas. *New England Journal of Medicine*, **288**, 78–89.

Maleville, J. & Heid, E. (1972) Skabies beim Menschen. Aktuelle klinische und epidemiologische Daten. *Münchener Medizinische Wochenschrift*, **114**, 27–32.

Metzger, M. & Smogor, W. (1969) Artificial immunisation of rabbits against syphilis. I. Effect of increasing doses of treponemes given by the intramuscular route. *British Journal of Venereal Diseases*, **45**, 308–312.

Miller, J. N. (1967) Immunity in experimental syphilis. V. The immunogenicity of *Treponema pallidum* attenuated by γ-irradiation. *Journal of Immunology*, **99**, 1012–1016.

Miller, J. N. (1972) Development of an experimental syphilis vaccine. *Medical Clinics of North America*, **56**, 1217–1220.

Morrison, A. W. (1969) Management of severe deafness in adults. The otologist's contribution. *Proceedings of the Royal Society of Medicine*, **62**, 959–965.

Morton, R. S. (1970) Male:female ratios in the VD clinics of England and Wales. *British Journal of Venereal Diseases*, **46**, 103–105.

Morton, R. S. (1971) *Sexual Freedom and Venereal Disease.* London: Peter Owen.

Nahmias, A. J., Dowdle, W. R., Naib, Z. M., Josey, W. E., McLone, D. & Domescik, G. (1969) Genital infection with type 2 *Herpesvirus hominis*: a commonly occurring venereal disease. *British Journal of Venereal Diseases*, **45**, 294–298.

Naib, Z. M., Nahmias, A. J., Josey, W. E. & Kramer, J. H. (1969) Genital herpetic infection: association with cervical dysplasia and carcinoma. *Cancer*, **23**, 940–945.

Nasemann, T. (1970) Neuere Behandlungsmethoden unterschiedlicher Herpes simplexinfektionen. *Archiv fur Klinische und Experimentelle Dermatologie*, **237**, 234–237.

Nicol, C. S. (1971) Other sexually transmitted diseases. II. *British Medical Journal*, **2**, 507–509.

Olsen, G. A. (1971) Value of vaginal and rectal cultures in the diagnosis of gonorrhoea. With special reference to areas with limited medical facilities. *British Journal of Venereal Diseases*, **47**, 102–106.

Olsen, G. A. & Lomholt, G. (1969) Gonorrhoea treated by a combination of probenecid and sodium penicillin G. *British Journal of Venereal Diseases*, **45**, 144–148.

Oriel, J. D. (1971) Natural history of genital warts. *British Journal of Venereal Diseases*, **47**, 1–13.

Oriel, J. D. & Almeida, J. D. (1970) Demonstration of virus particles in human genital warts. *British Journal of Venereal Diseases*, **46**, 37–42.

Oriel, J. D., Partridge, B. M., Denny, M. J. & Coleman, J. C. (1972) Genital yeast infections. *British Medical Journal*, **4**, 761–764.

Orkin, M. (1971) Resurgence of scabies. *Journal of the American Medical Association*, **217**, 593–597.

Ovčinnikov, N. M. & Delektorskij, V. V. (1971) Current concepts of the morphology and biology of *Treponema pallidum* based on electron microscopy. *British Journal of Venereal Diseases*, **47**, 315–328.

Pace, W. E. & Purres, J. (1971) Resurgence of scabies. *Canadian Medical Association Journal*, **104**, 719.

Pedersen, G. T. (1969) Yeast flora in mother and child: a mycological–clinical study of women followed up during pregnancy, the puerperium and 5–12 months after delivery, and of their children on the 7th day of life and at the age of 5–12 months. *Danish Medical Bulletin*, **16**, 207–220.

Perera, P. M. & Lim, K. S. (1975) Asymptomatic urethral gonorrhoea in men. *British Medical Journal*, **3**, 415–416.

Rees, E. & Annels, E. H. (1969) Gonococcal salpingitis. *British Journal of Venereal Diseases*, **45**, 205–215.

Reyn, A. (1969) Recent developments in the laboratory diagnosis of gonococcal infections. *Bulletin of the World Health Organisation*, **40**, 245–255.

Richmond, S. J., Hilton, A. L. & Clarke, S. K. R. (1972) Chlamydial infection: role of *Chlamydia* subgroup A in non-gonococcal and post-gonococcal urethritis. *British Journal of Venereal Diseases*, **48**, 437–444.

Rodin, P., Hare, M. J., Barwell, C. F. & Withers, M. J. (1971) Transport of herpes simplex virus in Stuart's medium. *British Journal of Venereal Diseases*, **47**, 198–199.

Rohatiner, J. J. (1966) Relationship of *Candida albicans* in the genital and anorectal tracts. *British Journal of Venereal Diseases*, **42**, 197–200.

Royston, I. & Aurelian, L. (1970) The association of genital herpesvirus with cervical atypia and carcinoma in situ. *American Journal of Epidemiology*, **91**, 531–538.

Schmidt, H. & Goldschmidt, E. (1972) Demonstration of motile treponemes in the aqueous humour in secondary syphilis. *British Journal of Venereal Diseases*, **48**, 400–401.

Scotti, A. T. & Logan, L. (1968) A specific IgM antibody test in neonatal congenital syphilis. *Journal of Pediatrics*, **73**, 242–243.

Shepard, M. C. (1956) T-form colonies of pleuropneumonia-like organisms. *Journal of Bacteriology*, **71**, 362–369.

Shepard, M. C. (1970) Non-gonococcal urethritis associated with human strains of 'T' mycoplasmas. *Journal of the American Medical Association*, **211**, 1335–1340.

Shrank, A. B. & Alexander, S. L. (1967) Scabies: another epidemic? *British Medical Journal*, **1**, 669–671.

Smith, I. W., Peutherer, J. F. & Robertson, D. H. H. (1973) Characterisation of genital strains of *Herpesvirus hominis*. *British Journal of Venereal Diseases*, **49**, 385–390.

Söltz-Szöts, J. (1971) Neue methoden bei der Behandlung der Viruserkrankungen. *Zeitschrift fur Haut- und Geschlechtskrankheiten*, **46**, 755–760.

Spangler, A. S., Jackson, J. H., Fiumara, N. J. & Warthin, T. A. (1964) Syphilis with a negative blood test reaction. *Journal of the American Medical Association*, **189**, 87–90.

Stolz, E. & Schuller, J. (1974) Gonococcal oro- and nasopharyngeal infection. *British Journal of Venereal Diseases*, **50**, 104–108.

Swanson, J., Kraus, S. J. & Gotschlich, E. C. (1971) Studies on gonococcus infection. I. Pili and zones of adhesion: their relation to gonococcal growth patterns. *Journal of Experimental Medicine*, **134**, 886–906.

Swanson, J. (1973) Studies on gonococcus infection. IV. Pili: their role in attachment of gonococci to tissue culture cells. *Journal of Experimental Medicine*, **137**, 571–589.

T'ang, F. F., Chang, H. L., Huang, Y. T. & Wang, K. C. (1957) Studies on the etiology of trachoma with special reference to isolation of the virus in chick embryo. *Chinese Medical Journal*, **75**, 429–447.

Valent, M. & Čatár, G. (1967) Concerning the problems of trichomoniasis in the Slovak opoulation. *Folia Facultatis Medicae, Universitatis Comenianae Bratislaviensis*, **5**, 101–147.

Wang, S.-P., Grayston, J. T. & Gale, J. L. (1973) Three new immunologic types of trachoma-inclusion conjunctivitis organisms. *Journal of Immunology*, **110**, 873–879.

Ward, M. E. & Watt, P. J. (1972) Adherence of *Neisseria gonorrhoeae* to urethral mucosal cells: an electron-microscopic study of human gonorrhoea. *Journal of Infectious Diseases*, **126**, 601–605.

Webster, B. (1972) Professional education and the control of the venereal diseases. *Medical Clinics of North America*, **56**, 1101–1104.

Weström, L. (1975) Effect of acute pelvic inflammatory disease on fertility. *American Journal of Obstetrics and Gynecology*, **121**, 707–713.

Willcox, R. R. (1972) A world look at the venereal diseases. *Medical Clinics of North America*, **56**, 1057–1071.

Willcox, R. R. & Goodwin, P. G. (1971) Nerve deafness in early syphilis. *British Journal of Venereal Diseases*, **47**, 401–406.

World Health Organisation (1975a) *Social and Health Aspects of Sexually Transmitted Diseases: Need for a Better Approach*. Geneva: WHO.

World Health Organisation (1975b) *World Health*. Geneva: WHO.

3
ARTHROPODS AND THE SKIN

Brian Bagnall   Arthur Rook

The medical importance to man of the arthropods in his environment has tended to increase in recent years, and the dermatologist who is not familiar with the life histories of those that molest his patients will leave many a case of 'prurigo' or 'papular urticaria' incompletely diagnosed and uncured.

Advances in immunology have led to a greater understanding of the wide range of different reactions which a single species of arthropod may evoke in different individuals, or in the same individual on different occasions. Drugs which suppress the immune response may profoundly modify the response to arthropod bites or to cutaneous parasitisation.

Increased suspicion has led to the development of improved techniques for sampling the patient's environment, at home, at work, and in his leisure activities. These techniques are as yet not used sufficiently frequently, but they have already shown that species of arthropod previously regarded as rarely attacking man can be quite often incriminated as causing a refractory and distressing pruritic eruption.

No attempt will be made to cover all the publications of the last 10 years. Recent advances in our knowledge of lice and human scabies are considered in some detail because these infestations are still common. Bees and wasps and their allies are important because of the occasional severity of the reactions to their stings. The other arthropods discussed have been selected because of their proven importance to the dermatologist or because publications concerning their effects on man have appeared mainly in the entomological journals and they have received little or no mention in the textbooks of dermatology. Only further research will establish their real medical significance.

The Investigation of the Patient with Prurigo

The patient attacked by a stinging insect is instantly aware of the fact; previous identification of the offending species is obviously desirable, but is essential only when hyposensitisation with specific venom is found to be necessary (p. 82). The very much commoner problem is the patient who is bitten by a non-stinging arthropod, and whose reaction—immediate weal or delayed papule, or both—is separated in time and often in space, from the unperceived 'bite'. The flying insects which do not sting, such as the thrips

(p. 80) can often be identified only on circumstantial evidence; the distribution of the eruption and its time of onset correlate with the known prevalence of the suspect species. The wingless arthropods which molest man provide the greatest diagnostic problem for the patient is usually totally unaware of their existence. In such cases the clinical picture may consist of a cluster of papules with central haemorrhagic puncta, but nature provides such diagnostic revelation only sparingly. More often the patient presents with a multitude of small papules, localised to one region of the body, generalised, or scattered apparently at random. If the lesions are strikingly asymmetrical and if they are grouped in lines or irregular clusters the probability of an exogenous cause is high; but reactions to 'insects' may be disconcertingly symmetrical, and in some cases pruritus, without visible lesions, may be the only symptom.

If the clinical features suggest that an eruption is probably caused by the activities of some arthropod, or if, after careful investigation and conclusive elimination of human scabies, a persistent or recurrent prurigo remains unexplained, the following procedure is recommended.

1. Any animals with which the patient comes into contact in his own home or in the homes of frequently visited relatives or friends should be examined. The presence of small numbers of fleas on cats and dogs can be detected by dislodging the small black flea 'dirts' (faeces) from the hair coat on to wetted white paper, where the blood pigments will cause red streaks (Fig. 3.1). *Cheyletiella* mites on dogs, cats and rabbits are just visible to the naked eye (Fig. 3.2) but can be easily detected by pressing a piece of transparent sticky tape (Sellotape) on to the skin surface several times and examining it under the microscope, applied to a glass slide. Examination of animal 'brushings' can also reveal flea faeces and *Cheyletiella* mites but is less accurate and more arduous. Dogs suffering from scabies present a characteristic clinical picture of pruritus (Fig. 3.3) but confirmation of the diagnosis rests with the veterinary surgeon who may find *Sarcoptes* mites in skin scrapings.

2. If there are no known animal contacts, or if these have been eliminated as sources of infection, samples of house dust should be collected. If the history suggests his place of work to be under suspicion, dust samples from there too should be obtained. Special attention should be paid to stored organic produce, such as cereals, flour, hay or dried fruits.

3. If no solution to the clinical problem has yet been obtained, then the patient's clothing, including any special clothing worn at work, should be turned inside out and vigorously shaken over an open polythene bag. The inner surface of each garment should then be brushed.

4. Lightly brushing the patient's skin, collecting the dust and debris in a polythene bag is occasionally informative.

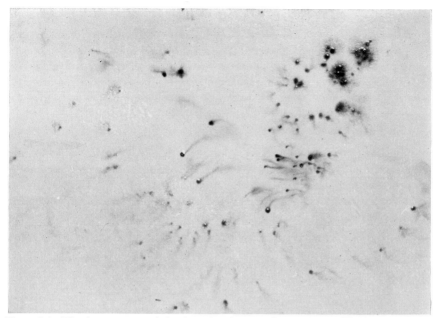

Figure 3.1 The 'wet paper test' for detecting fleas on dogs and cats. The backline fur is rubbed over a piece of wet white paper and any flea faeces are revealed by showing blood-stained streaks

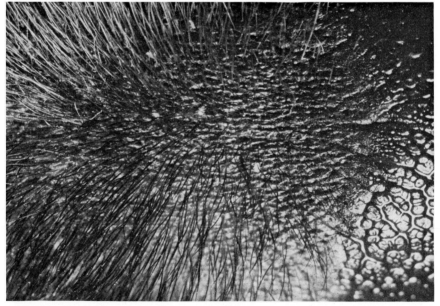

Figure 3.2 *Cheyletiella yasguri* mites moving about on the nasal skin of a dog. The parasites are about 0.5 mm long and can just be seen with the naked eye. Their presence is usually accompanied by marked scaling of the dog's skin ('scurf') but pruritus is not a prominent clinical sign

5. If these measures have all failed to provide evidence of the cause of a persistent and troublesome prurigo, apparently of external origin, the dermatologist may find it helpful to visit the patient's home or his place of work, accompanied if possible by an applied entomologist. Such visits have led the authors to the solution of many intractable problems, including the discovery of house-martins' nests under the house eaves outside the bedroom window of a woman tormented by papular urticaria.

In the majority of patients with skin lesions of parasitic origin a good history and a careful examination quickly suggest the probable source of infestation. In cases which remain mysteries the application of the apparently elaborate detective procedure suggested can be very rewarding (Hewitt, Walton and

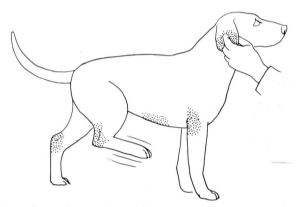

Figure 3.3 Dogs suffering from canine scabies present a clinical picture of continual itching and scratching. Rubbing their ear flaps with the fingers will often provoke a scratch reflex with the hind limb. Shaded zones show areas of the body most affected—ears, elbows, belly and hocks. Red papules and crusting are often masked by extensive self-inflicted skin trauma and hair loss so typical of the 'mangy dog'.

Waterhouse, 1971) and is ultimately less time-consuming than a succession of frustrating and therapeutically fruitless clinic consultations.

THE IMMUNE RESPONSE TO ARTHROPODS

Despite considerable recent advances in the understanding of immuno-logical responses to bacterial, viral and helminth infections, the responses to arthropods have been almost totally neglected by immunologists. This reluctance to study arthropod infestations can partly be explained by the difficulty in obtaining manageable supplies of parasites which fly, jump or crawl, and partly by the problem of securing sufficient quantities of their antigenic secretions. A major review of the subject has brought together much of the information obtained over many years (Benjamini and Feingold,

1970). Entomological aspects of host–ectoparasite relationships have also been recently reviewed (Nelson et al, 1975). As in many other immunological fields, little progress can be made unless experimental models using laboratory animals are developed. However, little has been published since the flea/guinea-pig work of Benjamini and co-workers in the early 1960s.

The immune response to arthropods can be as varied as the method of contact. Stinging insects may inject toxic substances into the skin, where the ability to form neutralising antibodies becomes important. Hypersensitivity reactions may result from the bites of arthropods which in non-sensitised individuals may pass unnoticed. Immunity to infestation or invasion by arthropod parasites (e.g. scabies) may show itself in the ability of the skin to reject them. Whether the parasite bites, stings, burrows or defaecates on the skin, the host response is none the less basically an attempt by the skin to defend itself against the parasite and its secretions or excretions. The responses, however, do not always have an immunological basis as they frequently involve non-specific inflammation or an itching induced merely by mechanical irritation to the skin, e.g. lice.

Parasite Feeding Mechanisms

With the exception of certain stinging insects and caterpillars or moths with urticating hairs, most arthropods leave an antigenic trail of their saliva in or on the skin where they have fed. The differing mechanisms by which arthropods feed can be expected to play a part in determining how and where this saliva is deposited, and consequently to influence any ensuing immune reactions. Little has been published on the feeding mechanisms of those parasites which feed on superficial skin scales and debris, e.g. the mites and biting lice. Their mouthparts may be adapted for chewing or they may secrete saliva on to the skin surface before sucking up the predigested material (Sweatman, 1957). Observations on surface-feeding *Cheyletiella* mites have shown that they are capable of firm attachment to the epidermis and can engorge clear fluid from the host (Foxx and Ewing, 1969).

Because of their important role as vectors of infectious disease, feeding mechanisms of the blood-sucking arthropods have been extensively reported, including two comprehensive reviews of the subject (Tatchell, 1969a; Hocking, 1971). There are two basically different types of blood-feeding mouthparts. The first has a single and usually broad channel extending distally from the mouth and serves to convey both the salivary secretion outwards and, alternately, the blood meal inwards. This type is found in the mites and ticks. The second type of feeding apparatus, found in most insects, has two channels extending forward and downward from the mouth—a small dorsal one through which blood is ingested and a ventral smaller one through which saliva is passed out into the skin. Arthropods which insert the tip of the food canal with some precision into a capillary blood vessel are referred to as vessel feeders and include sucking lice, bugs, fleas and most mosquitoes. Those which cut and stab with their mouthparts and feed on extravasated blood from damaged capillaries are known as pool feeders and include ticks, march flies, stable flies and tsetse flies. Their bites may be painful and accompanied by tissue damage which will be followed by inflammation and necrosis.

Functions of Arthropod Saliva

The role of saliva in the feeding process of arthropods is not fully understood. Hudson, Bowman and Orr (1960) showed that cutting the salivary duct of mosquitoes prevented the development of allergic reactions in man but did not stop successful feeding. Lester and Lloyd (1928) demonstrated that although the tsetse fly has an anticoagulant in its saliva it can feed successfully and repeatedly following the cutting of the salivary duct, again without causing allergic reactions in the host. From this work came clear evidence that it is the arthropod's saliva which contains antigens responsible for the development of hypersensitivity by the bitten individual. Recent studies have revealed a major function of the salivary glands of ixodid ticks as one of ion and water balance (Tatchell, 1969b; Kaufman and Phillips, 1973). Excess water and ions from ingested blood are largely returned to the host by the tick's salivary glands. Most insects eliminate this unwanted water via their Malpighian tubules. Many arthropods inject saliva or venom which contains pharmacologically active substances such as histamine, haemolysins, hyaluronidase and toxic polypeptides (Beard, 1963). These secretions may be injected for self-defence or to paralyse and kill the prey. Antivenenes for human use can be produced by vaccination of animals with extracts of some spider and tick venoms (Sutherland, 1974).

Types of Immune Responses to Arthropods

Apart from toxic skin reactions to venomous arthropods, the bites of most others are usually imperceptible to the non-sensitised human. Once sensitised to a particular parasite, however, immunological responses may give rise to a variety of clinical signs after subsequent bites. The most common reactions are those of cutaneous hypersensitivity, occurring either immediately after the bite when antibodies react with the insect antigens or delayed some 48 h when cell-mediated tissue responses become activated. Mixed hypersensitivity (immediate plus delayed) is not uncommon following arthropod bites—the weal arising within minutes fades in about an hour only to be replaced in the next day or two by an itching papule which may persist for days or even weeks before regressing. Many examples in the literature have shown that in both man and animals repeated exposures to the bites of a given arthropod can result in an alteration of the subject's skin reactivity. A sequence of events can be summarised by the progression through five stages: (1) no response,

(2) delayed hypersensitivity, (3) immediate plus delayed hypersensitivity, (4) immediate hypersensitivity only, (5) no response (tolerance). The elegant experiments of Benjamini, Feingold and Kartman (1961), who exposed guinea-pigs to the cat flea, demonstrated these stages convincingly but their work is greatly in need of updating in the light of modern immunology.

Systemic anaphylactic reactions are not uncommonly induced by the bites of toxin-secreting arthropods such as bees and wasps. These allergic reactions to stinging insects are probably the closest human analogue to experimental anaphylaxis in animals. Each subsequent sting in a sensitised patient may be accompanied by a reaction of increasing severity until the stage of acute anaphylactic shock is reached, perhaps causing death. Such serious consequences have naturally attracted much research attention which has been reviewed in detail (Benjamini and Feingold, 1970).

Persistent cutaneous granulomas sometimes occur at the sites of bites of arthropods, particularly of ticks (Yesudian and Thambiah, 1973). After excluding foreign-body reactions to retained insect mouthparts, these persistent lesions suggest a chronic immunological reaction which can often be aborted by intralesional injection of a corticosteroid. Further investigation is needed to explore the possibility that persistent granulomas are caused by arthropod antigens remaining at the bite site, perhaps bound to dermal collagen.

It appears that immunity to helminth parasites involves more than one element of the host's immune response and cooperation of both the humoral and cellular arms of the immune system in elimination of these parasites has been demonstrated (Ogilvie, 1974). It is unlikely, therefore, that responses to arthropods are going to be either exclusively antibody-mediated or cell-mediated but these traditional divisions are helpful in discussion of the clinical reactions.

The Antigens

There is a pressing need for increased study of the salivary and venom antigens of arthropods. Newer techniques of histological preparation should also allow a better idea of the structure and function of insect salivary glands and venom sacs which have been virtually ignored except for those of ticks (Meredith and Kaufman, 1973). Other parts of insect bodies have, however, also been proven to contain antigens which will react with serum antibodies from hypersensitive humans (Langlois, Shulman and Arbesman, 1965). Different species of insects may also share certain antigenic components, thus causing cross-sensitivity reactions between, for example, bees, wasps and hornets. Animal experiments have shown that at least three antigenic compounds are involved in the production of skin reactions to bites of the mosquito *Aedes aegypti*. One of these compounds occurs in all stages of the mosquito life cycle and is widely distributed in the body of the adult female, whereas the other two antigens are restricted to the thorax of adult female mosquitoes in which the salivary glands are situated (Wilson and Clements, 1965). Guinea-pigs exposed to the bites of one species of mosquito exhibited the phenomenon of cross-hypersensitivity to three other mosquito species, indicating that at least one common antigen was shared in the oral secretions of these different species (French and West, 1971).

No recent work has equalled the remarkable achievement of Benjamini et al (1963) in persuading large numbers of fleas to feed on distilled water through an artificial membrane, thus allowing the collection and fractionation of pure flea saliva. Results with this preparation were a considerable advance on those using whole-flea extracts which contain a number of constituents, the majority of which are not concerned with the bite hypersensitivity reaction. It was found that an adjuvant was required to induce immuno-genicity with the purified salivary extract in guinea-pigs, suggesting that the low-molecular weight active substance was a hapten which needed conjuga-tion with skin collagen to form a complete antigen (Feingold, Benjamini and Michaeli, 1968). A notable feature of many published reports on arthropod-induced immune reactions has been the very small amounts of antigenic material needed to induce a hypersensitivity response. This suggests that arthropod antigens are extremely potent immunogens worthy of more investigation for this fact alone.

Antibody-mediated Reactions

Certain antibodies detected in the serum of animals infected with a wide variety of metazoan parasites have been shown to provide a protective effect against the relevant invaders (Ogilvie, 1970). There remains a vast literature, however, on other antibodies which may be present in the serum but show no detectable protective effect, although they are sometimes useful in the sero-diagnosis of parasitic diseases (Kagan, 1974). Little information is available on the production or role of antibodies detected during arthropod infestations, with the exception of some work carried out on hypersensitivity to the bites of mosquitoes, fleas and some stinging insects (reviewed by Feingold et al, 1968). Serum antibodies associated with the immediate type of bite reaction have been demonstrated many times by transfer of the sensitivity to non-sensitive recipients with intradermal injections of serum from a hyper-sensitive individual. Precise characterisation of the antibodies has usually not been made in these reports although results often suggest IgE. Venom-specific IgE antibodies were detected in the serum of patients with histories of systemic anaphylactic reactions to stinging insects using the radioallergo-sorbent (RAST) method (Reisman, Wypych and Arbesman, 1975). Increased IgE levels have been described in many if not all helminth infections and it remains to be seen whether this is true also for arthropod infestations. Some helminths not only cause the formation of IgE antibodies against their own allergens but also have the ability non-specifically to potentiate the IgE response to unrelated antigens. This may be the explanation of elevated IgE levels in endemically parasitised populations (Ogilvie, 1974). Precipitating antibodies against arthropod antigenic extracts have frequently been detected in vitro by immunodiffusion in agar of serum from hypersensitive patients. Haemagglutinating antibodies were found also in patients sensitive to Hymenoptera stings (Langlois et al, 1965).

The immunological mechanisms of immediate-type antibody-mediated cutaneous hypersensitivity reactions (local anaphylaxis) are now well described (Parish, 1971). In man, skin mast cells and basophils sensitised by the attachment of IgE antibodies are injured when the appropriate antigen comes into contact with them, for example after an insect bite. These target cells release several pharmacologically active agents such as histamine which cause local and generalised tissue changes including contraction of smooth muscle, increased vascular permeability and oedema. The cell injury is usually transient and most of them recover. Antihistamine drugs will largely suppress the tissue changes but do not prevent the antigen–antibody reaction. Eosinophils usually accumulate at sites of local anaphylaxis but their function remains a matter for current speculation, possibly regulation that can limit the allergic reaction (Goetzl, Wasserman and Austen, 1975). Potentially fatal systemic anaphylactic reactions, as seen following Hymenoptera stings, are more intense versions of the same mechanisms, but sufficient histamine and other mediators are released to cause collapse and shock.

More inflammatory cutaneous reactions 2 to 4 h after arthropod bites indicate that another type of immune response, the Arthus reaction, may also be present. This reaction results from the parasite antigens reacting in the blood vessels or tissue spaces with free precipitating antibodies and forming aggregates which bind complement. This activated complement complex strongly attracts neutrophils, and considerable tissue damage may occur from enzymic action. Arthus-like reactions have been found following the bites of ticks (Berenberg, Ward and Sonenshine, 1972) and mosquitoes (Wilson and Clements, 1965) in experimental animals.

Cell-mediated Reactions

Delayed hypersensitivity reactions about 48 h after insect bites are characteristically indurated and erythematous, producing a raised itching skin papule. They follow the reaction of specifically sensitised lymphocytes in contact with the parasite antigens, as a result of which macrophages are activated and the typical histological picture of a mononuclear cell infiltrate appears. Many biologically active substances are released by sensitised lymphocytes during these reactions (Parish, 1971). The sequence of events is not altered by antihistamine agents but can be inhibited by corticosteroids. In experimental animals, delayed hypersensitivity reactions to arthropod bites can be transferred to previously unexposed donors by injection of lymphocytes from parasite-sensitised donors. The presence of large numbers of basophils and eosinophils in cutaneous hypersensitivity reactions to ticks has recently been reported in guinea-pigs (Allen, 1973; Bagnall, 1975). This may be significant in that these cells have been found to exert an antiparasitic effect in experimental helminth infections (Ogilvie, 1974).

Consequences of the Immune Response to Arthropods

Recent work has begun to outline the immunological basis of a beneficial phenomenon—the acquisition by animals of cutaneous 'resistance' to certain slow-feeding arthropods such as ticks (Roberts, 1968; Allen, 1973; Bagnall, 1975). The onset of hypersensitivity to the ticks leads to skin reactions at the site of feeding which are deleterious to the parasite and result in a substantial rejection of the total infestation. It appears that a similar phenomenon occurs in man; hypersensitivity reactions to larvae of the tick *Ixodes holocyclus* prevent the ticks from completing their blood meal from the skin, although the irritable papules give rise to a condition called 'scrub itch' (Sutherst and Moorhouse, 1971). There remains much to be done yet in investigation of the antiparasitic effects of allergic reactions to other arthropods in man. The hypothesis has been proposed that a major function of immediate hyper-sensitivity reactions is that of a defence against arthropods by inducing avoidance behaviour, protecting from antigen–antibody complexes and in-hibiting harmful delayed-type reactions (Stebbings, 1974). Unfortunately, the immune reactions to arthropods are usually considered a nuisance to man by causing pruritus and unsightly skin lesions. The bite reaction has not escaped the attention of microbiologists, however, who know that it can influence the ability of certain arthropod-transmitted pathogens to become established (Soulsby and Harvey, 1972).

Hyposensitisation

It is commonly recognised that an individual living in an area endemic for a specific insect may fail to react to bites after prolonged and repeated ex-posure. Such 'tolerance' has been reported for a variety of arthropod parasites including lice, sandflies, bedbugs, mosquitoes and fleas (Feingold et al, 1968). The injection of whole-body arthropod extracts as a clinical hyposensitisation procedure has been attempted many times. Results vary from enthusiastic claims of success to admissions of complete failure. The most notable feature of reports on hyposensitisation is the conflict in the claims. Attempts to reduce the serious reactions to Hymenoptera stings have, in general, met with some favourable results (reviewed by Benjamini and Feingold, 1970). In most cases the protection is short lived and the expense, time and risk of such therapy may not be justified by the modest degree of symptom relief that is obtained (see p. 82). The immunological basis for hyposensitisation is still unresolved but the development of 'blocking' antibodies and a reduction in the amount of specific antibody bound to tissue mast cells have been discussed (Lichtenstein, 1972).

Potentials for Immunodiagnosis

The major difficulties in obtaining even small amounts of pure arthropod antigens preclude their use for routine diagnostic purposes. The production of a concentrated *Sarcoptes* extract has been carried out using mites obtained from pigs and skin testing was able to detect the onset of hypersensitivity in these animals (Sheahan, 1975). Such an extract might be useful for investigating human patients with suspected scabies. The development of immunofluorescence techniques for detecting arthropod antigens and antibodies in skin is still awaited.

HUMAN SCABIES

Epidemiology

By the late 1950s human scabies had become an uncommon disease in dermatological clinics in many parts of the world. In 1963 the incidence began to increase, first in France, then in Britain (Orkin, 1971). At St John's Hospital London, scabies which had accounted for 0.1 per cent of new patients in 1963, accounted for 2.4 per cent in 1966. Much higher figures were reported from some other parts of Britain, e.g. Middlesbrough, 11.0 per cent of new outpatient attendances (Shrank and Alexander, 1967), and the West of Scotland, 7 per cent (Grant and Keczes, 1964). The disease spread rather more slowly throughout the rest of Europe and to a very variable degree. By 1968 scabies was present in about 1.5 per cent of dermatological patients in Cologne (Herrmann and Humann, 1970) but in 1969 accounted for over 12 per cent of such patients in Sardinia (Orkin, 1971). In Halle in Germany (Wozniak and Wienrich, 1972) the clinic incidence rose from 0.28 per cent in 1960 to 2.52 per cent in 1970, and in Jena (Barthelmes, Sönnichsen and Barthelmes, 1970) from 0.12 to 3.08 per cent over the same period. Over the period 1961 to 1970 the incidence in a region of Czechoslovakia (Palička and Merka, 1971) increased some twenty-fold to reach a morbidity rate of 418 cases per 100 000 of the population and 818 per 100 000 in the peak age group, 6 to 15 years.

This epidemic has provided the material for many studies of public health aspects of scabies and has led to some facile generalisations which are not supported when the international literature is critically reviewed. For example the sexual promiscuity which appears to have increased in some countries certainly favours the spread of scabies but in most communities, scabies is in most cases not predominantly a sexually transmitted disease. Figures based on the clientèle of a clinic for venereal diseases are biased and misleading.

Nair et al (1973) examined 2558 persons in an Indian village with a total population of 18 202. He found that 6 per cent of the population in 20 per cent of households had scabies. Over 50 per cent of those affected were under 5, and 31 per cent between 5 and 14. There was a steady decrease in incidence with increasing age. Overcrowding was an important factor, but the incidence showed little correlation with poverty and poor hygiene in the absence of overcrowding. In São Paulo, Brazil (Belda, 1973), also, the home was the chief source of infestation, and the peak age incidence was between one and nine years. Somewhat similar findings were reported by Schenone et al (1971), from Santiago, Chile, who found an incidence of 5.4 per cent in infants under 1 year, 15.7 per cent between the ages of 1 and 4, and 7.1 per cent in the age groups 5 to 9 years and 10 to 14 years. When the age distribution of 1047 cases was analysed 38 per cent were under 9, 45 per cent 10 to 19 and 9.9 per cent 20 to 29. Thereafter the incidence declined sharply. Spread within family groups was of far greater importance than spread within schools.

On the present evidence it would seem that about 15 years elapse between the end of one scabies epidemic and the beginning of another. A study carried out in the Kiel area of Germany (Schirren, 1970b) showed that persistent foci maintain the disease between epidemics. It is possible that undiagnosed cases of Norwegian scabies provide the core of such foci, since these patients harbour vast numbers of mites and have been proved to be the source of many small outbreaks (Haydon and Caplan, 1971). Given such a source of mites conditions are favourable for their epidemic spread when the proportion of non-immune subjects in the community reaches a necessary threshold level. When that level is reached crowded living conditions are usually the most important factor assisting wide dissemination of the disease, but sexual transmission also plays a role; the relative importance of these two factors varies according to the social conditions of each community. Such conditions and not variations in racial susceptibility account for observed differences in incidence between Bantu, Indian and Caucasoid subjects in South Africa (Richardson, 1972; Zumpt, 1972). A further factor which plays a far from negligible role in assisting the spread of scabies during the earlier stages of an epidemic is the failure of younger doctors, who have perhaps never encountered the disease, to diagnose it or to treat it adequately (Schirren, 1970a).

Sarcoptes scabiei

Relatively little has been added to our knowledge of the life-cycle and general biology of the scabies mite since the important monographs by Mellanby (1943, reprinted 1972), Heilesen (1946) and Borda (1955). Steigleder (1970) has provided a useful review. Only the female mite, 0.3 to 0.4 mm in length, forms burrows; the smaller males remain on the surface or in shallow pits. About 14 days are required for the development of the egg into a mature adult, passing through two larval stages. It appears to take some five weeks for the previously unexposed host to develop allergic sensitivity to the mite's allergen. It is at this stage that pruritus first develops. The course of the disease depends on the number of mites initially transferred, on the number of these and of their descendants removed by regular bathing, and on the immunological status of the host. Untreated, the mite infestation reaches its peak after 80 to 115 days and, except in Norwegian scabies, or in patients treated with systemic or topical immunosuppressive agents, the average population of adult males is about 11 and of adult females about 12. The interval between the original transfer of the mites and the development of symptoms is very variable in length and the tracing of source of infestation is therefore often difficult, but if sufficient effort be made the source can be traced in nearly 80 per cent of cases (Sönnichsen, Barthelmes and Barthelmes, 1971).

The distribution of scabies burrows has not been adequately explained. Madsen (1965) suggested that the acarus avoided areas such as the face because the density of hair follicles is 16 times greater than on the limbs. He was later able to show (Madsen, 1970) that on the rare occasions when burrows are formed on infants' faces or scalps, these burrows are in crusts and not in the horny layer itself.

Pathology

The histological appearance of the inflammatory lesions of scabies has been considered to be non-specific. Hejazi and Mehregan (1975) have found a combination of epidermal and dermal changes which is sufficiently distinctive to suggest the correct diagnosis. The epidermis shows acute spongiosis, and sometimes a mite is seen in the horny layer. The changes in the dermis simulate those of erythema multiforme. A conspicuous perivascular cellular infiltrate, extending deeply, consists mainly of eosinophils and lymphocytes, and there is some extravasation of red blood cells. Some capillaries are surrounded by fibrinoid, and their endothelial cells are swollen.

The immunoglobulins were measured in 100 patients with scabies, divided into 'early' (under three weeks' duration) and 'late' groups. IgA levels were significantly lower in both groups than in matched control subjects. IgE was normal. IgG and IgM levels were raised, which implies a humoral response to scabies or to possible secondary bacterial infection. It is suggested that low IgA levels may predispose to scabies (Hancock and Ward, 1974).

Clinical Features

The frequently long delay before the correct diagnosis is reached is explained in part by the lack of the classical clinical features in many cases, either because of high hygienic standards or because the abundant use of topical corticosteroids has modified the lesions. Even the classical presentation of scabies may be misdiagnosed in the early stages of an epidemic, and some authors have recalled some forgotten but still useful physical signs (Aruntjunov, 1970; Barthelmes and Barthelmes, 1971) such as the gluteal triangle syndrome and Hardy's sign.

Generalised urticaria may occasionally be the presenting manifestation of scabies. In a few such cases seen at Cambridge all but one had for some time been applying fluorinated corticosteroids to the lesions of hands and genitalia. The widespread application of such corticosteroids has resulted in a bizarre syndrome in which an infant was covered by thousands of burrows on all parts of the body (Macmillan, 1972). The response to Tetmosol was satisfactory.

Itching nodules persisting for weeks or months after adequate treatment of scabies were apparently first described in 1932; many recent authors have described them, but it is not clear whether or not they are now a more frequent complication than was formerly the case. Histologically the nodules show a dense infiltrate of lymphocytes, eosinophils and histiocytes, which may closely simulate a reticulosis (Thomson et al, 1974). Usually no mites or ova are found in the nodules, but they have been found occasionally, especially in papules of less than one month's duration.

It is believed that some immunological mechanism must account for the nodules, but its nature is obscure. In patients in whom the nodules have resolved spontaneously, they recurred in the previous sites and in new sites, when reinfestation with scabies took place (Marghescu and Ziethen, 1968).

Persistent nodules developed in 6.7 per cent of 2003 cases of scabies (Konstantinov and Stanowa, 1974). One to 15 were present in each patient. The commonest sites were the axillae 50 per cent, scrotum 40 per cent, abdomen 29 per cent, sides of chest 28 per cent, groins 26 per cent, penis 22 per cent. After treatment of the scabies 36 per cent resolved within a month, 44 per cent in one to three months, and only 20 per cent lasted more than three months. Resistance to treatment is often recorded, but these findings confirm the statement (Oberste-Lehn and Baggesen, 1968) that resolution eventually occurs. Excision has been advised (Berge and Krook, 1967) but is rarely necessary.

Acute Glomerulonephritis as a Complication of Scabies

That secondary streptococcal infection of the lesions of scabies may be followed by glomerulonephritis has long been recognised. Hersch (1967) of South Africa found that 44 of 75 consecutive patients admitted to hospital with acute glomerulonephritis had scabies. Svartman et al (1972) reported from Trinidad an epidemic of glomerulonephritis associated with scabies; the human scabies mite and streptococci were isolated from dogs in infected households. This report induced Allen (1972) to record from Edinburgh a single case of glomerulonephritis following scabies and to emphasise the rarity of this association, except in a tropical environment. Gordon (1972) found no increased incidence of nephritis in Cape Town, South Africa, in patients with scabies.

Venereal Diseases and Scabies

The statistics quoted on page 70 show that in most communities sexual contact is not the most frequent mode of transmission of scabies. Nevertheless it occurs and under some social conditions is important. The young adult with scabies must be carefully examined for coexistent venereal disease.

Norwegian Scabies

This unusual host response to infestation with the human scabies mite is gaining in importance, partly because of the epidemiological significance of these reservoirs of mites and partly because such cases increase our understanding of the normal host response to the mite.

Paterson, Allen and Berridge (1973) and Espy and Jolly (1976) reported Norwegian scabies in renal transplant patients receiving azathioprine and prednisolone. They reviewed the literature on the conditions predisposing to this disease. In addition to patients with known immune defects, those affected have had Down's syndrome or senile dementia, leukaemia, beri-beri, tuberculosis, leprosy, syringomyelia or tabes. An impaired cell-mediated response was probably present in many of these patients, but the sensory deficiency appears to be a common factor in others. Future cases deserve detailed immunological study. Schirren (1970b) also reviewed the literature, and expressed doubt about current views on the pathogenesis of this erythrodermic form of scabies.

A patient reported by Schmidt and Standan (1968) had both Down's syndrome and psoriasis. Kocsard (1974) basing his report on histological criteria and the response of some cases to methotrexate, suggested that Norwegian scabies is an abnormal response of the psoriatic skin.

ANIMAL SCABIES IN MAN

Mite infestations contracted from domestic animals are increasingly frequently diagnosed, but it is certain that a great many cases are still not being identified. Many species of mite have been reported to be transmitted from domestic animals to man, but only *Sarcoptes scabiei canis*, its feline counterpart *Notoedres cati*, and two species of the free-living mite *Cheyletiella* infest man sufficiently frequently to present important problems in diagnosis. Whether *Cheyletiella* should be regarded as a scabies mite (or mange mite in veterinary parlance) has been disputed, but from the dermatologist's point of view it is conveniently classified with them.

Sarcoptes scabiei is probably an evolving species; its subspecies show no morphological variations of taxonomic value, yet they are strongly host-specific (Fain, 1968). Kutzer and Grünberg (1969) demonstrated most effectively the inability of the canine mite to establish itself on man. They placed many mites, including 300 females, on their own skins. Irritable papules and scaling soon developed, but no mites could be detected after the twelfth day. In a similar experiment using *S. tapiei*, the mites were eliminated even more rapidly.

In its natural host the life cycle of *S. scabiei canis* has much in common with that of the human mite in man (Thomsett, 1968). The females form burrows preferentially in the thin-skinned areas, where an irritable papular eruption develops. Scratching leads to thickening, alopecia and secondary infection. Young dogs, not necessarily puppies, are most frequently infested, and chronic infestations, with little in the way of gross physical signs, may persist for years in some dogs which develop a degree of tolerance to the mites. In such cases thickening and crusting may be confined to the edges of the pinnae and to the lateral aspect of the elbows and hocks (see Fig. 3.3).

In man outbreaks of dog scabies (Beck, 1965; Smith and Claypoole, 1967; Norins, 1969) tend to centre around the family pet. There is a widespread eruption of discrete irritable papules and papulovesicles the distribution of which depends on the sites of closest contact with the dog. There are no burrows, but mites and eggs may be found in scrapings. The lesions subside in a week or two, even without treatment provided there is no further contact with the infested animal.

Notoedres cati infestation is very rare in Britain (Thomsett, 1968) but in many countries, e.g. Czechoslovakia (Nesvadba, 1967) and Japan (Ito et al, 1968), is not uncommon, and cat scabies in man is seen more frequently than dog scabies. The clinical features of the two infestations are similar and family or household outbreaks tend to occur (Haufe, Meyer and Haufe, 1966).

Cheyletiella. The free-living mites of this genus attach their eggs to the hairs of the species on which they normally spend all their lives. *Cheyletiella parasitivorax* was the species first described as causing lesions in man. It is a parasite of the rabbit which reached man from cats which had hunted rabbits. In 1965 *C. yasguri* was identified from dogs in the United States and subsequently all mites found on dogs and cats have been of the latter species. It is now generally accepted that there have been errors of identification in the past. The natural host of *C. parasitivorax* is the rabbit, but it may occur accidentally and probably transitorily in other mammals, in which it perhaps causes no lesions. The natural hosts of *C. yasguri* are the dog and cat (Gething and Walton, 1972; Hewitt and Turk, 1974).

Cheyletiella spp. have been regarded as predators and *C. parasitivorax* has been found on three separate occasions feeding on the rabbit flea (Rothschild, 1969). However *C. yasguri* could not be induced to prey on Otodectes and Psoroptes and is regarded by many authorities (Rack, 1971; Foxx and Ewing, 1969; Ewing, Mosier and Foxx, 1967) as a true scabies mite, moving freely in pseudoburrows in surface debris. Heavy infestations with *C. yasguri* occur particularly in puppies; in one breeding kennel there was conspicuous white scaling by the age of 12 weeks. The owners of the kennels developed an irritable papular eruption after handling the dogs (Dodd, 1970).

There have been numerous accounts of *Cheyletiella* infestations of man and although the species identification in earlier reports may be questionable there is no evidence that the lesions produced in man by *C. parasitivorax* and *C. yasguri* differ in any important respect. The clinical picture varies according to the route of exposure, the severity of the infestation, and probably also the degree and type of allergic sensitivity to the mite antigens. In experimental infestation the lesions were at first transitory, but later developed as persistent papules (Bjarke, Hellgren and Orstadins, 1973).

The eruption may be confined to the arms as small irritable papules (Moxham, Goldfinch and Heath, 1968; Taylor, 1969), but tends to be widespread on trunk and limbs and may simulate many dermatoses including dermatitis herpetiformis. Characteristically the papules have no visible puncta, but some may be necrotic (Bjarke et al, 1973). In generalised prurigo of unknown origin the mite was discovered in house dust and only thence traced to a dog (Bronswijk, Johnson and Ophof, 1972).

Other animal mites. 'Scabies without burrows' in persons in contact with species other than cats and dogs is always an indication for the examination of brushings from the animals concerned. For example 'scabies' occurred in workers handling mice infested by *Myobia musculi* and *Myocoptes musculinus* (Novitskaya, 1968).

DEMODICIOSIS (THE FOLLICLE MITES)

Entomology

A follicle mite of man, *Demodex folliculorum*, was described by Simon in 1843, but its pathogenicity in man although accepted by some authorities is doubted or even vigorously denied by others. In 1963 Akbulatova described a second species of mite, *Demodex brevis*, as also a frequent inhabitant of human follicles. Desch and Nutting (1972) confirmed that the two species are morphologically distinct. *D. folliculorum* lives in the hair follicles and *D. brevis* in the sebaceous glands, and both species may be present in the same individual. Studies in three groups of Australian aborigines (Nutting and Green, 1974) showed one or other species to be present in about two-thirds of the males in two of the groups, but absent in the third group. Only two individuals were found to harbour both species.

In the light of these investigations further workers will need to identify precisely the species concerned and it must be appreciated that in the literature up to the present the term '*D. folliculorum*' has been applied indiscriminately to all human follicle mites.

Pathogenicity

The presumption of the pathogenicity of *Demodex* in man was based in part on the proved pathogenicity of *Demodex* species in some domestic animals, in particular the dog. *D. canis* can occasionally be demonstrated in the follicles of normal dogs but those suffering from 'demodectic mange' show an overwhelming population of mites with distension and eventual rupture of the mite-filled follicles. Affected areas of skin may show lesions varying from mild hair loss and skin scaling to deep pustules and granuloma formation. Topical application of certain insecticides can resolve the disease which usually occurs in young dogs who are thought to be immunodeficient. The disease is non-contagious but the parasites are initially acquired from the skin of the nursing bitch during the postnatal period. Spontaneous cures are often seen after some months when the dogs mature. Large cystic hair follicles packed with *Demodex* mites are common in cattle, causing subsequent defects in leather production.

Rïechers and Kopf (1969) found *Demodex* on the face, neck and chest of all of nine human subjects thoroughly studied. They were never found in other regions of the body. This work suggests that the infestation rate of about 25 per cent (Gear, 1972) reported in some other surveys may be too low and that if the searcher is sufficiently diligent higher figures may be recorded. However, too little is known about possible geographical or racial variations.

Nutting and Green (1974) could detect no clinical differences in the appearance of the skin in individuals with or without follicle mites. However, by analogy with other species, the fact that in the great majority of hosts the *Demodex* evokes no clinically evident response does not exclude the possibility that it may do so in certain circumstances.

The evidence that *Demodex* may be pathogenic in man is largely circumstantial and is perhaps most convincing in the case of a papulopustular blepharitis with much scale formation. *Demodex* is present in large numbers in the pustules and the condition clears after treatment with sulphur (Ayres and Mihan, 1967).

Gear (1972) agrees in incriminating the *Demodex* in this form of blepharitis, and believes that it is responsible also for a variety of other follicular pustular eruptions of the face and scalp.

Working in Strasbourg, Grosshans, Kremer and Maleville (1974) cut serial sections of granulomatous papules in rosacea and found *Demodex* in areas of caseous necrosis. They suggest that the granulomas form as a delayed hypersensitivity reaction to the mite.

Conclusions

The role of the two *Demodex* parasites of man in the pathogenesis of skin lesions is not reliably established, but it seems probable that acute or chronic inflammatory follicular changes can sometimes be induced.

PEDICULOSIS CAPITIS

The incidence of head-louse infestation was high in city school children before 1939 and rose higher still during the Second World War. By 1960 it had been greatly reduced in the cities, and in most rural areas cases were uncommon. Before 1970, however, the infestation rate was already rising. In Glasgow for example (Wilson, 1969) 10 per cent of school entrants were infested, and by 1971 Coates found about 12 per cent of Teesside children to be infested when they returned to school at the end of the summer holidays. Similar figures have been reported from other parts of Britain (Department of Education and Science, 1974). This rise in incidence is no doubt to be attributed to a combination of factors including the relative lack of experience of pediculosis of young medical practitioners and school nurses.

Mellanby (1941) found up to 50 per cent of girls infested at all ages from 2 to 13. In boys the peak incidence of about 45 per cent occurred between the ages of two and four, and the percentage infested fell steadily through the school years. Wilson (1969) found a smaller difference between the infestation rates of boys and girls of school age, which suggests that the fashion for long hair in boys may be a factor in the increased incidence.

Pediculosis has for some years been treated either with DDT or with gammexane. Lice resistant to these chemicals have now been reported (Maunder, 1971). This resistance, unless it is quickly recognised, must further contribute to the spread of the disease. The treatment of choice in infestation by resistant lice is with Malathion 0.5 per cent in spirit. This should be applied liberally to the scalp, which should be thoroughly washed 24 h later, and combed with a fine comb to remove any remaining eggs.

Malathion was found to be effective in controlling an outbreak in Northern Ireland (Maguire and McNally, 1972). However only two months later about 20 per cent of the treated children were reinfested. This report emphasises the importance of examining all contacts of every case, and this examination should be conducted by someone familiar with the disease, since a variety of artefacts may mislead the unwary (Kutz, 1969; Gemrich et al, 1974). It is important to remember that pruritus depends on the presence of allergic hypersensitivity to the salivary antigens of the louse (Peck, Wright and Gant, 1943). A heavy infestation may occasionally be accompanied by little or no pruritus.

PHTHIRIASIS PUBIS

Pubic louse infestation is increasing in frequency in Britain (Fisher and Morton, 1970) and elsewhere. The age incidence parallels that of gonorrhoea with which it may coexist.

Infestation of the eyelashes (Korting, 1967) may occur in infants who contract the disease from their mother's breast hairs. Rarely the scalp may be colonised (Gartmann and Dickmans-Bermeister, 1970). The diagnosis of pubic lice infestation will be suggested by the presence of lice near the anterior scalp margin, and will be confirmed by microscopical identification of the broad crab-like insect. In such cases maculae caeruleae may be present on the shoulders and upper trunk, rather than the thighs and abdomen where they are commonly seen in infestations of the pubic region.

SIPHONAPTERA (FLEAS)

It is the experience of dermatologists who have diligently and systematically examined the brushings from the coats of the domestic pets of patients with unexplained pruritic dermatoses (e.g. Hewitt, Walton and Waterhouse, 1971) that flea infestations remain exceedingly common even in homes of the highest hygienic standards, and that this diagnostic possibility is frequently ignored. Four centuries ago Thomas Moufett wrote 'Though they trouble us much yet they neither stink as wall lice do, nor is it any disgrace to a man to be troubled with them as it is to be lousie' (Lehane, 1969). Contemporary man is less tolerant of the suggestion that he is flea-ridden and it is this squeamishness together with widespread ignorance of the life history of the fleas and of the variety of lesions they may cause in man, that is responsible for many missed diagnoses.

Ecology of the Fleas

(Busvine, 1966; Askew, 1971)

It has been said that the flea is nest-specific rather than host-specific; that is to say that the eggs and larvae of most fleas have a sharply defined range of temperature and humidity within which they can develop, but the adults will feed on a variety of hosts. Central heating now ensures suitable breeding conditions throughout the year in north temperate regions in which the winter formerly called a temporary halt to reproduction.

Pulex irritans, the human flea, feeds readily on pigs and breeds in pigsties. Although its primary host is man it is found on domestic animals and on some wild species. A recent study in Georgia, USA (Kalkofen and Greenberg, 1974), showed that over 80 per cent of fleas found on dogs were of this species. The average population was 167 fleas per dog, but some dogs carried over 500.

Ctenocephalides felis, the cat flea, and *Ct. canis*, the dog flea, each feed on both cats and dogs and readily feed on man. Of 21 infested houses in north-east England studied by Bolam and Burtt (1956), 15 harboured *Ct. felis*.

Ceratophyllus gallinae, the hen flea, is also a common parasite of wild birds, and will feed on man. *Ceratophyllus columbae*, the pigeon flea, has a more restricted range of bird hosts, but will feed on man. *Ceratophyllus* sp. were found in 5 of the 21 infested humans already mentioned (Bolam and Burtt, 1956).

Whatever the species, the life history is essentially the same. The female lays 3 to 18 eggs in the nest of the host, i.e. the basket of the cat or dog, the det's favourite chair, or beneath the edge of the fireside mat. The duration of incubation and of the latent stages varies from two weeks to many months, and in the favourable conditions of a modern house averages about three to four weeks. The adult can survive months without food.

Clinical Features

The clinical manifestations of flea infestation depend obviously on the extent and frequency of the fleas' activities, but also on the immunological status of the patient in relation to the fleas' antigens (see p. 64). An irregular line of irritable papules, each with a central haemorrhagic punctum, is unlikely to go unrecognised, but the clinical picture is likely to vary widely. In the patients studied by Hewitt et al (1971) even classical papular urticaria occurred in only about a third of affected children; the other children showed a much more extensive pleomorphic eruption. In adults the commonest changes were an extensive papular eruption with a tendency to lichenification, or a generalised papular prurigo. Variations sometimes seen were eruptions of the face with grouped papules, and clusters of papules on a background of diffuse erythema and oedema.

In most cases there is a tendency for new papules to appear in crops and clusters, often asymmetrically, but new lesions may also provoke increased activity in those that are already healing.

If the diagnosis is suspected, domestic animals should be examined as described on p. 60. If the patient has no pets, then the houses she regularly visits must be similarly investigated. We recently examined an air-line pilot alleged to have dermatitis herpetiformis of over a year's duration. His eruption suggested flea-bites but he owned no pets and dust samples from his home were free from parasites. He frequently visited the home of his fiancée who, to provide him with a comfortable seat, regularly turned her labrador dog off the couch in which it otherwise spent most of the day. Brushings from the dog and from the chair contained *Ct. felis* in abundance. It is of course common for many persons who may be heavily infested to develop no symptoms.

Treatment depends on efficient epidemiological investigation.

THRIPS

These small insects feed on plant juices, and some are troublesome pests of agricultural crops. As early as 1921 Williams reported that *Karnyothrips flavipes* would bite man. His report and others incriminating the same and different species appeared in entomological journals and there are few references in the medical literature. In 1968 Goldstein and Skipworth observed on the exposed skin of several hundred troops stationed in Hawaii, a profuse eruption of small pink papules, many of which were surrounded by pale halos. Circumstantial evidence suggested that thrips were responsible. Subsequently (Aeling, 1974) further cases were reported, also from Hawaii, and it was noted that the papules themselves were anaesthetic. Some doubt was thrown on the role of the thrips, and a mosquito was blamed. However, no proven mosquito bite has been described with these striking clinical features. Thrips are common insects in many parts of the world, and so are unexplained papular eruptions of exposed skin. A recent comprehensive study of thrips is therefore most welcome (Lewis, 1973).

According to Lewis, thrips tend to be troublesome to man in hot sultry weather when large numbers of these insects, on migration, may alight on bare skin. Most species cannot penetrate the epidermis, and the itching and prick- ing they produce are probably the results of their efforts to obtain water from the moist surface of the skin. In the course of these activities they may induce the formation of small pink papules. Species from many parts of the world, belonging to the genera Gynaikothrips, Caliothrips, Limothrips, and Thrips have been shown to behave in this fashion.

A few species have been shown to be capable of penetrating the human epidermis and sucking blood. These are *Karnyothrips flavipes* (Williams, 1921; Hood, 1927), *Thrips tabaci* and *Frankliniella moultoni* (Bailey, 1936). The bites are described by the entomologists concerned, as a 'blotchy papular rash' or as 'pink dots'. The blood meal is apparently lethal to the thrips.

HYMENOPTERA (Bees, Wasps, Ants)

This family of insects differs in several practical respects from others discussed in this chapter. Many species are capable of causing systemic reactions, which may be fatal, and because some of these species are common and also frequently sting man, such reactions have special importance, and attempts at hyposensitisation are unquestionably justifiable if not invariably successful. In those countries in which allergy and dermatology are separate specialties patients with sensitivity to Hymenoptera stings are more likely to find their way to the former. Nevertheless, many also consult dermatologists, and this highly selective review concentrates on those aspects of the problem of interest to the latter. Useful reviews include those of Barr (1971) and Feingold (1971).

Problems in Identification and Diagnosis

The sting of most of the Hymenoptera is sufficiently painful to attract the victim's immediate attention, and although he may not have seen the insect he is at least aware that he has been stung. However, the bites of horseflies and of the stable fly, *Stomoxys calcitrans*, may also be painful, and the latter tends to bite through clothing.

Problems in diagnosis arise when the insect has not been seen, because the victim was unconscious, or cannot be described, because the victim is an infant, or was not noticed because the 'sting' caused little or no discomfort.

Monomericum pharaonis, Pharoah's ant. This species, a native of warm regions, has been introduced into north-west Europe where it has become a pest, often particularly troublesome in large buildings such as hospitals, in which its trails tend to follow the pipes of the heating system. It may bite infants, especially around the eyelids (Busvine, 1966). These ants are attracted to suppurating wounds and as they also visit food preparation areas, the fact that they can carry *Salmonella* sp., *Staphylococcus* sp. and *Streptococcus* sp. (Beatson, 1972) makes them potentially hazardous.

Solenopsis saerissima. The fire ant also is a native of warmer regions which has been introduced from South America to many parts of the United States. It can be incriminated retrospectively as the attacker of an unconscious victim because after 24 h a small pustule develops in the centre of each weal (Smith and Smith, 1971).

Sclerodermus brevicornis is a small wasp of wide distribution which parasitises the 'wood worm', *Anobium punctatum*. The often multiple stings may not differ from those of other wasps, but in some cases there are irritable weals and papules (Ayula, 1967).

In stings inflicted by insects recognised by the patient only as bee-like or wasp-like, precise identification, however desirable for the purposes of desensitisation, may not be practicable, but the dermatologist familiar with the principal offending species in his area should be able to give some guidance. Books such as those of James (1961) and Smith (1973) are useful. Trinca (1964) listed the most frequent offenders in Australia, and Dao (1967) those of rural Venezuela. Scientific medicine is not advanced by those authors who use only the vernacular names of insects since such names are often applied to different species in different countries. In Britain, assistance with identification is provided by the Commonwealth Institute of Entomology, c/o British Museum (Natural History), Cromwell Road, London SW7 5BD.

The Patient

It has often been stated that allergic reactions to the stings of Hymenoptera occur more frequently in atopic subjects, but this assumption has been challenged. Of 2964 boy scouts of average age 13 years, 11 per cent suffered from asthma or hay fever. Allergy to bee stings occurred in 0.8 per cent of the atopics and in the same proportion of the remaining 89 per cent (Settipan, Newstead and Boyd, 1972). However Schwartz and Kahn (1970) found that of 41 individuals with systemic reactions to stings, only 14 gave no personal or family history of atopic disorders. The apparently lower incidence of systemic reactions in Negro than in white children (Sherry, North and Scott, 1969) certainly suggests that a genetic factor is implicated. In at least the majority of cases systemic reactions are mediated by IgE. Pure venoms were used to test leucocytic release of histamine, using cells from patients already assessed as having had systemic reactions. The test was positive in 13 of 16 patients (Sobotka et al, 1974). The study of autopsy records confirmed the increased vulnerability of atopic subjects (Barnard, 1967).

Over 30 deaths a year result from Hymenoptera stings in the United States alone, and 70 per cent of these deaths are due to respiratory tract obstruction from massive oedema and secretion (Barnard, 1973). Comparing fatal reactions with severe non-fatal reactions revealed no striking differences in the age of the patients, the number of stings and their sites, or in the speed of onset of the reactions (Barnard, 1970). The study of a larger series of severe reactions suggested that younger patients were more likely to survive such reactions. Only 2.8 per cent of generalised reactions were delayed, and these included thrombocytopenic purpura, the nephrotic syndrome (Barr, 1971) and necrotising angiitis (Fogel, Weinberg and Markowitz, 1967). During a severe non-fatal attack there were transitory changes in the electrocardiograph, followed by a rise in serum enzyme activity (Duble and Jackson, 1969).

In three patients who had suffered fatal reactions to bee stings, antibodies to bee antigens were demonstrable by immunofluorescence in sera, hearts and suprarenals (Huang et al, 1971). The procedure may have important forensic applications.

Hyposensitisation

Claims as to the effectiveness or otherwise of various desensitising procedures are conflicting. Whole body extracts are usually preferred as they are less costly than pure venom. Immunodiffusion studies of Hymenoptera antigens using rabbit antisera (O'Connor and Erickson, 1965, Langlois, Shulman and Arbesman, 1965) confirmed the presence of species specific and common antigens. Comparing whole body extracts and pure venom it could be shown that some of the venom antigens were detectable only in the corresponding antivenom sera. In principle treatment with pure venom would therefore seem preferable, but the frequent lack of previous identification of the species, together with the limited availability of certain venoms, may make the use of whole-body extracts unavoidable. Good results with such extracts are reported (Barr, 1971; Molkhou and Pinon, 1972). Moreover pure venom has proved effective when a whole-body extract has failed (Lichtenstein, Valentine and Sobotea, 1974).

The results of hyposensitisation to ants and some of the other less important Hymenoptera are said to be encouraging (Frazier, 1974) but detailed controlled trials have not been reported.

Skin tests starting with very high dilutions of antigen are valuable in planning a course of desensitising injections. They are of less value in confirming the presence of sensitivity, for many subjects with no clinical evidence of sensitivity give positive reactions (Bernton and Brown, 1965) and skin tests are sometimes negative in patients in whom clinical sensitivity is undoubtedly present.

LEPIDOPTERA (Butterflies and Moths)

Until relatively recently the butterflies and moths have occupied only a very modest corner in textbooks of dermatology. However, recent research, published mainly in the entomological journals, makes it clear that these insects are responsible for a wide range of clinical syndromes and that many of the species provoking these occur almost throughout the world. Most common are the syndromes caused by urticating hairs of either caterpillars or adults; of unknown incidence are infections spread by those species which feed on lacrymal or cutaneous secretions; finally there are certain species that can penetrate human skin and suck blood.

'Urticating' Hairs

The caterpillars of some moths and butterflies possess hairs which can puncture the skin allowing the penetration of a toxic substance often secreted by a gland at the base of each hair (Smith, 1973). The hairs retain their noxious properties after they have been shed; they may be present on the cocoon and on the adult, and may be carried considerable distances by the wind.

The pharmacological properties of the toxic substances require further investigation. They contain histamine-releasing agents, and sometimes anticoagulants. Extracts from the hairs of an unidentified Noctuid species showed fibrinolytic activity and activated human plasminogen (Arocha Piñango and Layrisse, 1969). There appear to be marked differences between the toxins of different species. Sensitisation also probably develops in many cases and modifies further responses (Ziprkowski and Rolant, 1966). Fragments of the hairs of some species (e.g. *Premolis semirufa*) provoke fibrosis and granulomatous reactions (Braga Dias and Cordeiro de Azevedo, 1973).

The clinical picture induced by contact with the caterpillar hairs obviously varies according to the nature of the toxin, the presence or absence of allergic sensitisation and the mode and degree of exposure. In 745 affected workers in tea gardens in East Pakistan (Akhand, 1969) there was a painful papulo-vesicular eruption of the legs and feet, with diffuse cellulitis; six patients developed cutaneous gangrene. In parts of Brazil up to 40 per cent of rubber plantation workers suffer from the effects of contact with the caterpillars of *Premolis semirufa;* weals and bullae and diffuse oedema are followed by fibrosis which may result in ankylosis (Braga Dias and Cordeiro de Azevedo, 1973).

A different type of severe reaction occurred in five persons in contact with the caterpillars of a Saturnid moth; there were extensive haemorrhagic lesions (Arocha Piñango and Layrisse, 1969).

Less severe manifestations are reported in 90 per cent of forestry workers in Oregon, USA, exposed to the tussock moth *Hemerocampa pseudotsugata;* pruritus, weals and oedema were of variable extent (Hoover and Nelson, 1974). However an Italian factory worker in contact with *Corethocampa pinivora* developed a widespread bullous eruption of the trunk and ulceration and scarring of the prepuce (Moschen, Policero and Savestano, 1967). Milder papulovesicular lesions of the face and neck were seen in two women in France, who had removed caterpillars from Christmas trees (Averighi, 1963). The Youta silk moth in Ghana caused outbreaks of urticaria (Clarke, 1966).

Urticating hairs are present in the adults of some species, e.g. of the Saturnid moth *Hybernia* (Allard and Allard, 1958). Moths swarming around lights caused troublesome papular dermatitis. Most of the crew of a tanker moored in the Orinoco river were affected when the hairs of another *Hybernia* species were disseminated by the ship's ventilator system (Goethe, Brett and Weidner, 1967).

In the eye the hairs of either caterpillars or adults may cause serious keratoconjunctivitis (Watson and Sevel, 1966; Bishop and Morton, 1968).

The 'Eye-frequenters'

It has been known since at least 1915 that some *Noctuid* species frequent the eyes of horses, cattle, pigs and other mammals, and feed on their lacrymal secretions. In a series of investigations it has been shown that various species of *Noctuidae, Pyralidae* and *Geometridae* in South-east Asia feed at the eyes, and on the pus and blood of these animals and of man (Bänziger and Büttiker, 1969). They may therefore possibly transmit infection.

The Blood Suckers

A *Noctuid* moth, *Calyptra eustrigata,* feeds on open wounds and on the blood excreted by replete mosquitoes feeding on cattle and other mammals. It has a strong proboscis and can suck blood from various species including man. In man a papule at the puncture site persists for several weeks (Bänziger, 1968).

REFERENCES

INTRODUCTION

Hewitt, M., Walton, G. S. & Waterhouse, M. (1971) Pet animal infestations and human skin lesions. *British Journal of Dermatology*, **85**, 215.

THE IMMUNE RESPONSE

Allen, J. R. (1973) Tick resistance: basophils in skin reactions of resistant guinea-pigs. *International Journal for Parasitology*, **3**, 195.

Bagnall, B. G. (1975) Cutaneous immunity to the tick *Ixodes holocyclus*. Ph.D. thesis, University of Sydney.

Beard, R. L. (1963) Insect toxins and venoms. *Annual Review of Entomology*, **8**, 1.

Benjamini, E., Feingold, B. F. & Kartman, L. (1961) Skin reactivity in guinea-pigs sensitised to flea bites. The sequence of reactions. *Proceedings of the Society for Experimental Biology and Medicine*, **108**, 700.

Benjamini, E., Feingold, B. F., Young, J. D., Kartman, L. & Shimizu, M. (1963) Allergy to flea bites. IV. In vitro collection and antigenic properties of the oral secretion of the cat flea *Ctenocephalides felis felis*. *Experimental Parasitology*, **13**, 143.

Benjamini, E. & Feingold, B. F. (1970) Immunity to arthropods. In *Immunity to Parasitic Animals*, ed. Jackson, G. J., Herman, R. & Singer, I. New York: Appleton-Century-Crofts.

Berenberg, J. L., Ward, P. A. & Sonenshine, D. E. (1972) Tick-bite injury: mediation by a complement-derived chemotictic chemotactic factor. *Journal of Immunology*, **109**, 451.

Feingold, B. F., Benjamini, E. & Michaeli, D. (1968) The allergic responses to insect bites. *Annual Review of Entomology*, **13**, 137.

Foxx, T. S. & Ewing, S. A. (1969) Morphologic features, behaviour and life history of *Cheyletiella yasguri*. *American Journal of Veterinary Research*, **30**, 269.

French, F. E. & West, A. S. (1971) Skin reaction specificity of guinea-pig immediate hypersensitivity to bites of four mosquito species. *Journal of Parasitology*, **57**, 396.

Goetzl, E. J., Wasserman, S. I. & Austen, K. F. (1975) Eosinophil polymorphonuclear leukocyte function in immediate hypersensitivity. *Archives of Pathology*, **99**, 1.

Hocking, B. (1971) Blood sucking behaviour of terrestrial arthropods. *Annual Review of Entomology*, **16**, 1.

Hudson, A., Bowman, L. & Orr, C. W. M. (1960) Effects of absence of saliva on blood feeding by mosquitoes. *Science*, **131**, 1730.

Kagan, I. G. (1974) Advances in immunodiagnosis of parasitic infections. *Zeitschrift für Parasitenkunde*, **45**, 163.

Kaufman, W. R. & Phillips, J. E. (1973) Ion and water balance in the ixodid tick *Dermacentor andersoni*. I–III. *Journal of Experimental Biology*, **58**, 523.

Langlois, C., Shulman, S. & Arbesman, C. E. (1965) The allergic response to stinging insects. II. Immunologic studies of human sera from allergic individuals. *Journal of Allergy*, **36**, 13.

Lester, H. M. O. & Lloyd, L. (1928) Notes on the process of digestion of tsetse flies. *Bulletin of Entomological Research*, **19**, 39.

Lichtenstein, L. M. (1972) Allergy. In *Clinical Immunobiology*, ed. Bach, F. H. & Good, R. A., Vol. 1. New York: Academic Press.

Meredith, J. & Kaufman, W. R. (1973) A proposed site of fluid secretion in the salivary gland of the ixodid tick *Dermacentor andersoni*. *Parasitology*, **67**, 205.

Nelson, W. A., Keirans, J. E., Bell, J. F. & Clifford, C. M. (1975) Host–ectoparasite relationships. *Journal of Medical Entomology*, **12**, 143.

Ogilvie, B. M. (1970) Immunoglobulin responses in parasitic infections. *Proceedings of the 2nd International Congress of Parasitology*, Part. III, p. 525.

Ogilvie, B. M. (1974) Immunity to parasites (helminths and arthropods). In *Progress in Immunology*, *II*, ed. Brent, L. & Holborow, J., Vol. 4. North-Holland Publishing Co.

Parish, W. E. (1971) Effectors of immunologic responses: their expression and modes of action in skin. In *Advances in Biology of Skin*, Vol. XI, *Immunology and the Skin*, ed. Montagna, W. & Billingham, R. E. New York: Appleton-Century-Crofts.

Reisman, R. E., Wypych, J. & Arbesman, C. E. (1975) Stinging insect allergy: detection and clinical significance of venom IgE antibodies. *Journal of Allergy and Clinical Immunology*, **56**, 443.
Roberts, J. A. (1968) Acquisition by the host of resistance to the cattle tick, *Boophilus microplus* (Canestrini). *Journal of Parasitology*, **54**, 657.
Sheahan, B. J. (1975) Pathology of *Sarcoptes scabiei* infection in pigs. 1. Naturally occurring and experimental induced lesions. *Journal of Comparative Pathology*, **85**, 87.
Soulsby, E. J. L. & Harvey, W. R. (1972) Disease transmission by arthropods. *Science*, **176**, 1153.
Stebbings, J. H. (1974) Immediate hypersensitivity: a defence against arthropods? *Perspectives in Biology and Medicine*, Winter 1974, 233.
Sutherland, S. K. (1974) Venomous Australian creatures: the action of their toxins and the care of the envenomated patient. *Anaesthesia and Intensive Care*, **2**, 316.
Sutherst, R. W. & Moorhouse, D. E. (1971) *Ixodes holocyclus* larvae and 'scrub itch' in south-east Queensland. *South-east Asian Journal of Tropical Medicine and Public Health*, **2**, 82.
Sweatman, G. K. (1957) Life history, non-specificity and revision of the genus *Chorioptes*, a parasitic mite of herbivores. *Canadian Journal of Zoology*, **35**, 641.
Tatchell, R. J. (1969a) Host–parasite interactions and the feeding of blood-sucking arthropods. *Parasitology*, **59**, 93.
Tatchell, R. J. (1969b) The ionic regulatory role of the salivary secretion of the cattle tick *Boophilus microplus*. *Journal of Insect Physiology*, **15**, 1421.
Wilson, A. B. & Clements, A. N. (1965) The nature of the skin reaction to mosquito bites in laboratory animals. *International Archives of Allergy*, **26**, 294.
Yesudian, P. & Thambiah, A. S. (1973) Persistent papules after tick-bites. *Dermatologica*, **147**, 214.

HUMAN SCABIES
Allen, B. R. (1972) Scabies and acute glomerulonephritis. *Lancet*, **1**, 434.
Aruntjunov, W. J. (1970) Ein neues Klinische Symptom der Skabies. *Dermatologische Monatsschrift*, **156**, 563.
Barthelmes, H. & Barthelmes, R. (1971) Untersuchungen zur Zunahme der Scabieser-krankungen. III. Die Therapie und ihre sozialhygienischen Aspekte. *Dermatologische Monatsschrift*, **157**, 725.
Barthelmes, R., Sönnichsen, N. & Barthelmes, H. (1970) Untersuchungen zur Zunahme der Scabieserkrankungen. I. Der zyklische Verlauf der Scabies humanus. *Dermatologische Monatsschrift*, **156**, 881.
Belda, W. (1973) Aspectos do Problema do Escabiosa no Estado de São Paolo. *Anais Brasilieros de Dermatologica e Sifilografia*, **48**, 61.
Berge, T. & Krook, G. (1967) Persistent nodules in scabies. *Acta dermato-venereologica*, **47**, 20.
Borda, J. M. (1955) *Sarna Humana*. Buenos Aires.
Epstein, E. (1966) Scabies ten years later. *Archives of Dermatology*, **93**, 60.
Espy, P. D. & Jolly, M. W. (1926) Norwegian scabies. *Archives of Dermatology*, **112**, 193.
Gordon, W. (1972) Epidemic scabies and acute glomerulonephritis. *Lancet*, **1**, 794.
Grant, P. W. & Keczes, K. (1964) Persistent nodules in scabies. *Archives of Dermatology*, **89**, 239.
Hancock, B. W. & Ward, A. N. (1974) Serum immunoglobulins in scabies. *Journal of Investigative Dermatology*, **63**, 482.
Haydon, J. R. & Caplan, R. M. (1971) Epidemic scabies. *Archives of Dermatology*, **103**, 168.
Heilesen, B. (1946) Studies on *Acarus scabiei* and scabies. *Acta dermato-venereologica*, **26**, Suppl. 14.
Hejazi, N. & Mehregan, A. H. (1975) Scabies: histological study of inflammatory lesions. *Archives of Dermatology*, **111**, 37.
Herrmann, W. P. & Humann, B. (1970) Jahreszeitliche Morbiditätsschwankungen bei der Scabies. *Hautarzt*, **20**, 467.
Hersch, C. (1967) Acute glomerulonephritis due to skin disease, with special reference to scabies. *South African Medical Journal*, **1**, 29.

Kocsard, E. (1974) Associated dermatoses and triggering factors in psoriasis. *Australian Journal of Dermatology*, **15**, 64.

Konstantinov, D. & Stanowa, L. (1974) Persistent scabies nodules. *Dermatologica*, **147**, 321.

Macmillan, A. L. (1972) Unusual features of scabies associated with topical fluorinated steroids. *British Journal of Dermatology*, **87**, 496.

Madsen, A. (1965) Why *Acarus scabiei* avoids the face. *Acta dermato-venereologica*, **45**, 167.

Madsen, A. (1970) Mite burrows in crusts from young infants. *Acta dermato-venereologica*, **50**, 391.

Marghescu, S. & Ziethen, H. (1968) Uber die nodöse Erscheinungsform der Skabies. *Dermatologische Wochenschrift*, **154**, 793.

Mellanby, K. (1943) *Scabies*. London: Oxford University Press. Reprinted 1972.

Nair, B. K. H., Joseph, A., Narayanan, P. I. & Chacko, K. V. (1973) Epidemiology of scabies. *Indian Journal of Dermatology and Venereology*, **39**, 101.

Oberste-Lehn, H. & Baggesen, I. (1968) Persistierende, rezidivierende juckende Papeln nach Skabies. *Dermatologische Wochenschrift*, **154**, 437.

Orkin, M. (1971) Resurgence of scabies. *Journal of the American Medical Association*, **217**, 593.

Palička, P. & Merka, V. (1971) Contemporary epidemiological problems of scabies. *Journal of Hygiene, Epidemiology, Microbiology and Immunology*, **15**, 457.

Paterson, W. D., Allen, B. R. & Berridge, G. W. (1973) Norwegian scabies during immunosuppression therapy. *British Medical Journal*, **4**, 211.

Richardson, B. D. (1972) *Sarcoptes scabiei*: the almost forgotten parasite. *Lancet*, **2**, 839.

Schenone, H., Falaha, F., Szekely, R. et al (1971) La sarna en pediatría. *Revista Chileana di Pediatría*, **42**, 561.

Schirren, J. M. (1970a) Die Scabies. Eine epidemiologische Studie. *Hautarzt*, **21**, 170.

Schirren, J. M. (1970b) Zur Kasuistik der Scabies norvegica sive crustosa. *Hautarzt*, **21**, 407.

Schmidt, U. & Standan, H. (1968) Ein Kasuistischer Beitrag zur Scabies norvegica. *Dermatologische Wochenschrift*, **154**, 1211.

Schrank, A. B. & Alexander, S. L. (1967) Scabies: another epidemic? *British Medical Journal*, **1**, 669.

Sönnichsen, N., Barthelmes, H. & Barthelmes, R. (1971) Untersuchungen zur Zunahme der Scabieserkrankungen. II. Klinik und Epidemiologie der gegenwartigen Scabiesepidemie. *Dermatologische Monatsschrift*, **157**, 418.

Steigleder, G. K. (1970) Epizootien, ihre Erkennung, Behandlung und Prophylaxie. *Fortschritte der praktischen Dermatologie und Venerelogie*, **6**, 272.

Svartman, M., Potter, E. V., Finkler, J. F., Poon-King, T. & Earle, D. P. (1972) Epidemic scabies and acute glomerulonephritis in Trinidad. *Lancet*, **1**, 249.

Thomson, J., Cochrane, T., Cochran, R. & McQueen, A. (1974) Histology simulating a reticulosis in persistent nodular scabies. *British Journal of Dermatology*, **90**, 421.

Wozniak, K. D. & Wienrich, I. (1972) Zur gegenwartigen Häufigkeit, Klinik und Therapie der Skabies. *Deutsche Gesundheitswesen*, **27**, 1188.

Zumpt, F. (1972) Scabies and sarcoptic mange. In *Essays in Tropical Dermatology*, ed. Marshall, J., Vol. 2, p. 198.

ANIMAL SCABIES IN MAN

Bakkers, E. J. M. & Fain, A. (1972) Dermatitis in man and in a dog caused by the mite *Cheyletiella yasguri*. *British Journal of Dermatology*, **87**, 245.

Beck, A. C. (1965) Animal scabies affecting man. *Archives of Dermatology*, **91**, 54.

Bjarke, T., Hellgren, L. & Orstadius, K. (1973) *Cheyletiella parasitovorax* dermatitis in man. *Acta dermato-venereologica*, **53**, 217.

Bronswijk, J. E. M. H. van, Jansen, L. H. & Ophof, A. J. (1972) Invasion of a human by the dog parasite *Cheyletiella yasguri* (Smiley, 1965): a mite causing prurigo in man. *Dermatologica*, **145**, 338.

Dodd, K. (1970) *Cheyletiella yasguri*: widespread infestation in a breeding kennel. *Veterinary Record*, **86**, 346.

Ewing, S. A., Mosier, J. E. & Foxx, T. S. (1967) Occurrence of *Cheyletiella* spp. on dogs with skin lesions. *Journal of the American Veterinary Medical Association*, **151**, 14.

Fain, A. (1968) Etude de la variabilité de *Sarcoptes scabiei* en une Réaction des Sarcoptidae. *Acta Zoologica Pathologica, Antwerp*, No. 47.

Foxx, T. S. & Ewing, S. A. (1969) Morphologic features, behaviour and life history of Cheyletiella yasguri. *American Journal of Veterinary Research*, **30**, 26.

Gething, M. A. & Walton, G. S. (1972) Possible host specificity of *Cheyletiella* mites. *Veterinary Record*, **88**, 512.

Haufe, U., Meyer, D. & Haufe, F. (1966) Katzenscabies beim Menschen, hervorgerufen durch eine an Sarcoptesräude und Trichophytie erkrankte Katze. *Dermatologische Wochenschrift*, **152**, 977.

Hewitt, M. & Turk, S. M. (1974) *Cheyletiella* sp. in the personal environment. *British Journal of Dermatology*, **90**, 679.

Ito, K., Ito, Y., Kondo, S. & Otani, M. (1968) Animal scabies in humans. *Bulletin of the Pharmacological Research Institute*, **77**, 1.

Kutzer, E. & Grünberg, W. (1969) Zur Frage der Ubertragung tierischer Sarcoptesräaden auf den Menschen. *Berliner und Münchenen Tierärztliche Wochenschrift*, **52**, 311.

Moxham, J. W., Goldfinch, T. T. & Heath, A. C. G. (1968) *Cheyletiella parasitivorax* infestation of cats associated with skin lesions of man. *New Zealand Veterinary Journal*, **16**, 50.

Nesvadba, J. (1967) Notedria Mange as a Parasitological Public Health and Economic Problem. *Acta Universitatis Agriculturea Brno Facultatis Veterinaria*, **36**, 526.

Norins, A. L. (1969) Canine scabies in children. *American Journal of Diseases of Children*, **117**, 239.

Novitskaya, S. A. (1968) Parasitism of man by the mites *Myobia musculi* and *Mycoptes musculinus*. *Meditsinskaya parazitologiya i parazitarnyl bolezni*, **37**, 113.

Rack, G. (1971) *Cheyletiella yasguri* Smiley 1965: ein fakultaten menschenpathogener Parasit des Hundes. *Zeitschrift für Parasitenkunde*, **36**, 321.

Rothschild, M. (1969) *Cheyletiella parasitivorax* feeding upon the rabbit flea. *Entomologists' Monthly Magazine*, **105**, 1262.

Smith, E. B. & Claypoole, T. F. (1967) Canine scabies in dog and in human. *Journal of the American Medical Association*, **199**, 59.

Taylor, R. M. (1969) *Cheyletiella parasitivorax* infection of a cat and associated skin lesions of man. *Amsterdam Veterinary Journal*, **45**, 435.

Thomsett, L. R. (1968) Mite infestations of man contracted from dogs and cats. *British Medical Journal*, **3**, 93.

DEMODICIOSIS

Ayres, S. & Mihan, R. (1967) Rosacea-like demodiciosis involving the eyelids. *American Medical Association Archives of Dermatology*, **95**, 63.

Desch, C. & Nutting, W. B. (1972) *Demodex folliculorum* (Simon) and *D. brevis* (Akbulatova) of man: redescription and reevaluation. *Journal of Parasitology*, **58**, 169.

Gear, J. W. (1972) The pathogenicity of *Demodex folliculorum*. In *Essays on Tropical Dermatology*, ed. Marshall, J., Vol. 2, p. 209.

Grosshans, E. M., Kremer, M. & Maleville, J. (1974) *Demodex folliculorum* und die Histogenese der granulomatösen Rosacea. *Hautarzt*, **25**, 166.

Nutting, W. B. & Green, A. C. (1974) Hair follicle mites (Acari–Demodicidon) from Australian aborigines. *Australian Journal of Dermatology*, **15**, 10.

Riechers, R. & Kopf, A. W. (1969) Cutaneous infestation with *Demodex follicularis* in man. *Journal of Investigative Dermatology*, **52**, 103.

PEDICULOSIS CAPITIS

Coates, K. G. (1971) Control of head infestation in school children. *Community Medicine*, **126**, 148.

Department of Education and Science (1974) *The Health of the School Child* 1971–72. London: HMSO.

Gemrich, E. G., Brady, J. G., Lee, B. L. & Parham, P. H. (1974) Outbreak of head lice in Michigan misdiagnosed. *American Journal of Public Health*, **64**, 805.

Kutz, F. W. (1969) A problem in the diagnosis of head lice. *Entomological News*, **80**, 27.

Maguire, J. & McNally, A. J. (1972) Head infestation in school children: extent of the problem and treatment. *Community Medicine*, **128**, 374.

Maunder, J. W. (1971) Resistance to organochlorine insecticides in head lice, and trials using alternative compounds. *Medical Officer*, **126**, 145.

Mellanby, K. (1941) The incidence of head lice in England. *Medical Officer*, **65**, 39.

Peck, S. M., Wright, W. H. & Gant, J. O. (1943) Cutaneous reactions due to the body louse (*Pediculus humanus*). *Journal of the American Medical Association*, **123**, 821.
Wilson, T. S. (1969) *Medical Officer*, **122**, 125.

PHTHIRIASIS PUBIS
Fisher, I. & Morton, R. S. (1970) *Phthirus pubis* infestation. *British Journal of Venereal Diseases*, **46**, 326.
Gartmann, H. & Dickmans-Bermeister ,D. (1970) Phthiri im Bereich der Kopfhaare, Augenbrauen und Wimpern bei einem 2½ jährigen Mädchen. *Hautarzt*, **21**, 279.
Korting, G. W. (1967) Phthiriasis palpebrarum und ihre ersten historischen Erwährungen. *Hautarzt*, **18**, 73.

SIPHONAPTERA
Askew, R. R. (1971) *Parasitic Insects*, p. 32. London: Heinemann.
Bolam, R. M. & Burtt, E. T. (1956) Flea infestation as a cause of papular urticaria. *British Medical Journal*, **1**, 1130.
Busvine, J. R. (1966) *Insects and Hygiene*, 3rd edn. London: Methuen.
Hewitt, M., Walton, G. S. & Waterhouse, M. (1971) Pet animal infestations and human skin lesions. *British Journal of Dermatology*, **85**, 215.
Kalkofen, U. P. & Greenberg, J. (1974) Public health implications of *Pulex irritans* infestation in dogs. *Journal of the American Veterinary Medical Association*, **165**, 903.
Lehane, B. (1969) *The Compleat Flea*. London: Murray.

THRIPS
Aeling, J. L. (1974) Hypoanaesthetic halos in Hawaii. *Cutis*, **14**, 541.
Bailey, S. F. (1936) Thrips attacking man. *Canadian Entomologist*, **60**, 201.
Goldstein, N. & Skipworth, G. B. (1968) Papular eruptions secondary to thrips bites. *Journal of the American Medical Association*, **203**, 53.
Hood, J. D. (1927) A blood-sucking thrips. *Entomologist*, **60**, 201.
Lewis, T. (1973) *Thrips, Their Biology, Ecology and Economic Importance*, p. 75. London and New York: Academic Press.
Williams, C. B. (1921) A blood-sucking thrips. *Entomologist*, **54**, 163.

HYMENOPTERA
Ayula, L. (1967) Su di una particolare dermatosi parassitaria da *Sclerodermus brevicornis*. *Minerva Dermatologica*, **42**, 593.
Barnard, J. H. (1967) Allergic and pathologic findings in fifty insect-sting fatalities. *Journal of Allergy*, **40**, 107.
Barnard, J. H. (1970) Non-fatal results in third-degree anaphylaxis from hymenoptera stings. *Journal of Allergy*, **45**, 92.
Barnard, J. H. (1973) Studies of 400 Hymenoptera sting deaths in the United States. *Journal of Allergy and Clinical Immunology*, **52**, 259.
Barr, S. E. (1971) Allergy to Hymenoptera stings. Review of the world literature 1953–70. *Annals of Allergy*, **29**, 49.
Beatson, S. H. (1972) Pharaoh's ants as pathogen vectors in hospitals. *Lancet*, **1**, 425.
Bernton, H. S. & Brown, H. (1965) Studies on the Hymenoptera. *Journal of Allergy*, **36**, 315.
Busvine, J. R. (1966) *Insects and Hygiene*, 3rd edn, p. 396. London: Methuen.
Dao, L. (1967) Picadura de Avispas en Zonas rurales de Venezuela. *Dermatologia Internationalis*, **6**, 144.
Duble, T. J. & Jackson, E. (1969) Stock, coma and electrocardiographic changes with enzyme release in cases of wasp-sting allergy. *British Medical Journal*, **3**, 761.
Feingold, B. F. (1971) Allergic reactions to Hymenoptera stings. *Journal of Asthma Research* **9**, 55.
Fogel, B. J., Weinberg, T. & Markowitz, M. (1967) A fatal connective tissue disease following a wasp sting. *American Journal of Diseases of Children*, **114**, 325.
Frazier, C. A. (1974) Biting insect survey: a statistical report. *Annals of Allergy*, **32**, 200.
Huang, I., Bernton, H. S., Stauch, J. & Brown, H. (1971) Fluorescent antibody studies in three patients dying from honey-bee sting. *Journal of Allergy*, **47**, 198.

James, H. & Harwood, R. (1969) Ticks and tick-borne diseases. In *Medical Entomology*, 6th rev. edn. New York: Macmillan.

Langlois, C., Shulman, S. & Arbesman, C. E. (1965) The allergic response to stinging insects. *Journal of Allergy*, **36**, 109, 147.

Lichtenstein, L. M., Valentine, M. D. & Sobotka, A. K. (1974) A case for venom treatment in anaphylactic sensitivity to Hymenoptera sting. *New England Journal of Medicine*, **290**, 1223.

Molkhou, P. & Pinon, C. (1972) Allergic aux hymenoptères. *Revue française d'Allergologie*, **12**, 333.

O'Connor, R. & Erickson, R. (1965) Hymenoptera antigens. *Annals of Allergy*, **23**, 151.

Schwartz, H. J. & Kahn, B. (1970) Hymenoptera sensitivity. II. The role of allergy in the development of clinical sensitivity. *Journal of Allergy*, **45**, 87.

Settipane, G. A., Newstead, G. J. & Boyd, G. K. (1972) Frequency of Hymenoptera allergy in an atopic and a normal population. *Journal of Allergy and Clinical Immunology*, **50**, 146.

Sherry, M. N., North, R. & Scott, R. B. (1969) Insect bites in white and Negro children: a comparison. *Annals of Allergy*, **27**, 547.

Smith, K. G. V. (1973) *Insects and Other Arthropods of Medical Importance*. London: British Museum.

Smith, J. D. & Smith, E. B. (1971) Multiple fire ant stings. *Archives of Dermatology*, **103**, 438.

Sobotka, A. K., Valentine, M. D., Benton, A. W. & Lichtenstein, L. M. (1974) Allergy to insect stings. I. Diagnosis of IgE-mediated Hymenoptera sensitivity by venom-induced histamine release. *Journal of Allergy and Clinical Immunology*, **53**, 170.

Trinca, J. C. (1964) Insect allergy in Australia: Results of a five year survey. *Medical Journal of Australia*, **2**, 659.

LEPIDOPTERA

Akhand, A. H. (1969) Caterpillar dermatitis. *Journal of the Pakistan Medical Association*, **19**, 65.

Allard, H. F. & Allard, H. A. (1958) Venomous moths and butterflies. *Journal of the Washington Academy of Sciences*, **48**, 18.

Arocha Piñango, C. L. & Layrisse, M. (1969) Fibrinolysis producida por contacto con una oruga. *Acta medica Venezolana*, **16**, 247.

Averighi, F. (1963) La dermatite méconnue des Arbres du Nord. *Bulletin de la Société française de Dermatologie et de Syphilographie*, **69**, 561.

Bänziger, H. (1968) Preliminary observations on a skin-piercing, blood-sucking moth (*Calyptra eustrigata* (HMPS) (Lep. Noctuidae)) in Malaya. *Bulletin of Entomological Research*, **58**, 159.

Bänziger, H. & Büttiker, W. (1969) Records of eye-frequenting Lepidoptera from man. *Journal of Medical Entomology*, **6**, 53.

Bishop, J. W. & Morton, R. R. (1968) Caterpillar-hair keratoconjunctivitis. *Medical Journal of Australia*, **2**, 995.

Braga, Dias, L. & Cordeiro de Azevedo, M. (1973) Pararama: a disease caused by moth larvae. *Bulletin of the Panamanian Health Organisation*, **7**, 9.

Clarke, M. G. (1966) Urticaria from moths. *British Journal of Dermatology*, **78**, 496.

Goethe, H., Brett, R. & Weidner, H. (1967) Butterfly itch: eine Schnetterliegsdermatose an Bord eines Tankers. *Zeitschrift für Tropenmedizin und Parasitologie*, **18**, 5.

Hoover, A. W. & Nelson, E. (1974) Skin symptoms attributed to tussock moth infestation. *Cutis*, **13**, 597.

Moschen, M., Policero, R. D. & Savestano, G. (1967) Insolita Dermatite bollosa de Processionaira del Pino. *Archivio Italiano di Dermatologia, Venereologia e Sessuologia*, **33**, 474.

Smith, K. G. V. (1973) Lepidoptera. In *Insects and Other Arthropods of Medical Importance*, p. 405. London: British Museum.

Watson, P. G. & Sevel, D. (1966) Ophthalmia nodosa. *British Journal of Ophthalmology*, **50**, 209.

Ziprkowski, L. & Rolant, F. (1966) Study of the toxin from the poison hairs of *Thaumetopoea wilkinsoni* caterpillars. *Journal of Investigative Dermatology*, **46**, 349.

4
TROPICAL SKIN DISEASES IN TEMPERATE CLIMATES

R. R. M. Harman

Introduction

Tropical dermatology defies strict definition. A recently published textbook on the subject wisely makes no attempt to define which skin diseases are tropical and which are not. Instead, it divides them into those which are prevalent in the tropical zone, and those which—though cosmopolitan—show special features when found there. The subject of tropical dermatology is best left ill-defined, for it merges with the theme of dermatology in temperate and arctic regions. Nevertheless, the zone between the tropics of Capricorn and Cancer contains some of the most interesting and lively of dermatoses, which are both preventable and curable: the speed of modern travel and huge population movements have brought them to enrich the clinical practice of dermatologists in so-called temperate countries though these, at least from a tropical viewpoint, have their arctic moments.

A very high proportion of diseases of the skin acquired in the tropics are infective. This reflects not only the climatic factors which favour transmission, but also the social and economic conditions under which so much of tropical mankind lives. These disorders are also subject to the genetic and developmental characteristics of the indigenous people. In the strictly geographical tropical zone the climatic factors are themselves inconstant. They vary greatly with altitude, proximity to oceans, the character of the land and other influences.

Systemic tropical diseases have assumed great importance in the jet, and now supersonic, age and there are numerous recent publications on them of interest to dermatologists. Among the most important of these diseases are malaria, smallpox, leishmaniasis, trypanosomiasis, amoebiasis, schistosomiasis, intestinal helminthic infestations and filariases, arboviral fevers and salmonelloses. Their main importance lies in their serious morbidity and all are of consequence to dermatologists. The laboratory diagnosis of tropical diseases is reviewed by Ridley (1974), and the difficulty of recognition under the ordinary conditions of the pathology laboratory in Britain is emphasised. The Vietnam War provoked a renewal of interest in tropical disease in the United States, and a considerable volume of publications has resulted. Diseases which are sexually transmitted are also affected by the mobility explosion and Catterall

(1975) presents evidence that there is a relationship between the number of tourists and other travellers and the prevalence of sexually transmitted diseases.

A list of recent general references to tropical disease and travel may be found at the end of this chapter.

Population Movements

Travellers may be divided into four groups. Temporary visitors on holiday or on business, students, workers who go to reside in a country for some years before eventually returning home and permanent emigrants.

In recent years the number of tourists has increased at an enormous rate. In 1950 there were approximately 17 million arriving at European frontiers, in 1973 the figure had risen to 156 million with the 1972 world expenditure on tourism 8 billion pounds. In 1950 0.523 million people passed through London Airport, whereas in 1973 the figure was 20.7 million. Of these approximately 1.5 million arrived in Britain from the geographic tropics, and between 2 and 3 millions from the Mediterranean region. Woodruff (1975) estimates that 1 in 10 to 15 persons in Britain at the moment has been exposed to disease in the tropics or subtropics within the incubation period of most of the infective disorders which may be acquired there.

The vulnerability of students and others travelling overland on minimum cost adventures are also emphasised by Woodruff (1975). Journeys to Africa and India associated with the taking of cannabis and hard drugs hold special terrors. The amount of ill health arising from these trips appears higher than in any other group of the travelling public.

Students from overseas in Britain averaged 71 000 during the last five years. Many are from the tropics and have spent long periods in rural areas with high prevalence rates of infective disease.

The European community has about 10 million foreign workers with their families mostly from Turkey, Yugoslavia, Greece, Portugal, Algeria and Morocco. In the whole of industrialised Europe there may be as many as 15 million if one includes the very large number of illegal workers and internal migrants from the south, such as Italians.

In Britain the estimated number of the population of New Commonwealth (NCW) ethnic origin at the 1971 census was 1.5 million. The 'coloured' component of this population is 1.3 million and excludes people from the Mediterranean Commonwealth of Cyprus, Gibraltar, Malta and Gozo. Estimates derived from that census lead to a figure of 1.75 million for the same population in mid-1974 (*Population Trends* No. 2, Winter 1975). NCW migrants come chiefly from the American New Commonwealth of the Caribbean, from India, Pakistan, Bangladesh, African and Mediterranean Commonwealth countries. At present 3.2 per cent of the whole population of Britain is of NCW ethnic origin, through these statistics are bedevilled by their being founded on place of birth of the subject or of his parents, rather than on his race.

The Changing Pattern of Tropical Diseases

Diseases that we now consider tropical were by no means always so. For example, in 1900 malaria was a world-wide disease, though the distribution has now shrunk to the tropics and subtropics (von Mohn, 1974). Environmental factors as well as advances in treatment have played a major part in this recession. Smallpox is now on the verge of eradication due to vaccination. This was practised initially only in temperate countries, but is now used in huge systematic programmes organised by WHO in tropical areas. In the not too distant past this formidable infection was not a tropical disease. In the Middle Ages the main areas of its distribution were the populous regions of Europe, where it was as common as influenza today. The disease has remained in tropical countries—not due to climatic conditions but to delay in the development of the economy and the absence of adequate public health measures (Zhdanov, 1968). Other examples could be cited such as typhoid, tuberculosis, leprosy, malnutrition and nutritional anaemias.

Dermatoses that Afflict Tropical Peoples

The dermatologist in Britain has come to recognise certain dermatoses and peculiarities of the skin which largely spare the Caucasian race, but may be quite common among tropical peoples. Subtle variations in the uniformity of pigmentation in Negroes give difficulty in diagnosis. So does a macular depigmentation composed of tiny points which has to be considered within the range of normal. The degree of normal pigmentation of soles, palms, eyes and buccal mucosa has to be learned by experience. The absence of lunules on the fingers of Negros, and the appearance of small pits in the palmar crease keratin are also remarkable. Voigt's line may be especially prominent in races of the Indian subcontinent and in the Japanese (Ito, K., 1965), but it is also clearly visible in African Negroes. The naevoid facial blemishes of dermatosis papulosa nigra are particularly common amongst adult Negroes, but are also seen in Asiatic patients.

Pityriasis rotunda is relatively common in the Far East, where it accounts for 0.2 per cent of dermatological cases (Ito and Tanaka, 1961). It also appears in South African Bantu and has been seen in West Indians in Britain (Sarkany and Hare, 1964). Similarly acrokerato-elastoidosis, which was originally described among Negroes and mulattoes in Brazil, has now been reported in Britain—both in Negroes born abroad and in Britain (Harman and Matthews, 1974). Pseudosycosis barbae, which affected 50 per cent of healthy male Negroes who shaved in Nigeria (Harman, 1967), is commonplace in a similar group in Britain. Sickle cell ulcers in Mediterranean and Negro races are also observed.

Unusual appearances of cutaneous sarcoid in West Indians may cause diagnostic confusion, and tuberculosis of the skin appearing as tuberculous lupus miliaris faciei deceives the European dermatologist's eye (Baker, 1976).

A new distinctive papular eruption of the face previously unreported in any climate has been described in Negro children. Marten et al (1974) described 22 cases in London and has seen others since.

On the other hand, dermatitis cruris pustulosa et atrophicans (sycosis cruris) which is commonly seen in Nigerian and Ghanaian outpatients (Harman, 1968, 1972; Clarke, 1952) has yet to be reported in a Caucasian and seems to be totally absent from West Africans living in Britain. Similarly, Mudi-Chood described by Sugathan and Nair (1972) on the nape of the neck and upper exposed back in girls and young women in South India has yet to be seen in Britain.

No doubt this list of skin peculiarities and fascinating disorders could and will be added to.

Those tropical diseases that the dermatologist in a cool climate encounters most frequently will be described in some detail: particularly their geographic distribution, diagnosis and occurrence in the temperate zone. Other tropical dermatoses are dealt with more briefly. Important viral fevers with cutaneous signs such as smallpox, and arboviral infections such as chikungunya are outside the scope of this chapter. Bilharziasis and trypanosomiasis are also considered overwhelmingly systemic and are not discussed. Certain cosmopolitan bacterial infections prevalent in the tropics, malnutrition and genetic disorders are also omitted.

BACTERIAL DISEASES

Leprosy (Hansen's disease)

The chronic contagious disease of leprosy, caused by *Mycobacterium leprae*, primarily affects the peripheral nervous system and involves, secondarily, the skin, mucosa of the mouth and upper respiratory tract, reticuloendothelial system, eyes, bones and testes.

GEOGRAPHIC DISTRIBUTION

Leprosy is endemic throughout the tropics and subtropics (Fig. 4.1). It is also endemic in countries bordering the Mediterranean, Adriatic and Black Seas, as well as in the islands of Malta and Cyprus.

Cases are being seen in temperate countries—both in the native population who have returned from working in the tropics, and in immigrant workers. In England these are mainly from Bangladesh, India, Africa, and the Mediterranean. Because of the insidious, hidden, yet ultimately serious nature of the disease, together with its mystique and social implications, it causes more alarm than any other of the imported tropical diseases.

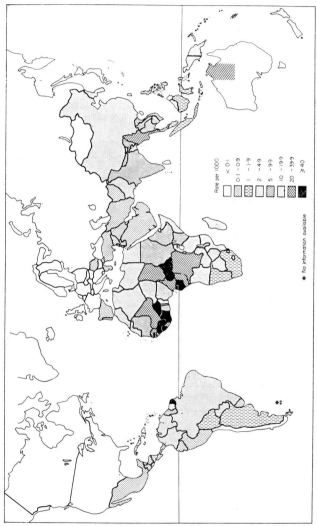

Figure 4.1 World distribution of leprosy. (WHO map, *Clinical Tropical Dermatology*, p. 110)

The world incidence of leprosy is estimated to be 11 000 000, but all the figures for national incidence, based on notification and case reports, are likely to be gross underestimates. A remarkable study of a well-known focus of leprosy in Louisiana from 1855 to 1970 showed a decrease in incidence, which began before the use of chemotherapy. With the advent of improved standards of life, the disease—which was once cosmopolitan—can now be regarded as tropical without endemic foci in Northern Europe and America (Feldman and Sturdivant, 1975). Non-endemic cases have been studied in France (Blanc and Nosny, 1970), and the psychological difficulties of treating immigrants with leprosy in a non-endemic country like West Germany have been emphasised by Abel and van Soest (1971), whilst the psychological stigma of leprosy in the continental United States has been studied by Gussow and Tracy (1972).

Schuppli (1972) concludes, from observations of the course of leprosy infections in Europe, that infections with the bacillus may occur in Europe, but rarely lead to clinical manifestations. He also (1971) discusses the use of the lepromin test in Middle Europe, and points out its usefulness in differentiating between sarcoidosis and tuberculoid leprosy.

Although it is customary to offer BCG inoculation to the families of persons found in this country to have leprosy, WHO trials are disappointing in providing evidence of its efficacy (Bechelli et al, 1974).

Progress in experimental work on the disease and its treatment has been made by the discovery that the organism can be cultured, not only in the foot-pads of mice (Shepard, 1960a, b), but also in armadillos (Kirchheimer and Storrs, 1971; Storrs, 1971) and newborn snakes (Kwapinski and Kwapinski, 1974).

Deformities are chiefly of the face and extremities (Fig. 4.2a, b), and their alleviation by plastic surgery is reviewed by Antia (1974).

An exhaustive description of leprosy is out of place in this context, and the reader is referred to publications by the following authors: Browne (undated), Jopling (1971), Canizares (1975) and Rook, Wilkinson and Ebling (1972).

However, certain points of importance to the dermatologist in a temperate climate must be emphasised. Patients with early leprosy are not ill, and suffer from no deformity. The disease is entirely silent. When considering the diagnosis, one must ascertain whether the patient has lived in an endemic area. Skin changes at first are so slight that they can well be missed. A good light for examination is essential and, when outdoors, direct sunshine falling obliquely across the skin is best. The earliest changes in a 'white' skin are subtle alterations of single or multiple areas, which are a little redder or duller or shinier than the surrounding skin. In the darker-skinned there may be very slight loss of pigment. The edges to the lesions are usually indistinct, but the pigmentary loss within the lesion is uniform. The back, forearms, buttocks, and thighs are the most commonly affected areas and, at this stage, there is no disturbance of sensation, sweating, or hair growth, and no bacilli may be

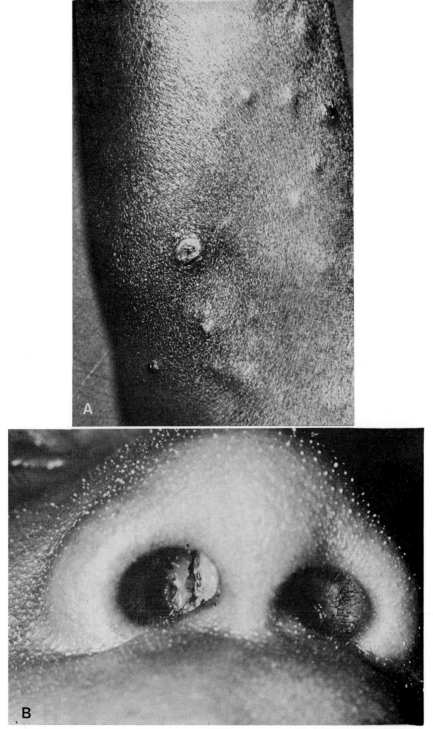

Figure 4.2 Lepromatous leprosy in a young woman from Gambia. (A) Ulcerating cutaneous nodules. (B) Crusting of the nasal mucosa. (Radcliffe Infirmary, Oxford)

Table 4.1 Leprosy, showing the principal clinical, bacteriological, histological and immunological features

Type	Skin and nerve changes	Bacteriology	Histology (dermis)	Immunology
T	Typically a single plaque (two or three at the most), anaesthetic, with dry surface well-defined edges, central flattening, and hair loss. Early nerve thickening	AFB absent	Foci of lymphocytes, epithelioid cells and giant cells in foci surrounding neurovascular elements and may not spare the subepidermal zone. Cutaneous nerves are destroyed by cellular reaction within and around them and cannot be identified	Lepromin reaction strongly positive
L	Typically macules, papules and nodules, very numerous, distributed bilaterally and symmetrically, having normal sensation and hair growth. Macules are shiny and have vague edges. Nerve thickening in late stages	AFB numerous, globi usual	Granuloma diffuse and consists largely of histiocytes and macrophages. Foamy change common. Free subepidermal zone. Cutaneous nerves contain AFB but no cellular infiltration	Lepromin reaction negative

T(TT) = tuberculoid; L = lepromatous; B = borderline; I = indeterminate; BT = borderline-tuberculoid; BB = mid-borderline; BL = borderline-lepromatous; AFB = acid fast bacilli.

Table 4.1 continued

Type	Skin and nerve changes	Bacteriology	Histology (dermis)	Immunology
B	Typically macules, plaques, annular lesions and punched-out lesions. Macules have well-defined edges; plaques have edges which are not consistently well defined and have little central flattening: annular and punched-out lesions are diagnostic. All show some degree of sensory loss; they are too numerous and not dry enough for tuberculoid: they are too few and not shiny enough for lepromatous. Early nerve thickening	AFB numerous or moderate in BL but globi unusual; moderate in BB; few or absent in BT	In BL there is a diffuse histiocytic granuloma, sometimes with lymphocytes in dense clumps. In BB there is a diffuse epithelioid cell granuloma. In BT there is a tuberculoid reaction more diffuse than in TT. In all three there is a free subepidermal zone. Cellular infiltrate within and around cutaneous nerves common in BB and BT, less so in BL	Lepromin reaction negative in BL and BB, weakly or moderately positive in BT
I	Lesions consist only of macules which are nondescript in character and asymmetrical in distribution	AFB absent (rarely present in cutaneous nerves)	Cellular reaction is of simple inflammatory type	Lepromin reaction unpredictable

T(TT) = tuberculoid; L = lepromatous; B = borderline; I = indeterminate; BT = borderline–tuberculoid; BB = mid-borderline; BL = borderline–lepromatous; AFB = acid fast bacilli.

Reproduced from Jopling and Harman (1972) In *Textbook of Dermatology*, 2nd edn, ed. Rook, A., Wilkinson, D. S. & Ebling, F. J. G. p. 688. Oxford: Blackwell.

demonstrable. This is indeterminate leprosy. It may remain localised and be self-healing, or may develop into one of the recognisable polar forms in which bacilli can be demonstrated. This type of leprosy is not uncommon in children who have been in household contact with an open case of leprosy, and the lesions have been called 'hazy patches'.

The main features of the four grades of leprosy—indeterminate, tuberculoid, dimorphous (borderline), and lepromatous—are summarised in Table 4.1.

DIFFERENTIAL DIAGNOSIS

The range of skin manifestations of leprosy is so wide, extending through every type of clinical lesion described in dermatology, that differential diagnosis is very extensive. Fortunately, however, the prognosis is very rarely affected by a short delay in diagnosis.

The distinctive clinical features of determinate leprosy should always be borne in mind, i.e.

1. *Skin:* A chronic lesion which may be hypopigmented, with impairment of sensation, hair growth, and sweating. Sensory testing should include perception of light touch, temperature, and pain.
2. *Nerve:* Thickening of a main nerve trunk in its superficial course, or of a branch close to a skin lesion.

Diagnostic histological findings are:

1. Acid fast bacilli in the dermis or nerve.
2. Tuberculoid changes in cutaneous or peripheral nerves.

TREATMENT

Dapsone remains the central drug for the treatment of leprosy, but there is not yet agreement amongst experts as to the best dosage schedule. Various ethnic and immunological factors no doubt influence the views of physicians who deal with leprosy in different parts of the world. For dosage schedules, the reader is referred to the volumes previously cited.

Rifampicin is bactericidal and is active against sulphone-resistant bacilli. Clinical response to it is very rapid, and in new lepromatous cases rifampicin, given for three to four weeks, followed by sulphone therapy is recommended.

Lamprene (B.663 Geigy—clofazimine) is a riminophenazine derivative found useful in lepromatous leprosy and leprous neuritis; particularly where dapsone has been unsatisfactory and there have been type II reactions with erythema nodosum leprosum. It has a specific anti-inflammatory effect, and a starting dosage of 100 mg once daily given after meals, decreasing to 100 mg three times a week is recommended. Dull red discoloration of the skin and sclerae occur with use of this drug, and higher doses cause gastrointestinal symptoms with abdominal pain and weight loss (Atkinson et al, 1967), such as occur in amyloidosis (Grigor, Lang and Nicholson, 1974).

Autopsy findings in a patient treated with clofazimine showed extreme congestion and oedema of the mucosa of the small intestine, together with deposits of clofazimine crystals (Desikan et al, 1975). A further case on prolonged high dosage of clofazimine was found at autopsy to have extensive destruction of mesenteric glands, as well as deposition of crystals in the intestinal mucosa (Harman, to be published).

Renal transplantation is reported in a patient with lepromatous leprosy (Adu et al, 1973). The deficiency of cell-mediated immune response in such patients results in a prolongation of survival of allogenic skin grafts, and this may well be of importance in organ transplantation. The immunologic aspects of leprosy have been discussed by Turk (1970).

Mycobacterial Ulceration

Mycobacterial ulceration, caused by *Mycobacterium ulcerans*, was first described in Australia. Credit for the recognition of it as a clinical entity goes to two general practitioners, Alsop and Searls, who found it in the vicinity of Bairnsdale, a country town in south-eastern Victoria at latitude 37° south, well outside the tropical belt. But now it is most commonly known as Buruli ulcer, after the area of Uganda where the greatest number of reports have originated. Other tropical areas of high incidence are in Zaire and Papua–New Guinea, where cases occur in clusters, and there are also reports in Indonesia, Malaysia, Nigeria and Mexico (Radford, 1975; Fig. 4.3). Keininger, Schubert and Ullmann (1972), in Germany, report the third case in an European. He had lived in Nigeria since his childhood.

Both sexes and all age groups are affected, and most patients present with an ulcer which is painless and has a characteristic, very deeply undermined edge. Lesions are usually on the arms or legs, and may rarely be seen at the earlier preulcerative stage when they are small, painless, subcutaneous swellings attached to the skin but not to the deep fascia. The tumours can resemble subcutaneous phycomycosis.

Microscopy of preulcerative lesions shows clumps of organisms surrounded by areas of necrosis of the subcutaneous tissues. This necrosis extends as the lesion progresses, cutting off the blood supply to overlying skin and resulting in large ulcers which can mutilate an entire limb. Extensive skin loss can lead to the death of a young child, but usually slow healing occurs, leaving ugly scars and contractures (Barker, 1974).

Krieg, Hockmeyer and Connor (1974) describe guinea-pig experiments with a heat-stable toxin produced by *M. ulcerans*—the only known toxin produced by a *Mycobacterium*. Stanford et al (1975) report a highly specific skin test antigen, named Burulin, prepared from *M. ulcerans*, and Schröder (1975) discusses the relationship of *M. buruli* to *M. ulcerans*. He states that *M. buruli* is not a legitimate species, but that some strains are identical with *M. ulcerans* whereas others show similarity to other mycobacterial species. *M. ulcerans* has

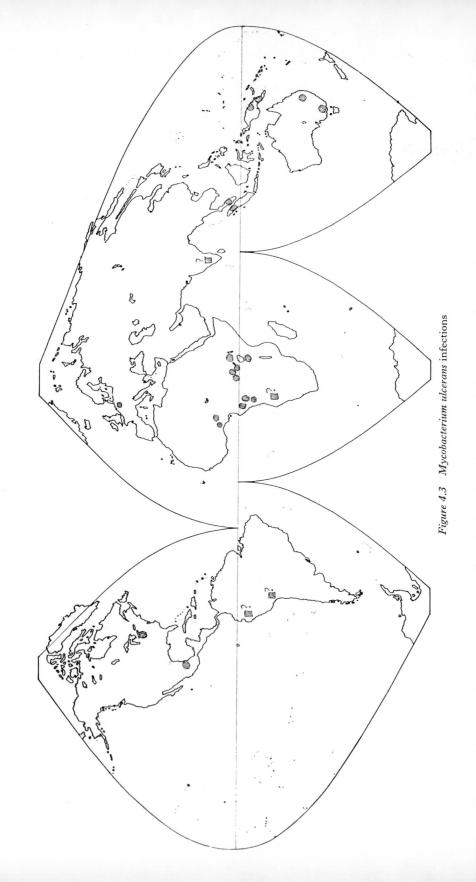

Figure 4.3   Mycobacterium ulcerans infections

never been isolated from a natural source, but intensive epidemiological research has firmly linked it with swamps and watercourses. Meyers et al (1974a) also establish the importance of trauma in the introduction of sub-cutaneous infection. BCG vaccination confers a 50 per cent protection rate against infection.

The *Mycobacterium* is sensitive to a number of drugs in vitro including clofazimine (Lamprene) and rifampicin, but the clinical results of treatment by chemotherapy have been disappointing. The disease remains one of the few infections for which the definitive treatment is agreed to be surgical. However, Meyers, Shelly and Connor (1974b) describe striking success in eight patients treated by the local application of heat to maintain a temperature of 40°C in the ulcerated area.

TROPICAL SUPERFICIAL FUNGUS INFECTIONS

Tinea nigra

Tinea nigra is a localised asymptomatic superficial fungus infection, usually causing a brown or black irregular, macular area on the palm. There is no scaling, and a dermal naevus is often mimicked. The causal fungus is *Cladosporium werneckii*. The complaint is found mainly in the tropics and subtropics of America, Asia and Australia, and has been seen occasionally in visitors returning from these areas (MacKenzie, personal communication; Tan, personal communication; Smith, Sams and Roth, 1958; Hitch, 1961; Chadfield and Campbell, 1972). Local treatment with benzoic acid compound ointment BPC is rapidly curative but tolnaftate is ineffective.

Tinea imbricata (tinea circinata tropica, tokelau ringworm)

Tinea imbricata is caused by *Trichophyton concentricum*. The geographic distribution is confined to the tropics in both the New and Old Worlds, including Oceania with the islands of Samoa, Fiji and Tokelau. The infection forms complicated patterns of finely scaling rings, usually begins on the trunk and spreads towards the extremities. Lesions are extremely itchy; hair and nail involvement are thought not to occur.

Occasional cases have been reported in Europeans who acquired the infection in the tropics and returned home (Church and Sneddon, 1962; Sharvill, 1952).

The fungus is griseofulvin sensitive, and the drug should be given in full dosage for between four and eight months. Relapses are common.

Piedra

Piedra is a Spanish word meaning a stone and refers to the nodules which the infection forms on hair shafts. It can be caused by two different fungi: black piedra by *Piedraia hortae* and white piedra by *Trichosporon beigelii*. Black piedra occurs in tropical America and Indonesia, while white piedra occurs principally in South America, but also in the temperate regions of central and eastern Europe and in Japan. Cases occurring in North America and Europe have usually been in those returning from the tropics, but there are occasional reports in those who have never been there (Hitch, 1959; Patterson Laine and Taylor, 1962; Kotovirta, Stubb and Salonen, 1975).

Favus

Favus due to *Trichophyton shoenleinii* most frequently affects the scalp, but may also invade nails and skin. It is common in the countries bordering the Mediterranean, the Middle East and Asia (Saracci, 1971), north-west India and China. There are foci in Mexico, Central America and Brazil, but it is rare in Black Africa. Though most common in the tropics and subtropics the disease is present in eastern Europe, and in Canada there are both native cases in rural areas and in Polish immigrants (Blank, 1962). Indigenous cases continue to appear in temperate climates and the infection is even stated to be common in Greenland (Beare, 1972). Pettit (1960) reported that 10 per cent of dermatology cases seen in Tabriz, Iran, had favus.

Other tropical dermatophytes are also being seen in cooler climates, mainly in immigrants, as are cosmopolitan fungal infections which assume special characteristics in the tropics.

Clayton (1975) has recorded the following scalp infections in London during the last 10 years:

Trichophyton soudanense	84
Trichophyton violaceum	59
Microsporon rivalieri	17
Trichophyton gourvilii	11
Microsporon langeronii	9
Trichophyton yaoundei	7
Microsporon ferrugineum	4
Trichophyton megninii	2
Trichophyton simii	1

Trichophyton soudanense

The clinical and cultural characteristics of infections due to *Trichophyton soudanense* were reviewed by Vanbreuseghem (1968). The fungus is prevalent in North and West Africa. Most cases in Europe have been in Africans previously resident in Africa, but there are isolated reports of patients who have never visited the tropics. Rippon and Medenica (1964) described a case in an American-born Negro woman, who had never been out of the United States, and a second American case in a white girl was reported by Johnson and Rosenthal (1968). Cases have been reported in Britain by Sarkany (1963) and in Germany by Kaben (1964).

Cases of nail involvement in Africans in England have been seen by Calnan, Djavahiszwili and Hodgson (1962) and English, Harman and Howell (to be published), and infections in African and West Indian children born in Britain are reported by Clayton (1968). Multiple infections in a family in Israel, which had migrated from Tunisia, were reported in 1973 (Harari, Sommer and Feinstein). A second affected family had been in contact at school with children of North African origin.

Trichophyton violaceum

Infections with this fungus are rare in the United Kingdom and in the United States, but common in the Middle East and Eastern Europe. It is an important cause of scalp ringworm in South America, India, Israel and North Africa, as well as in Spain and Portugal (Neves, 1960). The fungus is being isolated from immigrants to Britain of Indo-Pakistani origin (Campbell, personal communication).

Trichophyton yaoundei

This fungus causes an endothrix infection of hair and is endemic in Central and South-east Africa. Two cases of tinea capitis have been reported in Britain in boys arrived from Cameroun (Sarkany and Midgley, 1966).

Trichophyton megninii

Trichophyton megninii is an anthropophilic species found especially in Portugal, Sardinia and Sicily. It may also occur in Africa. Infections have been described in France in immigrant workers from Portugal (Puissant et al, 1969), and in Britain imported from Sicily and East Prussia (Sarkany, Clayton and Beck, 1963).

Trichophyton mentagrophytes

Widespread dermatomycoses occurred in American troops during the war in Vietnam. Very extensive plaques due to infections with *Trichophyton mentagrophytes* in servicemen in the Mekong Delta region, whose skin was wet for long periods, were reported (Blank, Taplin and Zaias, 1969). Military statistics show that skin problems were the commonest cause for outpatient visits, often exceeding the combined totals of the next two causes: diarrhoea and respiratory diseases. However, tropical acne was the major dermatologic cause for return to the temperate United States.

Hendersonula toruloidea

Gentles and Evans (1970) were the first to suggest that *Hendersonula toruloidea*, a wound parasite of trees in tropical regions (Wilson, 1947), could invade the skin and nails of man. They reported cases in immigrants to Britain from Pakistan, India, Kenya and Fiji, and since this time other cases have been reported in England (Campbell et al, 1973; Campbell, 1974). To date, this fungus has not been diagnosed as a cause of skin or nail disease in these tropical countries of origin.

TROPICAL DEEP FUNGUS INFECTIONS

Mycetoma (Maduromycosis, Madura Foot)

Mycetoma is caused by a number of species of fungi as well as by aerobic actinomycetes.

GEOGRAPHIC DISTRIBUTION

The distribution is essentially tropical, but exact data on the incidence and geographic distribution are lacking.

Throughout Central America and tropical South America, mycetoma is one of the most important of the deep mycoses. Cases are reported from tropical Africa—including Sudan, Asia and Oceania. Occasional cases have been seen in Europe, Canada and the United States.

Anning, La Touche and Hunter (1958), Chadfield (1964), Murray and Holt (1964), Murray, Dunkerley and Hughes (1964), and Baxter, Murray and Taylor (1966) reported cases seen in Britain, most of whom were immigrants who probably acquired the disease overseas. Cases have been reported from Germany (Reifferschied and Seeliger, 1955), and 24 cases from Roumania— only nine of them being actinomycotic—have been reported by Avram (1969). Mycetoma in Italy, caused by *Nocardia asteroides*, has been extensively reviewed by Leone (1974). *Madurella grisea* is reported as causing mycetoma in Northern California by Gould (1969). In Australia McClelland (1973) reports the condition in aborigines.

The first recorded cases in Iran are described by Griffiths, Kohout and Vessal (1975). Mycetoma formation in a patient in Pennsylvania with long-standing *Trichophyton rubrum* infection has also been reported, but without the mycetoma being proved due to *T. rubrum* (Burgoon et al, 1974). Findlay and Vismer (1974), in South Africa, have recently studied the chemistry, formation and significance of the tissue grains in mycetoma due to *Madurella mycetomi*. The whole subject has been covered extensively in an excellent monograph by Mahgoub and Murray (1973).

CLINICAL FEATURES

The feet are mainly affected by woody induration of skin and soft tissues, with multiple discharging sinuses that also penetrate bone. Other parts subject to trauma, such as the hand, are also prone. Agricultural workers who go barefoot are particularly at risk. The incubation period is uncertain, but appears to be from several days to a number of months. Early lesions are rarely seen. Extension is very slow, fortunately without severe pain.

Diagnosis is established by the histopathological identification of fungal grains, serology and characteristic x-ray bone changes. Chronic osteomyelitis and other deep fungal infections must be distinguished by pathological and mycological studies.

African Histoplasmosis

Involvement of the skin is a frequent feature of African histoplasmosis caused by *Histoplasma duboisii*. The disease is distinct from classical histoplasmosis due to *Histoplasma capsulatum*, which is primarily a lung condition and endemic in the Mississippi and Ohio Valleys of the United States of America.

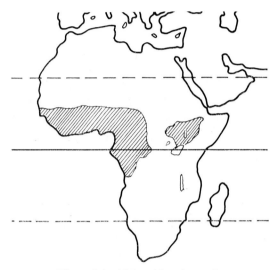

Figure 4.4   African histoplasmosis

It is chiefly confined to West Africa (Fig. 4.4), but is now being reported in travellers to Europe from this region (Hiltenbrand et al, 1971; Sureau, Berrod and Bardinon, 1973).

The clinical features comprising superficial cutaneous granulomata, subcutaneous granulomata and abscesses, osteomyelitic lesions, and secondary involvement of the skin are well reviewed and illustrated by Lucas (1970).

Medical treatment is with amphotericin B and slow-acting sulphonamides. An exhaustive bibliography (2300 titles) has been compiled by Cooke (1969).

Chromomycosis

Chromomycosis can be caused by three fungi—*Phialophora compactum*, *Phialophora dermatidis* and *Cladosporium carrionii*. Cases have been seen in the United Kingdom in coloured immigrants who have acquired the infection in their home country, in visitors from abroad, in British citizens who have worked abroad, and in those who have never left the country (Fountain, 1968). Cases have also been reported in Czechoslovakia (Horacek and Ulicna, 1969) and in Finland (Havu, 1970).

The lesions are usually on exposed sites, and present as slowly progressive warty papules and plaques, sometimes with ulceration. Diagnosis is made by biopsy and mycological culture. Clinical differential diagnosis from North American blastomycosis, tuberculosis verrucosa cutis, leishmaniasis, and syphilis may be very difficult. Successful treatment with oral and topical 5-fluorocytosine has been reported (Lopes et al, 1969, 1971; Morison, Connor and Clayton, 1974). Bayles (1971) throws some doubt on the validity of these reports, particularly regarding length of follow-up, and has found thiabendazole gives a cure rate of 36.4 per cent without recurrence over a period of four years follow-up.

South American Blastomycosis (Paracoccidioidomycosis)

The causal fungus is *Paracoccidioides braziliensis*. The disease is endemic in all parts of South America except Chile, and mainly affects agricultural workers, invading the skin, mucous membranes, lymph nodes and internal organs.

An autochthonous case has been reported from Africa (Lythcott and Edgcomb, 1964).

Pathological investigations will distinguish the disease from leishmaniasis, leprosy, endemic syphilis, and other deep mycoses.

Keloidal Blastomycosis (Lobo's Disease)

This tropical fungus disease, endemic in north-eastern Brazil, is caused by *Loboa loboi*. Lesions occur on exposed parts, usually following injury. Similar keloidal lesions are described in a patient from western France, caused by *Aureobasidium pullulans* (Vermeil et al, 1971).

Subcutaneous Phycomycosis

The causal fungus of this subcutaneous disease, in which rubbery, irregular, and extensive granulomata form, was originally thought to be *Basidiobolus ranarum*, but recent work has suggested that the causal agent is *B. haptosporus* (Srinivasan and Thirumalachar, 1965). The condition is essentially tropical and, since it was first described in Indonesia, has been reported in India, South America and Africa (Harman, Jackson and Willis, 1964). Cornic (1975) describes a new case in Senegal, and provides a table of all reports of the disease in Africa. A single possible case has been recorded in Britain (Symmers, 1960).

Diagnosis is by deep biopsy for histological and mycological examination. Treatment with potassium iodide by mouth and by intravenous amphotericin B have both been used with success. A similar granuloma, involving the nose and adjacent tissues caused by *Entomophthora coronata*, is described as rhinophycomycosis (Martinson and Clark, 1967).

TREPONEMATOSES

Endemic Syphilis

Syphilis caused by *Treponema pallidum* is normally sexually transmitted, but it exists in endemic non-venereal form in localised areas of the Old World (Bejel). Endemic syphilis is now regarded almost exclusively as a tropical or subtropical disease, acquired by children living under unhygienic conditions. Recent studies have been carried out by Grin (1962) and Guthe and Luger (1957, 1965). However, it was estimated that 6 per cent of the population of the Bosnia-Herzegovina area of Yugoslavia were affected by the disease (skerljevo) after the Second World War. As a result of mass campaigns by the World Health Organisation, which began in 1949, there is good reason to believe that this form of the disease has now been abolished from the area (Grin, 1953). Luger (1972) reported 'endemic' syphilis in a group of children living in one room in an asylum for the homeless in Vienna.

Yaws (Framboesia, Pian)

Yaws is a non-venereal treponematosis caused by the spirochaete *Treponema pertenue*. Morphologically and serologically the organism cannot be distinguished from the treponema of syphilis or pinta. Fifteen years ago it was estimated that there were 50 million people suffering from the disease in the tropical belt, and that over half of them lived in Central Africa (Pampiglione and Wilkinson, 1975). Other endemic regions are the Caribbean islands, India, North Australia (Garner et al, 1972) and Oceania (Foote, 1975).

Early yaws, with its framboesiform friable granulomas of skin (Figs. 4.5, 4.6) and mucocutaneous junctions teaming treponemas, has been seen rarely in Britain (King and Nicol, 1975). But the more frequent changes of late yaws also give rise to difficulty in diagnosis in immigrants from endemic areas. The clinical manifestations are:

1. Palmar and plantar keratoderma with contractures of the digits.
2. Arciform or serpiginous plaques with scarring resembling lesions of tertiary syphilis.
3. Gummatous lesions.
4. Osteoarticular lesions with periostitis, sabre tibia, and arthritis of large and small joints.
5. The central facial mutilation of gangosa and exostoses of goundou.

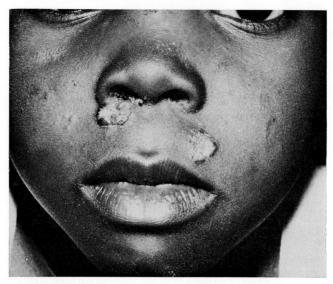

Figure 4.5 Framboesial yaws in a young patient from St Vincent. (Dr D. S. Wilkinson, Wycombe General Hospital, High Wycombe)

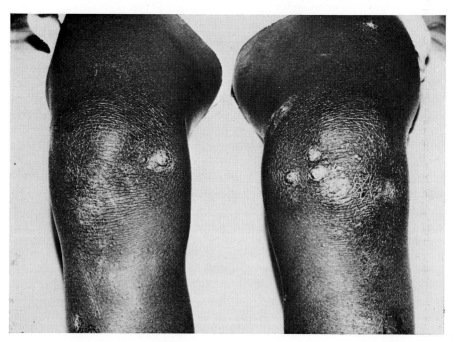

Figure *4.6* Early yaws granulomas in a West Indian child. (Dr D. S. Wilkinson, Wycombe General Hospital, High Wycombe)

As no pathological tests are available to distinguish the patient with positive serology due to syphilis from his brother with late yaws, there is real difficulty in differentiating the diseases in West Indians in Britain and in Samoans in New Zealand. History and physical examination must be relied on.

The disease is primarily one of primitive rural areas, and its decline has been hugely accelerated by WHO assisted mass penicillin therapy campaigns, in which some 50 million people have been treated. However, yaws—like pinta—confers some immunity against syphilis, and with its control syphilis is becoming a problem in some areas where previously it did not exist (Willcox, 1975).

Pinta

Pinta is a non-venereal treponematosis caused by *Treponema carateum*, and is found among the poor of Central and South America. It is acquired during childhood by direct contact through skin abrasions, and has been recognised amongst Aztec Indians since the early sixteenth century. Usually the skin alone is affected by dyschromic and achromic patches which mimic vitiligo. The face, hands and feet are favourite sites. Symmetrical hyperkeratoses, warty lesions and areas of atrophy also occur. Aortitis and juxta articular nodes have been reported rarely. Lawton Smith et al (1971) investigated 11 cases of late pinta in Venezuela, and found no ocular or neurological abnormalities except in one patient with bilateral interstitial keratitis.

The disease must be distinguished from erythema dyschromicum perstans in immigrants or visitors from endemic areas (Convit, Kerdel-Vegas and Rodriguez, 1961; Stevenson and Miura, 1966).

Tropical Ulcer (Phagedenic Ulcer)

Tropical ulcer is common in hot humid climates in children and youngsters in country districts. Lesions are single or multiple and usually occur on the lower leg or ankle. They are painful, deep, exuding and sloughing ulcers, infected with a variety of organisms including *Bacillus fusiformis* and *Treponema vincenti*. Malnutrition, anaemia, and a history of injury are commonly associated. Radiological changes with periosteal reaction occur (Ennis, Gueri and Sarjeant, 1972), and 7 out of 230 cases reported by Ariyan and Krizek (1975) developed squamous cell carcinomas.

The number of round scars on the legs of immigrants from Africa, the West Indies and, perhaps less commonly, from the Asian tropics are frequently remarkable and of considerable size. The contrast with the legs of a comparable European population is striking. History taking usually evokes a half remembered story of painful ulcers in childhood, probably with minor injury. Many of these scars will be the result of acute tropical ulcers in childhood.

Similar lesions were common in troops in South-East Asia and the Pacific during the Second World War, and tropical pyoderma a serious source of invalidism in American servicemen in Vietnam (McMillan and Hurwitz, 1969).

PROTOZOONOSES

Leishmaniasis

Three clinical forms of the condition are described, due to morphologically identical protozoa.

1. Cutaneous leishmaniasis–*Leishmania tropica.*
2. American cutaneous and mucocutaneous leishmaniasis—*L. braziliensis.*
3. Visceral leishmaniasis (kala-azar)—*L. donovani.*

A proportion of patients suffering from visceral leishmaniasis develop the cutaneous changes of post-kala-azar dermal leishmaniasis.

Cutaneous leishmaniasis (*Oriental, Quetta, or Lahore sore, Biskra button, Baghdad boil*)

Cutaneous leishmaniasis is an infective granuloma caused by *Leishmania tropica* transmitted by the bite of minute downy midges (sand flies)—commonly *Phlebotomus paptasii.*

GEOGRAPHIC DISTRIBUTION (Fig. 4.7)

The disease occurs in the tropics and subtropics, particularly in dry desert areas. It is endemic all round the Mediterranean coast—particularly North Africa, Asia Minor, and Asia, including China and Southern Russia (Saf' Janova and Aliev, 1973; Nazyrov, Yusupov and Dzhabarov, 1974). Infection usually occurs in childhood, with the subsequent development of immunity. Cases are recently described in Southern Europe by Guerra, Tosi and Molinelli (1974), Pasi and Saragoni (1970), and De Noronha (1970). An Italian immigrant, with an incubation period of three and a half years, is recorded in Australia by Charters and Staer (1970). Cases are being seen in Britain, both in immigrants and in visitors to the Mediterranean.

CLINICAL FEATURES

The incubation period is variable but is commonly about one month. Cases may, however, occur up to one year after infection. All uninoculated individuals are susceptible, and one or more lesions occur on unclothed parts of the body, which are easily bitten by *Phlebotomus*. The face, neck and arms are the prime targets. Lesions do not necessarily occur at exactly the same time, but in endemic areas one may see a family of children all with lesions at the same stage, and a history indicating infected sand-fly bites all acquired on the same night in the same room. Two distinctive forms are said to be distinguishable, but they may not be clear cut.

1. The wet, or early ulcerative form (rural). A red furuncle-like nodule

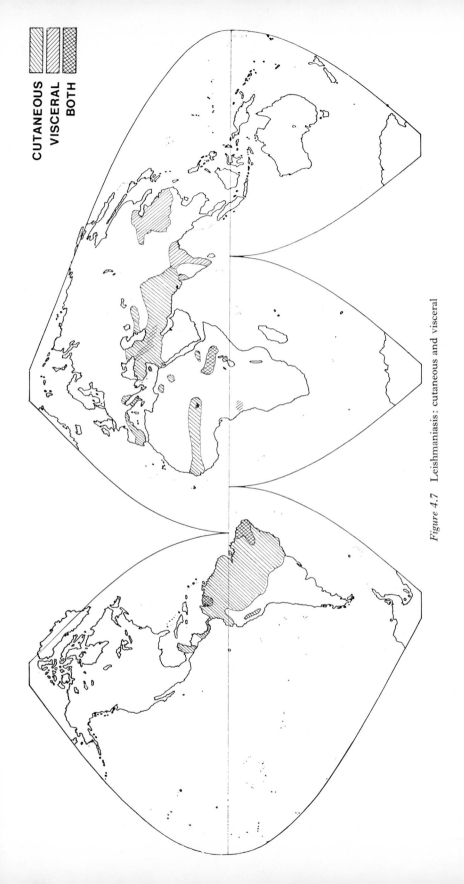

Figure 4.7 Leishmaniasis: cutaneous and visceral

appears at the site of inoculation and ulcerates rapidly as it enlarges. This continues for two to three months, and the lesion may become as large as 6 cm in diameter. Healing gradually takes place and usually takes about a year, leaving an ugly scar. In Iran the name for this lesion is 'solak' which means 'one year spot'.

2. The dry, or later ulcerative form (urban). After a similar incubation period, a small rounded nodule appears which slowly extends to become a plaque of about 2 cm in diameter within six months. At this stage, shallow ulceration appears in the centre, together with a crust. After 8 to 12 months the lesion beings to regress, and the ulcer heals leaving a scar. This process takes a longer time than the rural form and is considered due to *L. tropica* var. *minor*, whereas the wet form is caused by *L. tropica* var. *major*, and is an example of a zoonosis. The animal reservoir (Mutinga, 1975) varies in different parts of the world: dogs, foxes, squirrels, gerbils, hamsters and jackals are found responsible in various localities.

Chronic cutaneous leishmaniasis (*recidivans or lupoid*)

In about 10 per cent of cases of oriental sore a chronic lupoid stage develops. This tuberculoid granuloma without parasites may appear at the edge of a scar, or even some distance from it years after apparent clinical healing. The lesion is usually hard to distinguish from lupus vulgaris, but may form concentric rings. It persists for years, is highly disfiguring, and heals very slowly.

Other uncommon clinical varieties have been described, including a keloidal and verrucous type.

DIAGNOSIS

In the acute forms, smears of a suspected lesion are made and stained to demonstrate *Leishmania tropica*. These are best taken by scraping the edge of the lesion, avoiding secondary infection and necrotic tissue. Cultures are also made on NNN medium. A further useful sampling technique is with the use of a dental broach (Griffiths and Dutz, 1975). The intradermal test, using heat-killed parasites, gives a positive reaction consisting of a papule with surrounding erythema 1 to 2 cm in diameter at 48 h. But in endemic areas the test must be interpreted with caution, as a positive result may only mean that the adult had leishmaniasis in childhood.

TREATMENT

Antimonials still form the basis of treatment for all forms of leishmaniasis, but newer methods are being tried with variable results. In oriental sore, Kandil (1973) has recommended trimethoprim sulphamethoxazole. Long (1973) reported a single case as successfully treated with metronidazole, but personal experience and Griffiths (personal communication) do not support this observation. Repeated intralesional injections of a mixture of local anaesthetic and Glucantime appear effective when used in an endemic area, but success is also claimed for rifampicin—which at least has the merit of being painless. The best drug of a bad bunch remains pentavalent antimony (sodium stibogluconate, Pentostam, Glucantime) (Bryceson, 1976). Treatment of chronic cutaneous leishmaniasis is particularly disappointing, and there is no agreement as to the best remedy.

Disseminated cutaneous leishmaniasis (*disseminated anergic leishmaniasis, leishmaniasis cutanea pseudolepromatosa*)

This form of generalised cutaneous leishmaniasis was originally described in Venezuela (Convit, Kerdel-Vegas and Gordon, 1962), and shows very extensive skin involvement with infiltrated papules, nodules, and plaques containing abundant *L. brazilensis* parasites. More recently it has been found in Mexico, Brazil, Bolivia, Ethiopia and Japan. There is no visceral involvement, but discrete lesions occur on the nasal mucous membrane. These do not become destructive as do those of typical mucocutaneous leishmaniasis. The scalp, axillae, and inguino-crural regions of the skin are spared.

An incorrect clinical diagnosis of leprosy may well be made and, histopathologically, a granuloma formed by vacuolated macrophages adds further confusion. But the macrophages can be seen to be full of *Leishmania* parasites.

The diagnosis of leishmaniasis is established by the finding of *Leishmania* in impression smears and biopsy material. Cultures in NNN media give a high incidence of positivity. Montenegro's test, consisting of the intradermal injection of 0.10 ml of antigen, is positive in 97 per cent of cases.

American cutaneous and mucocutaneous leishmaniasis (*American leishmaniasis, South American leishmaniasis: espundia, mucous form; uta, cutaneous form, pianbois, chiclero's ulcer, forest yaws, bush yaws*)

American leishmaniasis is a specific disease caused by *Leishmania brazilensis*, which affects the skin and later the mucosa of the upper respiratory tract.

GEOGRAPHIC DISTRIBUTION

The disease is widely distributed throughout the tropics of the South American continent from Yucatan in Southern Mexico (Novales, 1974) to Northern Argentina 30° south of the Equator. Brazil and Peru have the highest incidence.

Damp rain forest areas encourage the spread of the disease, which is seasonal, being more prevalent in the rainy season, together with an increase in numbers of the vector *Phlebotomus*. Workers in the forests are particularly at risk, as well as chicle (gum) collectors. The pattern of the disease varies from one locality to another. In Southern Mexico a purely cutaneous form, similar to the oriental sore of the Old World, is found, whereas the espundia mucocutaneous type is more prevalent in low lying areas of South America.

IMMUNOLOGY

Cutaneous leishmaniasis of the Old World due to *Leishmania tropica* produces permanent immunity. But the American type due to *L. brazilensis* frequently results in late invasion of the upper respiratory tract, with the protozoa living in immunologically competent cells.

CLINICAL FEATURES

The primary lesion develops as a small papule on an exposed part following a *Phlebotomus* bite. The papule grows into a red nodule in from two weeks to two months or even longer. The nodule enlarges peripherally, whilst a bloody crust may form in the centre with ulceration. Lymphangitis or lymphadenopathy may occur in the drainage area. Vesicular and granulomatous (framboesoid) primary lesions are also described. Secondary infection is common. Secondary mucous membrane lesions form 1 to 10 years after the initial sore, producing deformity of the lip, palate, nasal septum, nasopharynx and larynx, including invasion of cartilage.

Chiclero's ulcer or Bay sore typically occurs in Mexican leishmaniasis, with gross destruction of cartilage.

DIAGNOSIS

Differential diagnosis is extensive, and includes tuberculosis, sporotrichosis, South American blastomycosis, syphilis, yaws, leprosy, and rhinoscleroma.

The causal organisms are found in smears from biopsy tissue stained with Wright's or Leishman's strain. Cultures of parasites may be made on NNN media.

The Montenegro intradermal test is reliable and positive in 98 per cent of cases.

TREATMENT

The primary lesion is treated with antimonials, as for cutaneous leishmaniasis. In the secondary stage of mucus involvement, treatment is as for visceral leishmaniasis, together with antibiotics to control secondary bacterial invasion. The relapse rate is high.

Amphotericin B, used under hospital conditions by intravenous drip, is also used successfully. Metronidazole (Flagyl) has been found effective in Mexican cutaneous leishmaniasis, but not in mucocutaneous forms.

Post-kala-azar dermal leishmaniasis (*dermal leishmanoid*)

Dermal involvement occurs in about 6 per cent of patients after they have contracted kala-azar (visceral leishmaniasis) in India, but does not occur in the Mediterranean variety (Busuttil, 1974) and rarely in South America. Skin lesions appear about two years after infection, but may be much longer delayed. The skin condition was first described in India by Brahmachari in 1922.

Cases have been diagnosed in temperate climates (Ecker and Lubitz, 1947; Munro, Du Vivier and Jopling, 1972).

Venereally acquired leishmaniasis from a patient with chronic kala-azar and post-kala-azar dermal leishmaniasis has been described in England (Symmers, 1960).

The clinical appearance is of hypopigmented macules, erythematous macules and of nodules, which may develop successively or in any combination. There may be a confusing thickening of the facial skin, with a strong suggestion of a lepromatous leonine facies due to inflammatory changes and some minimal impairment of sensation to temperature and light touch.

Differentiation from leprosy is helped by the absence of nodules or induration of the ears (Muir, 1930) and also the absence of madarosis. Biopsy of nodules shows chronic granulomatous changes without nerve bundle involvement and in active lesions, Leishman–Donovan bodies. Skin tests give a positive response to *L. donovani* protein antigen.

Treatment with amphotericin B has been reported successful in two patients by Yesudian and Thambiah (1974).

Cutaneous Amoebiasis

Amoebiasis, caused by *Entamoeba histolytica*, is a worldwide disease which is much more common in the tropics, where high proportions of individual populations may be affected (Fig. 4.8). Cutaneous complications of the intestinal disease are uncommon, but Stamm (1975) states that there are 200 new cases of clinical amoebiasis annually in England and Wales, with considerable morbidity caused by wrong treatment and delay in diagnosis.

Cutaneous amoebiasis most commonly arises in the perineal area by direct extension of disease of the bowel. Similar extension from an amoebic hepatic abscess also occurs. The skin may also become involved due to surgical intervention in both conditions, and from contact with infectious material from the patient's own colonic disease or from another's (Biagi and Martuscelli, 1963). Skin lesions consist of either deeply invading ulcers or ulcerating granulomas (amoebomas). The edges of ulcers are raised and often undermined, with foul discharge and intense pain. Diagnosis is made by the finding of organisms in fresh material taken from the edges. Trophozoites are also found in histological sections of ulcer edge.

Metronidazole (Flagyl) is considered by many as the treatment of choice in intestinal amoebiasis, but its effects in cutaneous amoebiasis are uncertain (Beirana, 1972). Biagi, Alvarez and Gonzalez (1974) report that etophamide gives parasitological cure in 95 per cent of children with acute intestinal amoebiasis.

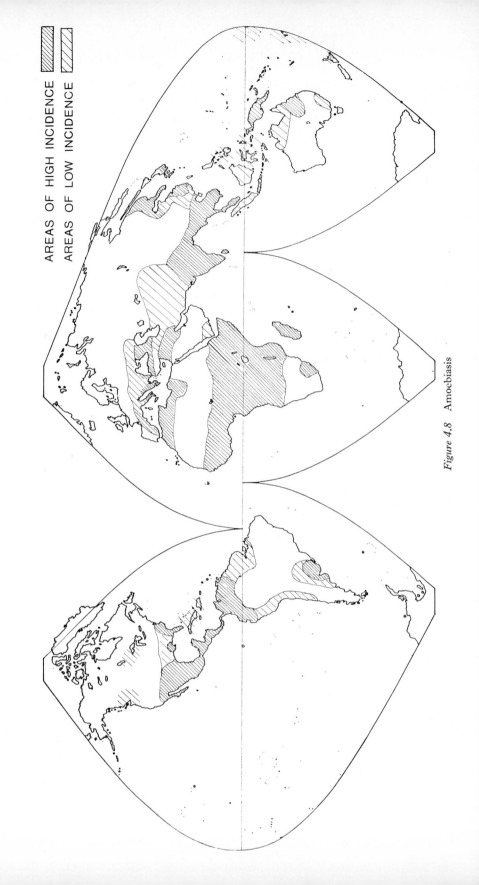

Figure 4.8 Amoebiasis

Toxoplasmosis

Toxoplasmosis is a multisystem disease with a world-wide distribution (Fig. 4.9). Nevertheless, the causal protozoon *Toxoplasma gondii* was first recognised in the North African rodent—the gondi—and in rabbits from the Brazilian tropics. Recent advances in knowledge are discussed by Shafer (1975) and Quinn et al (1975).

Successful treatment with trimethoprim and sulphamethoxazole instead of with the formerly used pyrimethamine in combination with sulphonamides, is described by Norrby et al (1975).

ALGAL DISEASE

Cutaneous Protothecosis

The first case of human cutaneous protothecosis, caused by an achlorotic member of the Chlorococcales, was reported by Davies, Spencer and Wakelin (1964), and amplified by Davies and Wilkinson (1967) in a rice farmer's foot in Sierra Leone. The alga in this case was designated *Prototheca segbwema* after the place where it was found, but is now named *P. zepfii*. Organisms of this genus are usually saprophytes. The disease presents as a chronic inflammatory plaque, and single cases have now been reported from the United States (Klintworth, Fetter and Nielson, 1968; Tindall and Fetter, 1971; Nosanchuk and Greenberg, 1973) and South Africa (Mars et al, 1971; Dogliotti et al, 1975). A case of systemic infection with *P. wickerhamii* in a Maori, with deficient cell-mediated immunity, is reported in New Zealand (Cox, Wilson and Brown, 1974).

Treatment is a problem. Surgical excision, potassium iodide, and amphotericin B have been tried with varying success. Spontaneous regression is also recorded.

HELMINTHIC DISEASES

Larva Migrans

Larva migrans is probably the commonest helminthic skin condition brought back to temperate climates by holidaymakers, who have walked and sunbathed on infected sands. The French describe it graphically as 'la dermatite vermineuse rampante'. The worms most frequently responsible are *Ancylostoma braziliensis*, *Ancylostoma caninum*, *Uncinaria stenocephala*, and *Ancylostoma ceylonicum*. These hookworms abound in the intestines of dogs and cats, and their eggs are deposited on the earth in their faeces. Filariform larvae emerge under favourable conditions and, if they are unlucky, penetrate the skin of a 'dead-end' host—man.

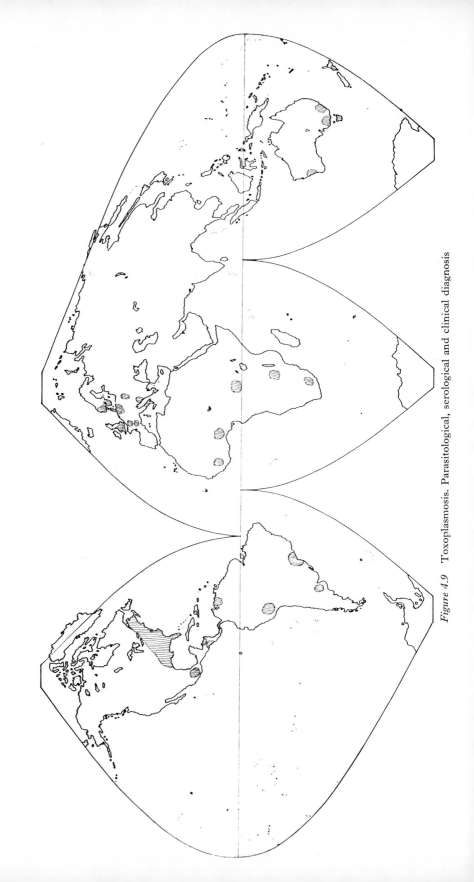

Figure 4.9　Toxoplasmosis. Parasitological, serological and clinical diagnosis

The human intestinal worm *Strongyloides stercoralis* is responsible for the much faster moving larva currens.

GEOGRAPHIC DISTRIBUTION

Infection is possible in all continents in the tropics and subtropics. Areas of high humidity are the most affected.

CLINICAL FEATURES

The parts of the body in contact with the ground are first affected—feet, buttocks and trunk in sunbathing holidaymakers (Fig. 4.10). Within 48 h a

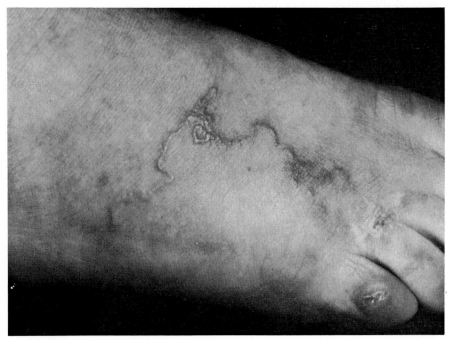

Figure 4.10 Larva migrans characteristically occurring on the foot. (Dr D. S. Wilkinson, Wycombe General Hospital, High Wycombe)

non-specific pruritic eruption develops at the site of entry of larvae (ground itch), and migration of the larvae begins within four days of penetration of the skin. They move at an erratic rate from 1 to 5 cm daily, whereas larva currens of *Strongyloides stercoralis* may move the same distance in half an hour. This activity does not always start within a few days of infection, but may be delayed for weeks or months. Lesions are aimless, red, raised, tortuous, thread-like tracks, and are very itchy. This diagnostic pattern may be obscured by scratching, with secondary infection—especially on the feet and toes. The wandering active eruption ceases when the larvae die without maturing, because they have entered an unsuitable host. The length of time this takes probably depends on the species inoculated, and estimates, of spontaneous cure times vary very considerably.

There are quite numerous reports of this readily identified eruption from dermatologists who have seen it in Europe recently: Josef (1972) in Germany, Huber (1972) in Switzerland, Da Fonseca (1968) in Portugal, Thomas et al (1969) in France, Rampini and Nunzi (1974) in Italy, and Niebauer and Reichel (1975) in Austria. But many cases must go unreported. Lehmuskallio (1975) in Finland reports moving hair fragments beneath the surface resembling larva migrans. Kahn and Johnson (1971) have investigated serum IgE levels in larva migrans, and report a trend towards raised levels—as found in other helminthic infections.

The rapidly moving tracks of larva currens from *Strongyloides stercoralis* intestinal infection fan out from the anus, and are mainly seen on buttocks, thighs and back. The disease may persist long after the patient has left tropical endemic areas (Stone, Newell and Mullins, 1972) and is effectively treated with thiabendazole (Doeglas and Tenberg, 1972; Thomas et al, 1971). The giving of prednisone in strongyloidiasis can give rise to a fatal ulcerative enteritis (Nagalotimath, Ramaprasad and Chandrashekhar, 1974). Immuno-suppression can also lead to occult strongyloidiasis becoming fulminant and lethal (Kuberski, Gabor and Boudreaux, 1975). Moqbel (1974) discusses the enormous increase in larval production after steroids under experimental conditions in rats. The diagnosis and management of strongyloidiasis is summarised by Grove, Warren and Mahmoud (1975).

TREATMENT

Treatment of larva migrans may be local, using freezing methods of solid carbon dioxide, liquid nitrogen, or ethyl chloride spray in the time-honoured way. Recently, topical applications of thiabendazole suspension, 2 per cent Gammexane cream, and 25 per cent piperazine ointment have been used successfully. Systemic thiabendazole is also successful, but its side effects may be unpleasant.

Visceral larva migrans, due to *Toxocara canis*, is of world-wide distribution and is also effectively treated with thiabendazole. The subject is reviewed by Rook and Staughton (1972).

Onchocerciasis (Onchocercosis, Blinding Filariasis, River Blindness, Coastal Erysipelas)

Onchocerciasis is a filarial disease caused by *Onchocerca volvulus*, and is transmitted to man by species of black flies of the genus Simuliidae (buffalo gnats). In Africa *Simulium damnosum* is mainly responsible—inflicting very painful bites as it does so. The world incidence of the complaint has been estimated as between 20 million and 50 million (Choyce, 1972).

GEOGRAPHIC DISTRIBUTION

Onchocerciasis is found in foci in Africa and America (Fig. 4.11). In tropical Africa it is found from coast to coast in a zone 15° north and south of the Equator stretching from Senegal (Imperato and Sow, 1971) to Ethiopia, and from Angola through Congo and Zaire to Tanzania (Wegesa, 1971). In the New World it occurs in Central America, Southern Mexico, Guatemala, Venezuela, and Colombia.

PATHOLOGY

Mature worms and microfilariae are found in dermal nodules (onchocercomata)—mainly on the scalp in Central America, but close to bony prominences on the trunk and limbs in Africa (Fig. 4.12). The nodules consist of an outer layer of fibroblasts, which contains the parasites in an organised fibrinous exudate. Inflammatory cells, including giant cells, accumulate round the worms. Calcification may occur. The life span of adult onchocercal worms is 10 to 15 years, and that of microfilariae 12 to 30 months.

Microfilariae congregate in the dermis and cause inflammatory changes recently studied by Connor et al (1969). In early onchocerciasis the skin may contain many microfilariae, but little, if any, inflammatory reaction. Later, acanthosis, hyperkeratosis, and parakeratosis appear, associated with an infiltrate of histiocytes, eosinophils, and lymphocytes in the dermis. Reticulum, elastic and collagen fibres proliferate, and the small dermal vessels become tortuous. Later the epidermis atrophies and the dermis becomes thickened with scar tissue. In some patients there are fibrinoid changes of dermal collagen and focal granulomas in the upper corium. The clinical varieties of onchocercal skin changes, known as elephant skin, lizard skin and leopard skin, can be matched with these microscopic findings.

Microfilariae also invade the eye causing keratitis, iritis and choroiditis, leading to blindness. Serious eye involvement is usually seen late in onchocerciasis in indigenous people who have lived for years in areas of high endemicity.

In Britain patients are seen mainly among those who have worked in tropical Africa and in their families, or in African students.

CLINICAL FEATURES

The incubation period is about one year.

The skin eruption of onchodermatitis in a European recently returned from the tropics with a light infection (Fig. 4.13), is usually on the back or buttocks with persistent itching and non-specific eczema-like changes. Later, lichenification varying with the severity of infection occurs, particularly round the pelvis, and in Africans on the thighs, with numerous tiny scars where papules have been scratched. Pigmentation increases, and a pattern of fine furrows develops—which is easily seen with a hand lens. The skin thickens progressively, lustre is lost, and the furrows deepen to form the so-called lizard skin

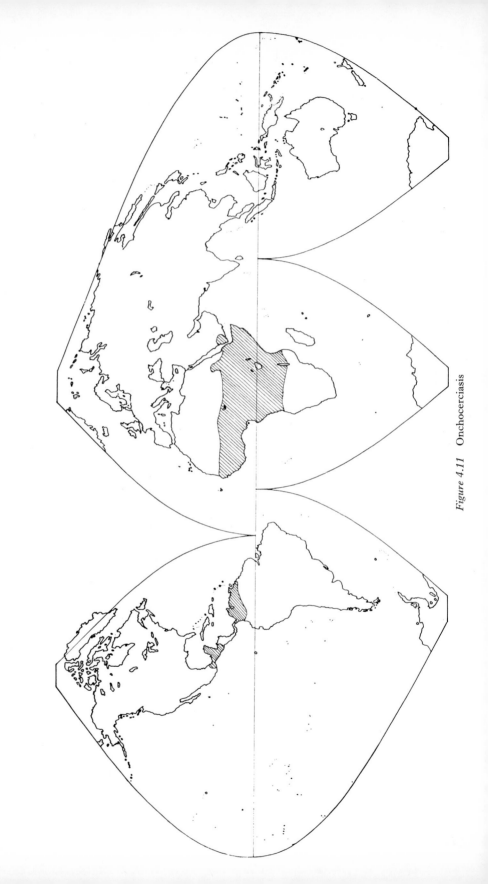

Figure 4.11 Onchocerciasis

and, in some severely affected patients, hanging groins (Nelson, 1958). Later, atrophic skin changes complete the clinical course with loss of elasticity, dryness, some scale formation and a delicate web-like pattern of soft ridges likened to crushed tissue-paper.

Onchocercal depigmentation also occurs in onchodermatitis of long duration in Africans, and may be accompanied by hypertrophic inguino-crural lymphadenopathy. This depigmentation is found most frequently bilaterally in the pretibial regions, but may occur in the groins, over bony

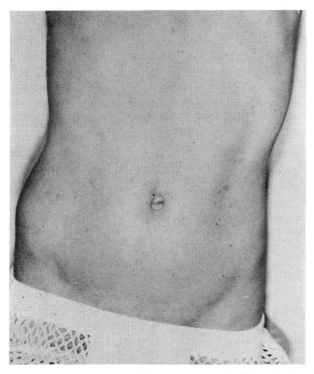

Figure 4.12 Onchocercal nodule above right anterior superior iliac spine in a boy who had lived in Cameroun. (Frenchay Hospital, Bristol)

prominences and in the pectoral region. In the early stages it is slight and punctate, but larger areas of depigmentation may develop, giving the pattern of leopard skin.

Onchocercomata are painless and mobile, of a variable size. In the early stages they may have to be felt for close to bony prominences, particularly pelvis and ribs.

In the American form an acute oedematous eruption of the face, with fever and malaise closely resembling erysipelas, occurs and is known as 'erisipela de la costa'.

Lymphatic involvement in onchocerciasis with unilateral swelling of a limb can occur, but is very much less frequent and pronounced than in filariasis caused by *Wuchereria bancroftii* and *W. malayi* (Jopling, 1960; Wolfe, 1974).

DIAGNOSIS

A certain diagnosis can be made by demonstrating microfilariae in skin snips, which may be difficult in light infections (Lagraulet, 1971), or by

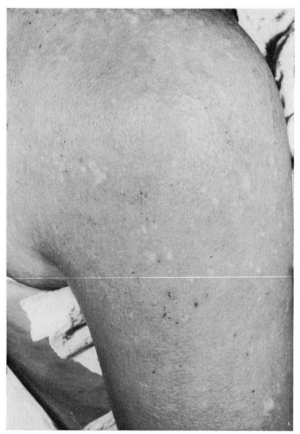

Figure 4.13 Onchocercal dermatitis with some swelling of the upper limb in a young woman who had lived in West Africa. (Dr R. P. Warin, Bristol Royal Infirmary)

removing a nodule and examining sections for adult worms. There should be a high index of suspicion in patients returned from tropical Africa with persistent pruritus of the trunk and buttocks. Microfilariae are not present in the blood. If skin snips are negative and nodules cannot be found, strong presumptive evidence is provided by a combination of a skin test, a serological test, and a white cell count. The skin test is a group test for all the filarial worms, and tends to remain positive for life. The complement fixation test and the fluorescent antibody test on serum are also group tests, but become negative several months after the infection has been cured. They are not positive in all cases of onchocerciasis, being negative in about one third. An eosinophilia is always present. It is important to establish that this is not due to intestinal helminths, and is a useful aid to diagnosis.

The Mazzotti test can be used where there is diagnostic difficulty. Here the patient is given one tablet of diethylcarbamazine (Banocide). The test is positive if, the following day, there has been an exacerbation of itching and rash. There may also be oedema, fever, and pain in the joints. Over 90 per cent of patients confirmed parasitologically give a positive Mazzotti test.

DIFFERENTIAL DIAGNOSIS

The acute oedematous changes must be distinguished from erysipelas, cellulitis, and lepra reaction. The chronic dermatitic changes may mimic scabies—particularly in Negroes where scabietic burrows are hard to find, atopic dermatitis, prurigo due to multiple insect bite reactions, and lichen simplex.

Nodules must be distinguished from fibromas, lipomas, sebaceous cysts, cysticercosis and, particularly in the American form, cylindromas. When present close to joints they may mimic the juxta articular nodes of yaws.

TREATMENT

Diethylcarbamazine (Banocide) kills the microfilariae and is given in the following doses:

First three days—1 mg/kg body weight three times a day.
Second four days—2 mg/kg body weight three times a day.
Second week—3 mg/kg body weight three times a day.
Third week—4 mg/kg body weight three times a day.

If there is a severe exacerbation of symptoms, a smaller dose and anti-histamines may be necessary in the first few days of treatment, and this is not unusual. Repeated courses are usually necessary until the patient is symptom-free and eosinophilia is lost.

Suramin (BP) kills mature worms, and is given to an adult as five intraven-ous injections of 1 g each at weekly intervals. The dosage for children is calculated on the basis of 20 mg/kg body weight weekly. It must be remem-bered that Suramin is a toxic drug, particularly to the kidneys, and must be given cautiously. The urine must be examined for protein, red cells, and casts before each injection. Nodules should be removed surgically where practicable.

Melarsonyl (Trimélarsan, Mel W) is also effective against adult worms, but not microfilariae.

Loiasis (Calabar Swellings, Fugitive Swellings, *Loa Loa* Filariasis)

Loiasis is an infestation with the filarial worm *Loa loa* transmitted to man by blood sucking tabanid flies of the genus *Chrysops* (deer fly, horse fly, and mangrove fly).

GEOGRAPHIC DISTRIBUTION

Loiasis occurs only in the rain forest regions of West and Central Africa, being found particularly in Eastern Nigeria, Cameroun, Congo and Zaire, from the Atlantic Coast to the Great Lakes (Fig. 4.14).

Cases in immigrants have been reported in Australia (Charters, Wellborn and Miller, 1972), in Rhodesia (Sparrow and Goldsmid, 1974), in London with

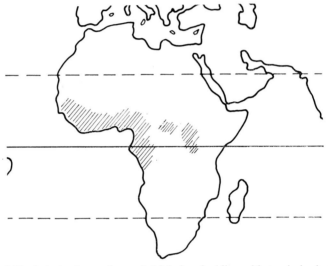

Figure 4.14   Loiasis. Areas of recorded loiasis coinciding with tropical rain forest

peripheral nerve involvement (Sarkany, 1959), and in North America in Pittsburgh in a visiting Nigerian (Vey, 1975).

CLINICAL FEATURES

Larvae are liberated from *Chrysops* as it takes a human blood meal, and enter the blood stream. About a year after the host has become infected, adult worms may appear in the conjunctiva, or be palpable under the skin, but microfilariae are not found in the blood until five months later. Adults wander through various body tissues and, while passing through subcutaneous tissues, cause transient shifting oedematous swellings—Calabar swellings. The microfilariae in the blood cause no symptoms and swellings may appear as early as three months after infection. There is usually one, but two or three may be seen. They may be preceded by pain and itching, but are themselves symptomless. They appear on any part of the body, but most commonly on the dorsa of the hands, arms, legs, and in the orbit. Severe pain and swelling may occur if the joints are affected, and the wrist, for example, may appear sprained. Where connective tissue is loose, such as in the eyelids, scrotum, or breast, the worm may be seen wandering about. When this occurs in the conjunctiva, discomfort and itching may be severe. Each swelling usually settles in less than a week.

Loa loa may also occur in the anterior chamber of the eye (Osuntokun and Olurin, 1975).

An eye worm *Thelazia californiensis* with some similar features occurs in California, but lately has been reported as far north as Seattle (Knierim and Jack, 1975).

DIAGNOSIS

Urticaria, urticarial reactions to insect bites, and contact urticaria must be considered in the differential diagnosis.

The history of a worm crossing the conjunctiva in a patient who has lived in West Africa is almost diagnostic, and the presence of an adult worm in loose connective tissue is highly suggestive. Support for the diagnosis is obtained by finding eosinophilia, a positive filaria skin test, and a positive filaria complement fixation test.

Microfilariae are identified in stained peripheral day blood samples, but they may be very few.

During treatment firm dead worms are sometimes palpable beneath the skin.

TREATMENT

One course of treatment with diethylcarbamazine (Banocide) is generally sufficient—given as for onchocerciasis. In the early stages of treatment an allergic reaction with further Calabar swellings, fever, headache, giddiness and vomiting may occur.

Dracontiasis (Dracunculosis, Guinea Worm, Medina Worm, Serpent Worm, Dragon Worm)

Dracontiasis is a chronic infestation of man due to the nematode worm *Dracunculus medinesis*. It causes extensive suffering and work loss, and is especially seen in rural people whose water supply is contaminated.

GEOGRAPHIC DISTRIBUTION

Dracontiasis occurs in West, Central and East Africa, as well as many areas of Asia—including Arabia, Iran, Turkey, Afghanistan, India, Burma and Southern Russia (Fig. 4.15). Also the northern parts of South America and the Caribbean islands. With the long incubation period of about one year, it is not only travellers by air who present with the disease in temperate areas.

The world incidence is estimated at more than 50 million cases, mostly in Asia, but this estimate is almost certainly much too low. In a Ghanaian study of Belcher et al (1975), less than 1 per cent of infected persons attended medical clinics. Adult male farmers using infected pond water as their drinking supply were most at risk. The disease is seasonal and coincides with peak agricultural activity.

AETIOLOGY AND CLINICAL FEATURES

The human disease is due to the determination of the metre-long adult female worm to break through the skin and deposit her larvae in water. For

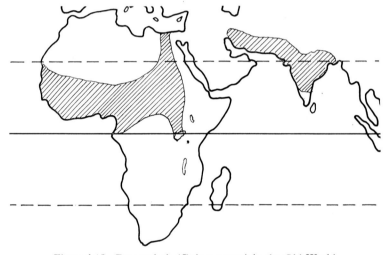

Figure 4.15   Dracontiasis (Guinea worm) in the Old World

survival and development the larvae must find the intermediate host, a crustacean *Cyclops*. Once within *Cyclops* the larvae take about 10 days before becoming infective to man in his drinking water. They burrow through his bowel wall into the loose retroperitoneal tissue, where they develop and mate. The female worm then wends her way down through tissue planes, usually reaching the lower limbs about a year after the drinking of infected water.

Before she penetrates the skin, there may be systemic prodromal symptoms of fever, urticaria and itchy, erythematous rashes, together with respiratory symptoms and diarrhoea. Later, a painful elevation of the skin is found, which blisters and ulcerates. In the centre is the prolapsed uterus of the worm, which protrudes and discharges free swimming embryos on contact with water. The clear fluid released from the blister becomes milky when this discharge of larvae takes place.

Toxic symptoms tend to disappear with rupture of the blister, but secondary infection frequently enters through the broken skin causing cellulitis, lymphangitis, regional adenitis, and oedema. Other rarer complications are severe local foreign body reaction, ankylosing arthritis, periostitis, neuritis and tetanus. More than one worm may appear, and other parts of the body—such as the scrotum—can be affected. The worm may become palpable in the tissues as a firm, tortuous cord, and larval ejection takes several weeks. When it is complete the worm dies and is gradually absorbed or calcifies. The development of a chronic pruritic lichenified dermatitis of the legs is also described by Hodgson and Barrett (1964).

DIAGNOSIS

Once the worm has appeared the diagnosis is self-evident. Douching the ulcer with water to elicit a milky discharge is a helpful pointer; intradermal tests are of doubtful value. X-ray examination may show old dead calcified worms. There is a moderate eosinophilia.

In the prodromal phase of systemic symptoms, pneumonia or malaria may be closely mimicked.

TREATMENT

Spraying the skin with ethyl chloride encourages the female to discharge all her larvae, after which she may be left to be absorbed. This rarely causes any harm to the patient. Alternatively, it is tempting to try to extract the worm without breaking her. This is done by holding the protruding end between finger and thumb and gently pulling repeatedly. At the same time the overlying skin is massaged towards the opening. When no more progress can be made, the worm is wound round a stick and left for half an hour before repeating the action.

Diethylcarbamazine (Banocide) is effective in the early stages (Hawking, 1956). Niridazole (Ambilhar) in a dosage of 25 mg/kg/day for 10 days, thiabendazole 50 to 100 mg/kg/day and metronidazole (Flagyl) in three 200 mg doses for seven days are also recommended (Cole, 1973). But at least one recent study has shown the latter two drugs to be ineffective when used prophylactically (Belcher et al, 1975).

Bancroftian and Malayan Filariases

Bancroftian filariasis is caused by infection with the nematode *Wuchereria bancrofti*, and Malayan filariasis by *Brugia malayi*. Similar symptoms are produced by both worms, but *B. malayi* is confined to the Malayan peninsula and its microfilariae have certain minor morphologic distinctions. The disease is transmitted by at least 50 different species of mosquitoes. The adult worms are parasites of the human lymphatic system, and may be found in any part of it, but especially in the limbs, scrotum and inguinal regions. The microfilariae are found in blood, lymph and in the urine if there is accompanying chyluria.

It takes from three to six months or longer before the development of inoculated larvae allows them to begin to multiply.

GEOGRAPHIC DISTRIBUTION

The distribution is tropical and subtropical between latitudes 45° north and 25° south, with Africa (Satti and Nur, 1974), the northern parts of South America, India, Malaysia, Indonesia, Oceania (Desowitz and Hitchcock, 1974), and the northern territories of Australia bearing the brunt (Fig. 4.16).

The world incidence exceeds 300 million, and many Latin American citizens of the United States come from endemic zones, but few cases are detected. American interest in filarial infections reached a peak towards the end of the Second World War. Several hundred thousand soldiers had been exposed to the disease and 15 000 were known to have had circulating microfilariae. Elaborate plans were laid to cope with the expected hordes developing scrotal and pedal elephantiasis, but these conditions were almost never seen (Cahill, 1964).

CLINICAL FEATURES

The incubation period usually lasts a year or longer, and the disease may be divided into three phases (Kerdel-Vegas, 1975): —

1. Asymptomatic.
2. Early acute inflammatory.
3. Late chronic and obstructive.

Asymptomatic phase. This phase may last months or very many years. Eosinophilia, positive intradermal and serological tests, together with microfilariae in the blood are found.

The early acute inflammatory phase. Attacks of fever, resembling malaria, last a few days to a week. They are accompanied by severe systemic symptoms, and are followed by periods of remission. Gradually localising signs arise, due to acute inflammation in the region of lymphatics. At other times local symptoms may predominate, or may be exclusively present, with painful erythematous swelling of arm, leg or scrotum and moderate adenopathy. Also, acute lymphangitis and adenitis with tensely oedematous overlying skin, fever and rigors. Suppuration may occur. Genital involvement with severe pain, inflammation and enlargement is common in Bancroftian filariasis, but rare in the Malayan variety.

Late chronic obstructive phase. This develops in parts of the body previously affected by acute early symptoms. Elephantiasis of the lower limbs—so characteristic of the complaint—is the most common, together with scrotal enlargement and hydrocele. The upper limbs, breasts and vulva may also be distended.

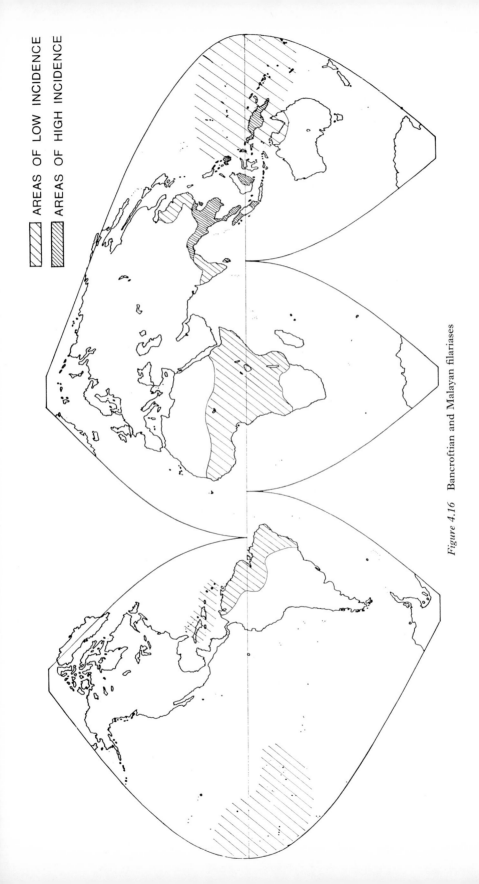

Figure 4.16 Bancroftian and Malayan filariases

Lymphatic varices occur affecting the superficial vessels of the pudendal region, and lymph scrotum with the scrotal skin thickened and studded with tiny vesicles, which contain milky or clear fluid. These may rupture, leading to maceration, secondary infection and sinus formation. Deep lymphatics may also rupture into serous cavities.

DIAGNOSIS

Differential diagnosis includes other causes of lymphangitis—especially bacterial, which is also common in the tropics; also, rarely, onchocerciasis.

The diagnosis is made on the clinical picture, together with the geographic history, the demonstration of microfilariae in the night blood, positive intra-dermal and complement fixation tests. The Mazzotti test—using diethyl-carbamazine in the same way as in onchocerciasis, in which a sharp allergic reaction occurs within 24 h of giving the drug—is also useful. Methods of isolation of microfilariae have been reported by Ah, McCall and Thompson (1974), and quantitative methods are described by Gubler and Bhattacharya (1974) and Southgate (1974).

Biopsy of an enlarged lymph node provides support for diagnosis.

TREATMENT

Diethylcarbamazine (Banocide) is the drug of choice, and is given in the same dosage as for onchocerciasis.

It may be necessary to repeat the course of treatment after a few months if microfilariae reappear in the blood. Unpleasant side effects occur, but not fatal complications. Examination one year after treatment showed that 60 per cent of patients with acute symptoms had had no recurrences, and there was partial or total regression of the presenting signs. Elephantiasis is not affected by medical treatment.

Gnathostomiasis

Gnathostomiasis is an infestation with larval worms of the genus *Gnatho-stoma*. It is well recognised in Thailand, and infections occur throughout the Far East. It is also reported in Israel, and occasional imported cases are diagnosed in colder countries (Whimster, personal communication). Miyazaki (1966) reported the disease in Japan.

The adult nematode was originally described in 1836 in the intestine of a tiger in a London zoo, but it is found in the guts of cats and dogs as well as in wild canivores. Eggs are excreted in the faeces, and man is infected by eating fresh-water fish, crabs or frogs which have ingested the first intermediate host, a small crustacean.

The disease is marked by migrating, localised, painful swellings, which may also be itchy. They occur most frequently on the chest and abdomen with abscess formation, small haemorrhagic spots and cord-like masses in the swellings. A pattern of migrating oedema is known in China as Yangtze oedema.

Recent work by Daengsvang (1971) has extended knowledge of the infectivity of *Gnathostoma spinigerum*. Urinary gnathostomiasis is described by Nitidandhaprabhas et al (1975). Otological involvement is discussed by Prasansuk and Hinchcliffe (1975), and work on the infestation of pigs in China is described by Chiu and Lin (1974).

Sparganosis

Sparganosis is caused by tapeworm larvae (spargana) of the genus *Spirometra*. The term 'sparganosis' refers to the sparganum of plerocercoid larva which is usually ribbon-like (Greek 'sparganon' means 'swaddling clothes').

The disease is most frequent in Asia and China, where it was first described, but its distribution is world-wide. Canadian cases have been recorded recently, and approximately 50 cases have been officially reported from the United States (Ali-Khan et al, 1973).

Man is infected by:

1. Drinking infected water.
2. Eating raw or very lightly cooked infected flesh of frogs, snakes, birds and mammals.
3. The application of a poultice of raw split frog to an inflamed surface. This oriental habit is unlikely to be seen in a temperate climate.

Infection by ingestion results in oedematous painful lumps which are usually in the subcutis. There is intense inflammation with necrosis, and the lesions may tend to migrate. Lymphatic invasion causes localised elephantiasis.

Diagnosis is made from the history, and by the recovery of spargana from lesions. The subject has been reviewed recently by Daly, Baker and Johnson (1975).

Dirofilariasis

Dirofilariasis is a subcutaneous infection by worms of the genus *Dirofilaria*. The great majority of cases described have been single worm infections presenting as a tender nodule, but the worm has also been found in the conjunctiva and eyelid. The infestation is described in Italy by Passaglia, Sacchi and De Carneri (1974), but most patients have been found in subtropical Florida (Beaver and Orihel, 1965). The causal organism, *Dirofilaria tenuis*, is fairly common in wild raccoons (Orihel and Beaver, 1965), and the salt-water marsh mosquito *Aedes taeniorhynchus* is considered the vector. Infections are more common in females by a ratio of five to one, and two-thirds of the worms in the nodules are dead when removed.

As pavement and condominiums replace the natural habitat of the raccoon, the worm must learn to adopt man as host or perish from this earth (Powell and Grossnickle, 1971).

DISEASES CAUSED BY ARTHROPODS

Myiasis

Cutaneous myiasis is the infestation of any part of the skin by larvae of *Diptera*, and is liable to be seen in patients who have very recently left the tropics. The most important tropical flies causing the condition are listed in Table 4.2.

Table 4.2 Common tropical myiases

Type of lesion	Common name	Scientific name	Geographic distribution
Furunculoid	Tumbu fly	*Cordylobia anthropophaga*	Tropical Africa
Furunculoid	Human bot fly	*Dermatobia hominis*	Tropical America
Bites with local reaction	Congo floor maggot	*Aucheromyia luteola*	Tropical Africa
Invasion of ulcers, wounds, etc.	New World screwworm fly	*Cochliomyia hominovorax*	American tropics
Invasion of ulcers, wounds, etc.	Old World screwworm fly	*Cochliomyia bezziana*	African and Asian tropics

Adapted from Canizares, O. (1975) *Clinical Tropical Dermatology.*

Cordylobiasis

Cordylobia anthropophaga the Tumbu or mango fly, is found in Africa, south of the Sahara. Eggs are deposited by the adult female on clothing contaminated by urine or faeces, or on sand and soil in the shade. The disease is quite frequent in urban areas of tropical Africa, where the infection is acquired by sitting or lying on contaminated sand or ground. Babies are likely to be infected from eggs deposited on nappies or other clothing. Children seem particularly susceptible and may present not only with skin lesions, but also fever and lymphadenopathy shortly after leaving tropical Africa (Calvert, 1961; Chaddah and Warin, 1966; Feverstein, Aspock and Wiedermann, 1969; Tio, 1975).

Cordylobia rodhaini is a similar parasite which is harboured in an animal reservoir, i.e. antelope and the African giant rat (Kremer et al, 1970).

CLINICAL FEATURES

Larvae penetrate the skin without irritation, but within two or three days multiple papules appear, gradually enlarge and become very painful (Fig.

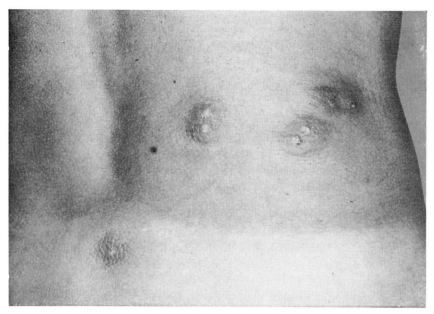

Figure 4.17 Cordylobiasis from West Africa. Boil-like lesions containing larvae. (Dr R. P. Warin, Bristol Royal Infirmary)

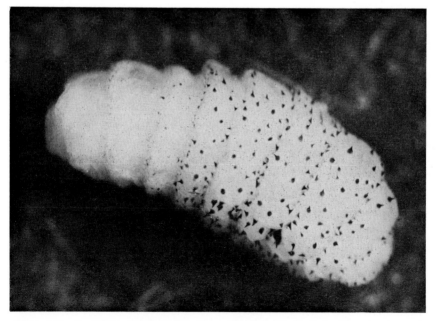

Figure 4.18 Cordylobia anthropophaga larva. (Dr R. P. Warin, Bristol Royal Infirmary)

4.17). As the larvae develop in the skin they can be seen wriggling (Fig. 4.18), and two little black dots (the spiracles) are visible, moving in the centres of lesions resembling boils.

The application of liquid paraffin kills the larvae by blocking respiration. Individual lesions may have to be incised and larvae expressed or curetted out. If very numerous, a general anaesthetic is necessary.

Dermatobia hominis Infestation (the Tropical or Human Bot Fly)

Dermatobia hominis is confined to South and Central America, including Mexico, but human infestations are seen beyond these limits (Smart, 1965; Prasad and Beck, 1969; Salomon, Catts and Knox, 1970; Macias et al, 1973).

The fly is a parasite of domestic cattle and man. The adult is large, non-blood sucking, and has a blue metallic sheen. The female glues her eggs to a mosquito which she catches, and when the mosquito takes a human blood meal, larvae emerge from the eggs and penetrate the human skin. Painful boil-like swellings, as seen in cordylobiasis, slowly develop, and the larvae which they contain emerge and drop to the ground two to four months after penetration. Exposed parts of the body are most affected, and the conjunctivae are often involved in children.

Treatment is as for cordylobiasis.

Genital myiasis occurs (Aspock and Leodolter, 1970; De Miranda, 1971), but does not seem to have been reported recently due to imported tropical infestation.

Tungiasis (Jiggers or Chigoe)

Jiggers is caused by the female flea *Tunga penetrans*. The disease is endemic in Mexico, Central America, the West Indies and South America, and the flea also found its way to tropical Africa in sand carried as ballast by a ship in 1872 (Londono, 1972). Tunga fleas live in sandy, shaded soil, and attack the feet of those who walk about without shoes. The pregnant female burrows into the skin without penetrating it completely, causing particularly painful lesions—which are often round the lateral margins of the toes. Occasional imported cases have been reported by Faust and Maxwell (1930), Reiss (1966) in the United States of America, and Borelli and Mueller (1962) in Germany.

Bites and Stings

Bites and stings in travellers returning from the tropics may be merely a nuisance, or can have serious consequences (Harman, 1971) (see Table 4.3). On land there are hazards including envenoming by scorpions, spiders, ticks, centipedes, bees, hornets, wasps, caterpillars and snakes. For the bather there are venomous fish stings, sea-urchin injuries (Fig. 4.19), jelly-fish stings

Table 4.3 Systemic tropical diseases transmitted by bites and stings

Vector	Disease
Insecta	
Mosquitoes	Malaria, filariasis, arboviral infections, e.g. Denge, chikungunya
Sandflies	Leishmaniasis, bartonellosis
Blackflies	Onchocerciasis
Midges	Filariasis
Tsetse flies	African trypanosomiasis
Horseflies	Loiasis, tularaemia
Lice	Typhus, Q fever
Fleas	Plague, typhus
Bugs	American trypanosomiasis
Arachnida	
Mites	Typhus
Soft ticks	Relapsing fever
Hard ticks	Typhus, arboviral infections
Dogs and bats	Rabies

Adapted from Reid, 1975.

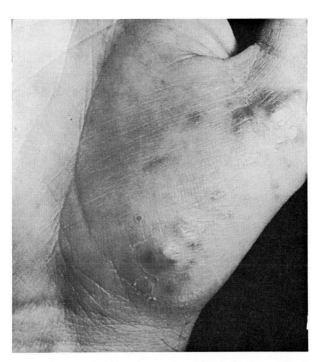

Figure 4.19 Sea urchin granulomas of the palm following injury. (Dr E. Waddington University Hospital of Wales, Cardiff)

and, in Asian waters of the Pacific, sea-snake bites (Reid, 1975). The subject of the therapy and pathophysiology of arthropod bites and stings has been well summarised recently (Harves and Millikan, 1975).

The silk trade brought irritant hairs of the wild silk moth of Nigeria back to Britain to cause irritation of the skin (Pomeroy, 1921; Rothschild et al, 1970).

TUMOURS

Kaposi's Sarcoma (Multiple Idiopathic Pigmented Haemangiosarcoma)

Although Kaposi's sarcoma is rare in Europe and the Americas, it constitutes 9 per cent of malignant tumours in indigenous males in Uganda (Taylor et al, 1971). The disease, presenting as multiple subcutaneous nodules often on the upper and lower extremities (Fig. 4.20), has been reported from many temperate parts of the world, but is most commonly found in Central and East Africa. Cases in Negro immigrants have been seen in Britain, and the subject is reviewed by Palmer (1972).

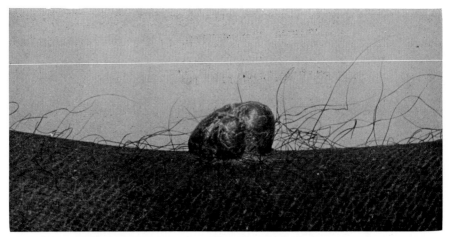

Figure 4.20   Kaposi's sarcoma nodule in a West Indian. (Dr Bernard Thomas, Royal Gwent Hospital, Newport)

The possibility of lesions occurring in unusual sites in Negroes must be borne in mind. Cox, Halprin and Akerman (1970) described a case localised to the penis.

The first case in an Eskimo was described recently (Masse and Glazebrook, 1974).

ACKNOWLEDGEMENT

All the maps other than Figure 4.1 are drawn from those on display in the Wellcome Museum of Medical Science, London.

REFERENCES

INTRODUCTION

Baker, H. (1976) Tuberculous lupus miliaris faciei. *Proceedings of the Royal Society of Medicine*, **69** (1), 4.

Catterall, R. D. (1975) Sexually transmitted diseases and the mobility explosion. *Postgraduate Medical Journal*, **51**, 838–842.

Clarke, G. H. V. (1952) A note on dermatitis cruris pustulosa et atrophicans. *Transactions of the Royal Society of Tropical Medicine and Hygiene*, **46**, 558.

Harman, R. R. M. (1967) A survey of diseases of the skin in medical students at University College, Ibadan, Nigeria. *Dermatologia Internationalis*, **6**, 35–38.

Harman, R. R. M. (1968) Dermatitis cruris pustulosa et atrophicans, the Nigerian shin disease. *British Journal of Dermatology*, **80**, 97–107.

Harman, R. R. M. (1972) Ghana Medical School and dermatology. *Transactions of the St John's Hospital Dermatological Society*, **58** (2), 290–297.

Harman, R. R. M. & Matthews, C. N. A. (1974) Acrokeratoelastoidosis (without elastorrhexis). *Proceedings of the Royal Society of Medicine*, **67**, 1237.

Ito, K. (1965) The peculiar demarcation of pigmentation along the so-called Voigt's line among the Japanese. *Dermatologia Internationalis*, **4** (i), 45–47.

Ito, M. & Tanaka, T. (1961) Pseudo-ichthyosis acquisita en taches circulaires proposed as a better name for pityriasis circinata Toyama. *Japanese Journal of Dermatology*, **71**, 586–588.

Marten, R. H., Presbury, D. G. C., Adamson, J. E. & Cardell, B. S. (1974) An unusual papular and acneform facial eruption in the Negro child. *British Journal of Dermatology*, **91**, 435–438.

Mohn, W. von (1974) Tropenkrankheiten in Europa. *Wiener Medizinische Wochenschrift*, **123**, 191–198.

Population Trends No. 2, Winter 1975. Office of Population Censuses and Surveys. London: HMSO.

Ridley, D. S. (1974) The laboratory diagnosis of tropical diseases with special reference to Britain: a review. *Journal of Clinical Pathology*, **27** (b), 435–444.

Sarkany, I. & Hare, P. J. (1964) Pityriasis rotunda (pityriasis circinata). *British Journal of Dermatology*, **76**, 223–228.

Sugathan, P. & Nair, M. B. (1972) Mudi-Chood—a new dermatosis. In *Essays in Tropical Dermatology*, ed. Marshall, J., Vol. 2, pp. 183–188. Amsterdam: Excerpta Medica.

Woodruff, A. W. (1975) Diseases of travel with particular reference to tropical diseases. *Postgraduate Medical Journal*, **51**, 825–829.

Zhdanov, V. M. (1968) Tropical diseases. *Israel Journal of Medical Sciences*, **4**, 390–401.

LEPROSY

Abel, G. & van Soest, A. H. (1971) Psychologic difficulties in the treatment of leprosy patients in a non-endemic country. *International Journal of Leprosy*, **39** (2), 429–432.

Adu, D., Evans, D. B., Millard, P. R., Calne, R. Y., Shwe, T. & Jopling, W. H. (1973) Renal transplantation in leprosy. *British Medical Journal*, **1**, 280–281.

Antia, N. R. (1974) The scope of plastic surgery in leprosy: a ten-year progress report. *Clinics in Plastic Surgery*, **1** (1), 69–82.

Atkinson, A. J., Sheagren, J. N., Rubio, J. B. & Knight, V. (1967) Evaluation of B.663 in human leprosy. *International Journal of Leprosy*, **35**, 119–126.
Bechelli, L. M., Lwin, K., Garbajosa, P. G., Gyi, M. M., Uemura, K., Sundaresan, T., Tamondong, C., Matejka, M., Sansarricq, H. & Walter, J. (1974) B. C. G. vaccination of children against leprosy: nine-year findings of the controlled W.H.O. trial in Burma. *Bulletin of the World Health Organisation*, **51**, 93–99.
Blanc, F. & Nosny, Y. (1970) Le lèpre et les lepreux à Marseille. *Bulletin de la Societé de Pathologie Exotique*, **63**, 417–429.
Browne, S. G. (not dated) *The Diagnosis and Management of Early Leprosy for Medical Practitioners*. London: The Leprosy Mission.
Canizares, O. (Ed.) (1975) *Clinical Tropical Dermatology*. Oxford: Blackwell.
Desikan, K. V., Ramanujam, K., Ramu, G. & Balakrishnan, S. (1975) Autopsy findings in a case of lepromatous leprosy treated with clofazimine. *Leprosy Review*, **46**, 181–189.
Feldman, R. A. & Sturdivant, M. (1975) Leprosy in Louisiana 1855–1970. An epidemiologic study of long-term trends. *American Journal of Epidemiology*, **102** (4), 303–310.
Grigor, R. R., Lang, W. R. & Nicholson, G. I. (1974) Gut amyloidosis in lepromatous leprosy regressing with therapy. *Leprosy Review*, **45**, 313–320.
Gussow, Z. & Tracy, G. S. (1972) The phenomenon of leprosy stigma in the continental United States. *Leprosy Review*, **43**, 85–93.
Harman, R. R. M. (To be published).
Jopling, W. H. (1971) *Handbook of Leprosy*. London: Heinemann.
Kirchheimer, W. F. & Storrs, E. E. (1971) Attempts to establish the armadillo (*Dasypus novemcinctus* Linn.) as a model for the study of leprosy. 1. Report of lepromatoid leprosy in an experimentally infected armadillo. *International Journal of Leprosy*, **39**, 693–702.
Kwapinski, J. B. G. & Kwapinski, E. H. (1974) Pathobiological relationships between *Mycobacterium leprae* and its primitive host. *Bulletin of the World Health Organisation*, **50** (5), 473–474.
Rook, A., Wilkinson, D. S. & Ebling, F. J. G. (Eds.) (1972) *Textbook of Dermatology*, 2nd edn. Oxford: Blackwell.
Schuppli, R. (1971) On the significance of the lepromin test in Middle Europe. *International Journal of Leprosy*, **39** (2), 608.
Schuppli, R. (1972) Zur frage der infektionsitat der lepra in Europa. *Dermatologica*, **145**, 102–105.
Shepard, C. C. (1960a) Acid fast bacilli in nasal excretions in mice, and results of inoculations of mice. *American Journal of Hygiene*, **71**, 147–157.
Shepard, C. C. (1960b) The experimental disease that follows the infection of human leprosy bacilli into foot pads of mice. *Journal of Experimental Medicine*, **112**, 445–454.
Storrs, E. E. (1971) The nine-banded armadillo: a model for leprosy and other biomedical research. *International Journal of Leprosy*, **39**, 703–714.
Turk, J. L. (1970) Immunological aspects of clinical leprosy. *Proceedings of the Royal Society of Medicine*, **63**, 1053–1056.

MYCOBACTERIAL ULCERATION
Barker, D. J. P. (1974) Mycobacterial skin ulcers. *British Journal of Dermatology*, **91**, 473–474.
Keininger, G., Schubert, G. E. & Ullmann, U. (1972) Das buruliulkus. *Zeitschrift für Tropenmedizin und Parasitologie*, **23**, 342–353.
Krieg, R. E., Hockmeyer, W. T. & Connor, D. H. (1974) Toxin of *Mycobacterium ulcerans*. Production and effects on guinea-pig skin. *Archives of Dermatology*, **110**, 783–788.
Meyers, W. M., Shelly, W. M., Connor, D. H. & Meyers, E. K. (1974a) Human *Mycobacterium ulcerans* infections developing at sites of trauma to skin. *American Journal of Tropical Medicine and Hygiene*, **23**, 919–923.
Meyers, W. M., Shelly, W. M. & Connor, D. H. (1974b) Heat treatment of *Mycobacterium ulcerans* infection without surgical excision. *American Journal of Tropical Medicine and Hygiene*, **23**, 924–929.
Radford, A. J. (1975) *Mycobacterium ulcerans* in Australia. *Australia and New Zealand Journal of Medicine*, **5**, 162–169.
Schröder, K. H. (1975) Investigation into the relationship of *Mycobacterium ulcerans* to *M. buruli* and other mycobacteria. *American Review of Respiratory Disease*, **3**, 559–562.

Stanford, J. L., Revill, W. D. L., Gunthorpe, W. J. & Grange, J. M. (1975) The production and preliminary investigation of Burulin, a new skin test reagent for *Mycobacterium ulcerans* infection. *Journal of Hygiene (Cambridge)*, **74**, 7.

TINEA NIGRA

Chadfield, H. W. & Campbell, C. K. (1972) A case of tinea nigra in Britain. *British Journal of Dermatology*, **87**, 505–508.
Hitch, J. M. (1961) Tinea nigra palmaris; report of a case originating in North Carolina. *Archives of Dermatology*, **84**, 318–320.
MacKenzie, D. W. R. Personal communication.
Smith, J. G., Jr, Sams, W. M. & Roth, F. J., Jr (1958) Tinea nigra palmaris; a disorder easily confused with junction naevus of the palm. *Journal of the American Medical Association*, **167**, 312–314.
Tan, R. S. Personal communication.

TINEA IMBRICATA

Church, R. & Sneddon, I. (1962) Tinea imbricata: a report of two cases treated with griseofulvin. *Lancet*, **1**, 1215–1216.
Sharvill, D. (1952) Tinea imbricata in a European: double infection with *Trichophyton concenticum* and *Trichophyton rubrum*. *British Journal of Dermatology*, **64**, 373–377.

PIEDRA

Hitch, J. M. (1959) Piedra: report of a fifth case originating in the U.S.A. *Archives of Dermatology*, **79**, 99–100.
Kotovirta, M.-L., Stubb, S. & Salonen, A. (1975) Trichosporosis (white piedra), a case report from Finland. *Acta dermato-venereologica (Stockholm)*, **55**, 218–220.
Patterson, J. C., Laine, S. L. & Taylor, W. B. (1962) White piedra occurring on the pubic hair of a native caucasian North American. *Archives of Dermatology*, **85**, 534–536.

FAVUS

Beare, J. M. (1972) In *Textbook of Dermatology*, ed. Rook, A., Wilkinson, D. S. & Ebling, F. J. G., p. 736. Oxford: Blackwell.
Blank, F. (1962) Human favus in Quebec. *Dermatologica*, **125**, 369–381.
Pettit, J. H. S. (1960) Griseofulvin in favus; a report on work in progress. *British Journal of Dermatology*, **72**, 179–184.
Saracci, T. (1971) Skin diseases in children in Eastern Turkey. *Turkish Journal of Paediatrics*, **13**, 51–58.

TRICHOPHYTON SOUDANENSE

Calnan, C. D., Djavahiszwili, N. & Hodgson, C. J. (1962) *Trichophyton soudanense* in Britain. *British Journal of Dermatology*, **74**, 144–148.
Clayton, Y. M. (1968) Studies in mycology. IV. *Trichophyton soudanense*. *Transactions and Reports of the St John's Hospital Dermatological Society*, **54** (2), 197–199.
Clayton, Y. M. (1975) Personal communication.
English, M. P., Harman, R. R. M. & Howell, R. (To be published).
Harari, Z., Sommer, B. & Feinstein, A. (1973) *Trichophyton soudanense* infection in two white families. *British Journal of Dermatology*, **88**, 243–244.
Johnson, J. A. & Rosenthal, S. A. (1968) Superficial cutaneous infection with *Trichophyton soudanense*. *Archives of Dermatology*, **97**, 428–431.
Kaben, U. (1964) Erstmalige isolierung von *Trichophyton soudanense* joyeaux in Deutschland. *Mykosen*, **7**, 82–85.
Rippon, J. W. & Medenica, M. (1964) Isolation of *Trichophyton soudanense* in the United States. *Sabouraudia*, **3**, 301–302.
Sarkany, I. (1963) Infection with *Trichophyton soudanense* in a white girl. *British Journal of Dermatology*, **75**, 408–410.
Vanbreuseghem, R. (1968) *Trichophyton soudanense* in and outside Africa. *British Journal of Dermatology*, **80**, 140–147.

TRICHOPHYTON VIOLACEUM
Campbell, C. Personal communication.
Neves, H. (1960) Mycological study of 519 cases of ringworm infections in Portugal. Signifi-
cance of multiple localisations. Tinea as a single infection. *Mycopathologica*, **13**, 121–132.

TRICHOPHYTON YAOUENDI
Sarkany, I. & Midgley, G. (1966) *Trichophyton yaoundei* infection in Britain. *British Journal of
Dermatology*, **78**, 225–226.

TRICHOPHYTON MEGNINII
Puissant, A., Drouhet, E., Badillet, G., David, V. & Malard, A. (1969) Extensive mycosis from
Trichophyton rosaceum (*Trichophyton megninii*). *Annales de Dermatologie et Syphiligraphie
(Paris)*, **96**, 271–278.
Sarkany, I., Clayton, Y. M. & Beck, G. A. (1963) *Trichophyton megninii* in Britain. *British
Journal of Dermatology*, **75**, 388–391.

TRICHOPHYTON MENTAGROPHYTES
Blank, H., Taplin, D. & Zaias, N. (1969) Cutaneous *Trichophyton mentagraphytes* infections in
Vietnam. *Archives of Dermatology*, **99**, 135–143.

HENDERSONULA TORULOIDEA
Campbell, C. K., Kurwa, A., Abdel-Aziz, A.-H. M. & Hodgson, C. (1973) Fungal infections
of the skin and nails by *Hendersonula toruloidea*. *British Journal of Dermatology*, **89**, 45–52.
Campbell, C. K. (1974) Studies on *Hendersonula toruloidea* isolated from human skin and nail.
Sabouraudia, **12**, 150–156.
Gentles, J. C. & Evans, E. G. V. (1970) Infection of the feet and nails with *Hendersonula
toruloidea*. *Sabouraudia*, **8**, 72–75.
Wilson, E. E. (1947) The branch wilt of Persian walnut trees and its cause. *Hilgardia*, **17**,
413–430.

MYCETOMA
Anning, S. T., La Touche & Hunter (1958) Madura foot (mycetoma). *British Journal of
Dermatology*, **70**, 309.
Avram, A. (1969) Quelques particularités concernant les mycétomes d'une contrée à climat
tempéré: la Roumanie. *Dermatologica*, **139**, 390–398.
Baxter, M., Murray, I. G. & Taylor, J. J. (1966) A case of mycetoma with serological diagnosis
of *Allescheria boydii*. *Sabouraudia*, **5**, 138–140.
Burgoon, C. F., Blank, F., Johnson, W. C. & Grattel, S. F. (1974) Mycetoma formation in
Trichophyton rubrum infection. *British Journal of Dermatology*, **90**, 155–162.
Chadfield, H. W. (1964) Mycetoma of the foot. *Mycopathologia et Mycologia applicata*, **24**,
130–136.
Findlay, G. H. & Vismer, H. F. (1974) Black grain mycetoma. A study of the chemistry,
formation and significance of the tissue grain in *Madurella mycetomi* infections. *British
Journal of Dermatology*, **91**, 297–303.
Gould, W. M. (1969) Black grain mycetoma originating in Northern California. A case caused
by *Madurella grisea*. *Archives of Dermatology*, **99**, 426–428.
Griffiths, W. A. D., Kohout, E. & Vessal, K. (1975) Mycetoma in Iran. *International Journal
of Dermatology*, **14**, 209–213.
Leone, R. (1974) Micetoma da *Nocardia asteroides*. *Giornale Italiano di Dermatologia Minerva
Dermatologica*, **109**, 197–217.
McClelland, K. (1973) Pseudomycete mycetoma. *Medical Journal of Australia*, **1**, 388–390.
Mahgoub, E. S. & Murray, I. G. (1973) *Mycetoma*, p. 132. London: Heinemann.
Murray, I. G., Dunkerley, G. E. & Hughes, K. E. A. (1964) A case of madura foot caused by
Phialophora jeanselmei. *Sabouraudia*, **3**, 175–177.
Murray, I. G. & Holt, H. D. (1964) Is *Cephalosporium acremonium* capable of producing
maduromycosis? *Mycopathologia et Mycologia applicata*, **22**, 335–338.
Reifferschied, M. & Seeliger, H. (1955) Monosporiose und maduromycose. *Deutsche medizin-
ische Wochenschrift*, **80**, 1841.

AFRICAN HISTOPLASMOSIS

Cooke, W. B. (1969) A bibliography of histoplasmosis. *Mycopathologia*, **39**, 1–94.

Hiltenbrand, C., Antoini, H.-M., Durosoir, J.-L., Misson, R., Guenard, C., Garrel, J. & Millet, P. (1971) African histoplasmosis of cutaneous, osseous, lymphnodal and pulmonary type. Report of a case. *Bulletin de la Société française de Dermatologie et de syphiligraphie*, **78**, 600–602.

Lucas, A. O. (1970) Cutaneous manifestations of African histoplasmosis. *British Journal of Dermatology*, **82**, 435–447.

Sureau, B., Berrod, J. & Bardinon, M.-P. (1973) Imported histoplasmosis—a new disease in Europe. *Materia medica polonica*, **5**, 277–287.

CHROMOMYCOSIS

Bayles, M. A. H. (1971) Chromomycosis: treatment with thiabendazole. *Archives of Dermatology*, **104**, 476–485.

Fountain, R. B. (1968) The chromomycoses in England. *Transactions and Reports of the St John's Hospital Dermatological Society*, **54**, 187–196.

Havu, V. K. (1970) Chromoblastomycosis. A new case with diagnostic problems. *Duodecim (Helsinki)*, **86**, 291–296.

Horacek, J. & Ulicna, D. (1969) Third case of chromomycosis in Czechoslovakia. *Česká Dermatologie*, **44**, 118–120.

Lopes, C. F., Alvarenga, R. J., Cisalpino, E. O., Armond, S., Porto, R. V., Maia, F. A. & Peixoto, Y. (1969) Treatment of chromoblastomycosis with 5-fluorocytosine. *Hospital (Rio)*, **75**, 1335–1342.

Lopes, C. F., Cisalpino, E. O., Alvarenga, R. J., Armond, S., Porto, R. V., Maia, F. A. & Peixoto, Y. (1971) Treatment of chromomycosis with 5-fluorocytosine. *International Journal of Dermatology*, **10**, 182–191.

Morison, W. L., Connor, B. & Clayton, Y. (1974) Successful treatment of chromoblastomycosis with 5-fluorocytosine. *British Journal of Dermatology*, **90**, 445–449.

SOUTH AMERICAN BLASTOMYCOSIS

Lythcott, G. I. & Edgcomb, J. H. (1964) The occurrence of South American blastomycosis in Accra, Ghana. *Lancet*, **1**, 916–917.

KELOIDAL BLASTOMYCOSIS

Vermeil, C., Gordeff, A., Leroux, M.-J., Morin, O. & Bouc, M. (1971) Blastomycose cheloidienne à *Aureobasidium pullulans* (De bary) Arnaud en Bretagne. *Mycopathologia et mycologia applicata*, **43**, 35–39.

SUBCUTANEOUS PHYCOMYCOSIS

Cornic, J. P. (1975) A report of a new case of phycomyosis in Senegal. *Médecine Tropicale*, **35**, 248.

Harman, R. R. M., Jackson, H. & Willis, A. J. (1964) Subcutaneous phycomycosis in Nigeria. *British Journal of Dermatology*, **76**, 408–420.

Martinson, F. D. & Clark, B. M. (1967) Rhinophycomycosis entomophthorae in Nigeria. *American Journal of Tropical Medicine and Hygiene*, **16**, 40–47.

Srinivasan, M. C. & Thirumalachar, M. J. (1965) Basidiobolus species pathogenic for man. *Sabouraudia*, **4**, 32–34.

Symmers, W. St. C. (1960) Mucormycotic granuloma possibly due to *Basidiobolus ranarum*. *British Medical Journal*, **1**, 1331–1333.

ENDEMIC SYPHILIS

Grin, E. I. (1953) Epidemiology and control of endemic syphilis. Geneva. *World Health Organisation Monograph Series*, No. 11.

Grin, E. I. (1962) Endemic treponematoses. *Transactions of the St John's Hospital Dermatological Society*, **48**, 11–26.

Guthe, T. & Luger, A. (1957) Epidemiological aspects of non-venereal endemic syphilis. *Dermatologica (Basle)*, **115**, 248–272.

Guthe, T. & Luger, A. (1965) The control of endemic syphilis of childhood. *I.N.T./V.D.T.*, **203**, 65.

Luger, A. (1972) Non-venereally transmitted 'endemic' syphilis in Vienna. *British Journal of Venereal Diseases*, **48**, 356–359.

YAWS

Foote, G. A. (1975) Case of the spring season. *Seminars in Roentgenology*, **10** (2), 97–98.
Garner, M. F., Backhouse, J. L., Moodie, P. M. & Tibbs, G. J. (1972) Treponemal infection in the Australian Northern Territory aborigines. *Bulletin of the World Health Organisation*, **46**, 285–293.
King, A. & Nicol, C. (1975) *Venereal Diseases*, 3rd edn. London: Baillière Tindall.
Pampiglione, S. & Wilkinson, A. E. (1975) A study of yaws among pigmies in Camaroon and Zaire. *British Journal of Venereal Diseases*, **51**, 165–169.
Willcox, R. R. (1975) International aspects of venereal diseases and non-venereal treponematoses. *Clinical Obstetrics and Gynaecology*, **18** (1), 207–222. Harper & Row Inc.

PINTA

Convit, J., Kerdel-Vegas, F. & Rodriguez, G. (1961) Erythema dyschromicum perstans. A hitherto undescribed skin disease. *Journal of Investigative Dermatology*, **6**, 457–462.
Lawton Smith, J., David, N. J., Indgin, S., Israel, E. W., Levine, B. M., Justice, J. Jr, McCrary, J. A., III, Medina, R., Paez, P., Santana, E., Sarkar, M., Schatz, N. J., Spitzer, M. L., Spitzer, W. O. & Walter, E. K. (1971) Neuro-ophthalmological study of late yaws and pinta. II. The Caracas project. *British Journal of Venereal Diseases*, **47**, 226–251.
Stevenson, J. B. & Miura, M. (1966) Erythema dyschromicum perstans (ashy dermatosis). *Archives of Dermatology*, **94**, 196–199.

TROPICAL ULCER

Ariyan, S. & Krizek, T. (1975) Tropical ulcers. *Plastic and Reconstructive Surgery*, **55**, 324–329.
Ennis, J. T., Gueri, M. C. & Sarjeant, G. R. (1972) Radiological changes associated with leg ulcers in the tropics. *British Journal of Radiology*, **45**, 8–14.
McMillan, M. R. & Hurwitz, R. M. (1969) Tropical bacterial pyoderma in Vietnam. *Journal of the American Medical Association* **210** (9), 1734–1737.

LEISHMANIASIS

Brahmachari, U. N. (1922) Dermoid leishmanoid. *Indian Medical Gazette*, **57**, 125–127.
Bryceson, A. (1976) Tropical dermatology—cutaneous leishmaniasis. *British Journal of Dermatology*, **94**, 223–226.
Busuttil, A. (1974) Kala-azar in the Maltese islands. *Transactions of the Royal Society of Tropical Medicine and Hygiene*, **78**, 236–240.
Charters, A. D. & Staer, P. A. (1970) Cutaneous leishmaniasis of long incubation period in an Italian immigrant in Western Australia. *Medical Journal of Australia*, **2**, 278–279.
Convit, J., Kerdel-Vegas, F. & Gordon, B. (1962) Disseminated anergic cutaneous leishmaniasis. *British Journal of Dermatology*, **74**, 132–135.
De Noronha, T. (1970) Clinical aspects of endemic cutaneous leishmaniasis in Portugal: an endemic case of malignant cutaneous leishmaniasis. *Revista de Diagnóstico Biológico (Madrid)*, **19**, 599–618.
Ecker, H. D. & Lubitz, J. M. (1947) Kala-azar in the United States: review of the literature and report of two cases: stilbamidine treatment. *Annals of Internal Medicine*, **26**, 720–733.
Griffiths, W. A. D. Personal communication.
Griffiths, W. A. D. & Dutz, W. (1975) Repeated tissue sampling with a dental broach; a trial in cutaneous leishmaniasis. *British Journal of Dermatology*, **93**, 43–45.
Guerra, R., Tosi, P. & Molinelli, G. (1974) Leishmaniasis of the lid in Tuscany. *Ophthalmologica*, **168**, 193–196.
Kandil, E. (1973) Treatment of cutaneous leishmaniasis with trimethoprim sulphamethoxazole combination. *Dermatologica*, **146**, 303–309.
Long, P. I. (1973) Cutaneous leishmaniasis treated with metronidazole. *Journal of the American Medical Association*, **223**, 1378–1379.
Muir, E. (1930) The differential diagnosis of leprosy and dermal leishmaniasis. *Indian Medical Gazette*, **64**, 257–258.

Munro, D. D., Du Vivier, A. & Jopling, W. H. (1972) Post Kala-azar dermal leishmaniasis. *British Journal of Dermatology*, **87**, 374–378.

Mutinga, M. J. (1975) The animal reservoir of cutaneous leishmaniasis on Mount Elgon, Kenya. *East African Medical Journal*, **52**, 142–151.

Nazyrov, F., Yusupov, K. A. & Dzhabarov, L. N. (1974) Cutaneous leishmaniasis in Termez, U.S.S.R. *Meditsinskaya Parazitologiya i Parazitarnye Bolezni*, **43**, 653–655.

Novales, J. (1974) Cutaneous leishmaniasis in Mexico. *International Journal of Dermatology*, **13**, 283–286.

Pasi, F. & Saragoni, A. (1970) Consideration on the cutaneous leishmaniasis in the inhabitants of Forli. *Romagna Medica*, **22**, 242–246.

Saf'Janova, V. M. & Aliev, E. I. (1973) Comparative study of biological characteristics of the causal agents of zoonotic and anthroponotic cutaneous leishmaniasis in the U.S.S.R. *Bulletin of the World Health Organisation*, **49**, 499–506.

Symmers, W. St C. (1960) Leishmaniasis acquired by contagion. A case of marital infection in Britain. *Lancet*, **1**, 127–132.

Yesudian, P. & Thambiah, A. S. (1974) Amphotericin B therapy in dermal leishmanoid. *Archives of Dermatology*, **109**, 720–722.

CUTANEOUS AMOEBIASIS

Beirana, L. (1972) In *Dermatologia Clinica*, 2nd edn, ed. Cortes, J. L., p. 877. Mexico: Union Grafica, S.A.

Biagi, F. & Martuscelli, A. (1963) Cutaneous amoebiasis in Mexico. *Dermatologia Tropica*, **2**, 129–136.

Biagi, F., Alvarez, R. & Gonzalez, M. (1974) Anti-amoebic action of etophamide in children. *Transactions of the Royal Society of Tropical Medicine and Hygiene*, **68** (5), 368–369.

Stamm, W. P. (1975) Amoebiasis in England and Wales. *British Medical Journal*, **2**, 452–453.

TOXOPLASMOSIS

Norrby, R., Eilard, T., Svedhem, A. & Lycke, E. (1975) Treatment of toxoplasmosis with trimethoprim-sulphamethoxazole. *Scandinavian Journal of Infectious Diseases*, **7**, 72–75.

Quinn, E. L., Fisher, E. J., Cox, F. & Madhavan, T. (1975) The clinical spectrum of toxoplasmosis in the adult. *Cleveland Clinic Quarterly*, **42**, 71–81.

Shafer, M. (1975) Toxoplasmosis. *New York State Journal of Medicine*, **75**, 1049–1061.

CUTANEOUS PROTOTHECOSIS

Cox, G. E., Wilson, J. D. & Brown, P. (1974) Prototothecosis: a case of disseminated algal infection. *Lancet*, **2**, 379–382.

Davies, R. R., Spencer, H. & Wakelin, P. O. (1964) A case of human protothecosis. *Proceedings of the Royal Society of Tropical Medicine and Hygiene*, **58**, 448–451.

Davies, R. R. & Wilkinson, J. L. (1967) Human protothecosis: supplementary studies. *Annals of Tropical Medicine and Parasitology*, **61**, 112–114.

Dogliotti, M., Mars, P. W., Rabson, A. R. & Rippey, J. J. (1975) Cutaneous protothecosis. *British Journal of Dermatology*, **93**, 473–474.

Klintworth, G. K., Fetter, B. F. & Nielson, H. S. (1968) Protothecosis, an algal infection. Report of a case in man. *Journal of Medical Microbiology*, **1**, 211–216.

Mars, P. W., Rabson, A. R., Rippey, J. J. & Ajello, L. (1971) Cutaneous protothecosis. *British Journal of Dermatology*, **85**, Suppl. 7, 76–84.

Nosanchuk, J. S. & Greenberg, R. D. (1973) Protothecosis of the olecranon bursa caused by achloric algae. *American Journal of Clinical Pathology*, **59**, 567–573.

Tindall, J. P. & Fetter, B. F. (1971) Infections caused by achloric algae (protothecosis). *Archives of Dermatology*, **104**, 490–500.

LARVA MIGRANS AND CURRENS

Da Fonseca, M. (1968) Larva migrans in metropolitan Portugal. *Trabalhos da Sociedad de Dermatologia*, **26**, 189.

Doeglas, H. M. G. & Tenberg, J. A. G. (1972) Larva currens (migrans) casued by *Strongyloides stercoralis*. *Dermatologica*, **144**, 350–352.

Grove, D. I., Warren, K. S. & Mahmoud, A. A. F. (1975) Algorithms in the diagnosis and management of exotic diseases. III. Strongyloidiasis. *Journal of Infectious Diseases*, **131** (6), 755–758.

Huber, H. P. (1972) Epidemic appearance of creeping eruption. *Dermatologica*, **145**, 88–91.

Josef, C. (1972) Oral treatment of myiasis linearis migrans (creeping disease) with thiabendazole. *Hautarzt*, **23**, 511–512.

Kahn, G. & Johnson, J. A. (1971) Serum IgE levels in cutaneous larva migrans. *International Journal of Dermatology*, **10**, 201–203.

Kuberski, T. T., Gabor, E. P. & Boudreaux, D. (1975) Disseminated strongyloidiasis. A complication of the immunosuppressed host. *Western Journal of Medicine*, **122**, 504–508.

Lehmuskallio, E. A. (1975) Hair fragment in the skin resembling larva migrans. *British Journal of Dermatology*, **93**, 349–350.

Moqbel, R. (1974) Effect of steroids on experimental strongyloidiasis. *Proceedings of the British Society for Parasitology*, **69** (2), xviii.

Nagalotimath, S. J., Ramaprasad, A. V. & Chandrashekhar, N. K. (1974) Fatal strongyloidiasis in a patient receiving corticosteroids. *Indian Journal of Pathology and Bacteriology*, **17** (3), 190–192.

Niebauer, G. & Reichel, K. (1975) Creeping disease (larva migrans). *Wiener klinische Wochenschrift*, **87**, 177–180.

Rampini, E. & Nunzi, K. (1974) A case of larva migrans. *Giornale Italiano di Dermatologia Minerva Dermatologica*, **110**, 10–12.

Rook, A. & Staughton, R. (1972) The cutaneous manifestation of toxocariasis. *Dermatologica*, **144**, 129–143.

Stone, O. J., Newell, G. B. & Mullins, J. S. (1972) Cutaneous strongyloidiasis: larva currens. *Archives of Dermatology*, **106**, 734–736.

Thomas, J., Lugagne, J., Rosso, A.-M., Heraut, L., Sagnet, H., Revil, H. & Mafart, Y. (1969) Treatment of creeping eruption with thiabendazole: report of 50 cases. *Marseilles Médical (France)*, **106**, 717–721.

Thomas, J., Renambot, J., Barbotin, M., Rigaud, J. & Saint-Andre, P. (1971) Urticaire lineaire recidivante mobile, au cours de la strongyloidose: guérison par le thiabendazole. *Bulletin de la Société de pathologie exotique et de ses Filiales*, **64**, 486–498.

ONCHOCERCIASIS

Choyce, D. P. (1972) Epidemiology and natural history of onchocerciasis. *Israel Journal of Medical Science*, **8**, 1143.

Connor, D. H., Williams, P. H., Helwig, E. B. & Winslow, D. J. (1969) Dermal changes in onchocerciasis. *Archives of Pathology*, **87**, 193–200.

Imperato, T. J. & Sow, O. (1971) Incidence of and beliefs about onchocerciasis in the Senegal river basin. *Tropical and Geographical Medicine*, **23**, 385–389.

Jopling, W. H. (1960) Onchocerciasis presenting without dermatitis. *British Medical Journal*, **1**, 861.

Lagraulet, J. (1971) Etude des biopsies cutanées et de la réaction de Mazzotti chez les onchocerquiens examinés en France. *Bulletin de la Société de pathologie exotique et de ses Filiales*, **64**, 231–235.

Nelson, G. S. (1958) 'Hanging groins' and hernia, complications of onchocerciasis. *Transactions of the Royal Society of Tropical Medicine and Hygiene*, **52**, 272–275.

Wegesa, P. (1971) The present status of onchocerciasis in Tanzania: a review of the distribution and prevalence of the disease. *Tropical and Geographical Medicine*, **22**, 345–351.

Wolfe, M. S. (1974) Onchocerciasis presenting with swelling of one limb. *American Journal of Tropical Medicine and Hygiene*, **23**, 361–368.

LOIASIS

Charters, A. D., Wellborn, T. A. & Miller, P. (1972) Calabar swellings in immigrants in Western Australia. *Medical Journal of Australia*, **1**, 268–271.

Knierim, R. & Jack, M. K. (1975) Conjunctivitis due to *Thelazia californiensis*. *Archives of Ophthalmology*, **93**, 522–523.

Osuntokun, O. & Olurin, O. (1975) Filarial worm (*Loa loa*) in the anterior chamber. *British Journal of Ophthalmology*, **59**, 166–167.

Sarkany, I. (1959) Loiasis with involvement of peripheral nerves. *Transactions of the St John's Hospital Dermatological Society*, **42**, 149.
Sparrow, C. H. & Goldsmid, J. M. (1974) Imported loiasis in Rhodesia. *Central African Journal of Medicine*, **20**, 143–146.
Vey, E. K. (1975) Filaria—*Loa loa:* case report. *Annals of Ophthalmology*, **7**, 389–392.

DRACONTIASIS
Belcher, B. W., Wurapa, F. K., Ward, W. B. & Lourie, I. M. (1975) Guinea worm in Southern Ghana: its epidemiology and impact on agricultural productivity. *American Journal of Tropical Medicine and Hygiene*, **24**, 243–249.
Cole, A. C. E. (1973) Advances in tropical medicine. *Practitioner*, **211**, 528–534.
Hawking, F. (1956) Treatment of filariasis. *Tropical Diseases Bulletin*, **53**, 829–834.
Hodgson, C. & Barrett, D. F. (1964) Chronic dracunculosis. *British Journal of Dermatology*, **76**, 211–217.

FILARIASIS
Ah, H.-S., McCall, J. W. & Thompson, P. E. (1974) A simple method for isolation of *Brugia pahangi* and *Brugia malayi* microfilariae. *International Journal for Parasitology*, **4**, 677–679.
Cahill, K. M. (1964) *Tropical Diseases in Temperate Climates*. Philadelphia: Lippincott.
Desowitz, R. F. & Hitchcock, J. C. (1974) Hyperendemic Bancroftian filariasis in the kingdom of Tonga: the application of the membrane filter concentration technique to an age-stratified blood survey. *American Journal of Tropical Medicine and Hygiene*, **23**, 877–879.
Gubler, D. J. & Bhattacharya, N. C. (1974) A quantitative approach to the study of Bancroftian filariasis. *American Journal of Tropical Medicine and Hygiene*, **23**, 1027–1036.
Kerdel-Vegas, F. (1975) In *Clinical Tropical Dermatology*, ed. Canizares, O. Oxford: Blackwell.
Sasa, M. (1974) Anti-filariasis campaign: its history and future prospects. *Progress in Drug Research*, **18**, 259–268.
Satti, M. H. & Abdel Nur, O. M. (1974) Bancroftian filariasis in the Sudan. *Bulletin of the World Health Organisation*, **51**, 314–315.
Southgate, B. A. (1974) A quantitative approach to parasitological techniques in Bancroftian filariasis and its effect on epidemiological understanding. *Transactions of the Royal Society of Tropical Medicine and Hygiene*, **68**, 177–185.

GNATHOSTOMIASIS
Chiu, J. K. & Lin, Y. T. (1974) *Gnathostoma dolloresi* from pigs in Taiwan. *Chinese Journal of Microbiology*, **7**, 107–108.
Daengsvang, S. (1971) Infectivity of *Gnathostoma spinigerum* larvae in primates. *Journal of Parasitology*, **57**, 476–478.
Miyazaki, I. (1966) *Gnathostoma* and gnathostomiasis in Japan. *Progress in Medical Parasitology in Japan*, **3**, 531–586.
Nitidandhaprabhas, P., Sirikarna, A., Harnsomburana, K. & Thepsitthar, P. (1975) Human urinary gnathostomiasis: a case report from Thailand. *American Journal of Tropical Medicine and Hygiene*, **24**, 49–51.
Prasansuk, S. & Hinchcliffe, R. (1975) Gnathostomiasis. A case of otological interest. *Archives of Otolaryngology*, **101**, 254–258.
Whimster, I. W. (1975) Personal communication.

SPARGANOSIS
Ali-Khan, Z., Irving, R. T., Wignall, N. & Bowmer, E. J. (1973) Imported sparganosis in Canada. *Canadian Medical Association Journal*, **108**, 592–593.
Daly, J. J., Baker, G. F. & Johnson, B. R. (1975) Human sparganosis in Arkansas. *Journal of the Arkansas Medical Society*, **71**, 397–402.

DIROFILARIASIS
Beaver, P. C. & Orihel, T. C. (1965) Human infections with filariae of animals in the United States. *American Journal of Tropical Medicine and Hygiene*, **14**, 1010–1029.

Orihel, T. C. & Beaver, P. C. (1965) Morphology and relationship of *Dirofilaria tenuis* and *Dirofilaria conjunctivae*. *American Journal of Tropical Medicine and Hygiene*, **14**, 1030–1043.
Passaglia, A., Sacchi, S. & De Carneri, I. (1974) Un affezione cutanea non rara in Italia: la dirofilariosi due nuovi casi padvesi. *Giornale Italiano de Dermatologia*, **109**, 218–224.
Powell, L. W. Jr & Grossnickle, J. W. (1971) Subcutaneous filarial worms in Florida. *Journal of the Florida Medical Association*, **58**, 26.

CORDYLOBIASIS
Calvert, H. (1961) Myiasis from the tumbu fly: two cases recorded in Britain. *British Medical Journal*, **1**, 1513–1514.
Chaddah, V. K. & Warin, R. P. (1966) Cutaneous myiasis due to the tumbu fly. *British Journal of Clinical Practice*, **20**, 215–218.
Feverstein, W., Aspock, H. & Wiedermann, G. (1969) Haut-myiasis durch *Cordylobia antropophaga*. *Wiener klinische Wochenshrift*, **81**, 634–635.
Kremer, M., Lenys, J., Basset, M., Rombourg, H. & Molet, B. (1970) Two cases of myiasis by *Cordylobia rodhaini* contracted in Camaroun and diagnosed in Alsace. *Bulletin de la Société de pathologie exotique*, **63**, 592–596.
Tio, Tiong Ho (1975) Cordylobiasis in the Netherlands. *Nederlandsch tijdschrift voor geneeskunde*, **119**, 137–140.

DERMATOBIA HOMINIS INFESTATION
Aspock, H. & Leodolter, I. (1970) Vaginal myiasis from *Sarcophaga argyrostoma*. *Wiener klinische Wochenshrift*, **82**, 518–521.
De Miranda, D. V. P. (1971) Vulval myiasis. Case report and biologic study of the causative Diptera *Callotropa americana*. *Journal Brasiliaro de Gynecologia*, **72**, 309–318.
Macias, E. G., Graham, A. J., Green, M. & Pierce, A. W. (1973) Cutaneous myiasis in South Texas. *New England Journal of Medicine*, **289**, 1239–1241.
Prasad, C. & Beck, A. R. (1969) Myiasis of the scalp from *Dermatobia hominis*. *Journal of the American Medical Association*, **210**, 133.
Salomon, P. F., Catts, E. P. & Knox, W. G. (1970) Human dermal myiasis caused by rabbit bot fly in Connecticut. *Journal of the American Medical Association*, **213**, 1035–1036.
Smart, J. (1965) *Insects of Medical Importance*, 4th edn, ed. Smart, J. London: British Museum.

TUNGIASIS
Borelli, S. & Mueller, E. (1962) Tungiasis in polyclinical practice in Munich. *Hautarzt*, **13**, 23–25.
Faust, C. E. & Maxwell, T. A. (1930) The finding of the larvae of the chigoe, *Tunga penetrans*, in scrapings from human skin. *Archives of Dermatology and Syphilogy (Chicago)*, **22**, 94–97.
Londono, F. (1972) Tungiasis. In: *Essays on Tropical Dermatology*, ed. Marshall, J., Vol. 2, pp. 216–221. Amsterdam: Excerpta Medica.
Reiss, F. (1966) Tungiasis in New York City. *Archives of Dermatology*, **93**, 404–407.

BITES AND STINGS
Harman, R. R. M. (1971) Insect bites and stings. *Practitioner*, **206**, 595–602.
Harves, A. D. & Millikan, L. E. (1975) Current concepts of therapy and pathophysiology of arthropod bites and stings. *International Journal of Dermatology*, **14** (8), 543–562; (9), 621–634.
Pomeroy, A. W. J. (1921) The irritating hairs of the wild silk moths of Nigeria. *Bulletin of the Imperial Institute*, **19**, 311.
Reid, H. A. (1975) Bites and stings in travellers. *Postgraduate Medical Journal*, **51**, 830–837.
Rothschild, M., Reichstein, T., von Euw, J., Aplin, R. & Harman, R. R. M. (1970) Toxic lepidoptera. *Toxicon*, **8**, 293–299.

TUMOURS
Cox, J. W., Halprin, K. & Akerman, A. B. (1970) Kaposi's sarcoma localised to the penis. *Archives of Dermatology*, **102**, 461–462.

Masse, S. R. & Glazebrook, G. A. (1974) Kaposi's sarcoma in an Eskimo. *Canadian Medical Association Journal*, **111**, 809–811.

Palmer, P. E. S. (1972) Haemangiosarcoma of Kaposi. *Acta radiologica*, Suppl. 316, 52.

Taylor, J. F., Templeton, A. C., Votel, C. L., Ziegler, J. L. & Kalwazi, S. K. (1971) Kaposi's sarcoma in Uganda: a clinicopathological study. *International Journal of Cancer*, **8**, 122–135.

FURTHER READING
Tropical Dermatology

RECENT GENERAL REFERENCES

Canizares, O. (1975) Dermatology in Mexico. *International Journal of Dermatology*, **13**, 244–247.

Charters, A. D. (1975) A review of tropical skin diseases seen in Western Australia 1966–1973. *Australian Journal of Dermatology*, **16**, 83.

Harman, R. R. M. (1972) Ghana Medical School and dermatology. *Transactions of the St John's Hospital Dermatological Society*, **58** (2), 290–297.

Jopling, W. H. (1973) The patient from the tropics presents with skin trouble. *British Clinical Journal*, **1** (7), 5–11.

Kerdel-Vegas, F. (1973) The challenge of tropical dermatology. *Transactions of the St John's Hospital Dermatological Society*, **59** (1), 1–9.

Marshall, J. (1970) New skin diseases in Africa. *Transactions of the St John's Hospital Dermatological Society*, **56** (1), 3–10.

Marshall, J. (1973) Tropical dermatoses. *Practitioner*, **211**, 620–624.

Okoro, A. N. (1973) Skin disease in Nigeria. *Transactions of the St John's Hospital Dermatological Society*, **59** (1), 68–72.

Vollum, D. I. (1973) An impression of dermatology in Uganda. *Transactions of the St John's Hospital Dermatological Society*, **59** (1), 120–125.

Vollum, D. I. (1973) Pityriasis rosea in the African. *Transactions of the St John's Hospital Dermatological Society*, **59** (2), 269–271.

RECENT BOOKS

Canizares, O. (Ed.) (1975) *Clinical Tropical Dermatology*. Oxford: Blackwell.

Marshall, J. (Ed.) (1972) *Essays on Tropical Dermatology*, Vol. 2. Amsterdam: Excerpta Medica.

Rook, A., Wilkinson, D. S. & Ebling, F. J. G. (Eds.) (1972) *Textbook of Dermatology*, 2nd edn. Oxford: Blackwell.

Simons, R. D. G. P. & Marshall, J. (Eds.) (1969) *Essays on Tropical Dermatology*. Amsterdam: Excerpta Medica Foundation.

Tropical Diseases and Travel

GENERAL REFERENCES

Cahill, K. M. (1971) Tropical medicine and Ireland. *Journal of the Irish Medical Association*, **64**, 507–510.

Cole, A. C. E. (1973) Advances in tropical medicine. *Practitioner*, **211**, 528–534.

Dorolle, P. (1968) Old plagues in the jet age. International aspects of present and future control of communicable disease. *British Medical Journal*, **4**, 789–792.

Edington, V. M. (1971) Progress in tropical pathology with special reference to Nigeria. *Journal of the National Medical Association*, **63** (3), 181–191.

Editorial (1971) Exotic disease. *British Medical Journal*, **3**, 1–2.

Editorial (1974) La pathologie des retours de voyages en pays exotiques. *Médecine Pratique*, **3**, 1561–1562.

Flentje, B. von, Doll, H. & Steinecke, K. (1972) Intestinal parasites in citizens of the G.D.R. travelling abroad. *Deutsche Gesundheitswesen*, **27**, 90–92.

Gilbert, D. N., Moore, W. L., Hedberg, C. L. & Sanford, J. P. (1968) Potential medical problems in personnel returning from Vietnam. *Annals of Internal Medicine*, **68** (3), 662–678.

Gilles, H. M. (1975) The ecology of disease in the tropics. *Bulletin of the New York Academy of Medicine*, **51**, 621–630.

Gillis, H. M., Browne, S. G., Shrank, A. B. & Davis, A. (1975) Tropical diseases. *Medicine*, 2nd series, Part 4.

Hauser, W. (1970) Localisation of exanthemata in tropical skin diseases. *Archiv für klinische Experimentelle Dermatologie*, **237**, 330–331.

Huisman, J. & Wolthuis, F. H. (1971) Importation of exotic diseases into the Netherlands. *Folia medica neerlandica*, **14**, 1–3.

Imperato, P. J. & Wing, G. (1974) A study of patient populations in New York City Tropical Diseases Clinics. *Acta Tropica (Basle)* **31**, 97–107.

Janssens, P. G. (1970) Tropical diseases brought by travellers and immigrants. *Bruxelles Médical*, **50**, 361–369.

Joseph, S. C. (1975) Pyomyositis. A 'tropical' disease? *American Journal of Diseases of Children*, **129**, 775–776.

Kyronseppa, H. (1971) Tropiikkituristin Tautiprofylaksi. *Duodecim*, **87**, 1353–55.

Laverdant, M. C., André, L. J., Charmot, G., Gentilini, M. & Pene, P. (1974) Practical problems posed by imported tropical diseases. *Cahiers de Médecine*, **15**, 711–729.

Le Riche, W. H. & Lenczner, M. M. (1973) New migration pattern increases incidence in Canada of diseases common in tropical areas. *Canadian Medical Association Journal*, **109**, 546–548.

Maegraith, B. G. (1969) Tropical medicine today (Presidential Address of 63rd session of the Society). *Transactions of the Royal Society of Tropical Medicine and Hygiene*, **63**, 689–707.

Maegraith, B. G. (1974) Tropical medicine: trends and progress. *Journal of Tropical Medicine and Hygiene*, **77**, Suppl. 4, 4–7.

Malcolm, N. (1972) Fitness for the tropics. *Practitioner*, **208**, 268.

Medical Staff Conference (1969) Diseases from Vietnam. *California Medicine*, **111**, 461–466.

Mello, S. (1968) The superiority of tropical man. *Revista Brasileira de Medicina (Rio de Janeiro)*, **24**, 446–449.

Penman, H. G. (1971) Tropical pathology by post: a Fijian experience. *New Zealand Medical Journal*, **73**, 83–85.

Ridley, D. S. (1974) The laboratory diagnosis of tropical diseases with special reference to Britain: a review. *Journal of Clinical Pathology*, **57**, 435–444.

Rowland, H. A. K. (1970) Management of patients recently arrived from the tropics. *British Medical Journal*, **3**, 447–449.

Seah, S. K. K. (1974) Tropical medicine in Canada—problems and prospects. *Canadian Journal of Public Health*, **65**, 269–272.

Starkey, D. H. (1973) Problems of tropical and exotic diseases affecting Canadian medicine: a perspective. *Canadian Journal of Public Health*, **64**, 103–106.

Stevenson, D. (1974) Tropical medicine and international health. *Central African Journal of Medicine*, **20**, 9–12.

Woodruff, A. W. (1958) Tropical diseases in Great Britain. *Transactions of the Medical Society of London*, 185th session, **74**, 140–151.

Woodruff, A. W. (1968) Advances in the treatment of tropical diseases. *The Practitioner*, **201**, 638–645.

Woodruff, A. W. (1968) Current practice in tropical medicine (Lettsomian lectures). *Transactions of the Medical Society of London*, **85**, 111–143.

Woodruff, A. W. (1972) Tropical ophthalmology: ocular involvement in tropical disease. *Proceedings of the Royal Society of Medicine*, **65**, 953.

Woodruff, A. W. (1973) The clinical unit in tropical medicine and epidemiology. *Transactions of the Royal Society of Tropical Medicine and Hygiene*, **67**, 755–769.

Woodruff, A. W. (1975) Diseases of travel with particular reference to tropical diseases. *Postgraduate Medical Journal*, **51**, 825–829.

BOOKS

Cahill, K. M. (1964) *Tropical Diseases in Temperate Climates*. Philadelphia: Lippincott.

Jopling, W. H. (1968) *The Treatment of Tropical Diseases*, 2nd edn. Bristol: Wright.

Maegraith, B. G. (1965) *Exotic Diseases in Practice*. London: Heinemann.

Maegraith, B. G. & Gillis, H. M. (1971) *Management and Treatment of Tropical Diseases*. Oxford: Blackwell.

USEFUL BOOKLETS

Department of Health and Social Security (1972) *Communicable Diseases Contracted Outside Great Britain.* London: HMSO.

Maegraith, B. G. (1971) *Imported Diseases in Europe*, p. 34. Basle: Ciba-Geigy.

Central Office of Information (1975) *Notice to Travellers. Health Protection.* London: HMSO.

Preservation of Personal Health in Warm Climates (1974) 7th edn. London: The Ross Institute of Tropical Hygiene.

5

SWEAT GLANDS AND THEIR DISORDERS

Katherine Grice   Julian Verbov

The sweat gland in mammals has been described as a protective organ (Jenkinson, 1969, 1973). Sweat secretion protects the body against high environmental temperature, helps keep the horny layer pliable and prevents frictional damage to special areas such as the palm and eyelid. Sweat glands excrete waste products and possibly by acting as scent glands may be partially responsible for the perpetuation of the species. Animals may use sweat to mark the limit of territorial ownership.

Classification of sweat glands

All sweat glands have probably evolved from an unidentified but primitive sweat gland. Human sweat glands are usually classified into eccrine and apocrine and these are easily separated as they differ in distribution, structure and function (Ellis, 1968). For man and other mammals a different method of classification has been suggested, depending on anatomical or functional differences in sweat glands.

1. *Anatomical.* Apocrine ducts open into hair follicles or occasionally just beside the follicle; they have been renamed epitrichial (associated with a hair follicle) sweat glands. Eccine ducts open directly on to the skin surface and have been renamed atrichial (not connected or related to a hair follicle) glands (Bligh, 1967). This is probably the safest classification to use while awaiting the complete understanding of sweat gland physiology in the animal kingdom (Jenkinson, 1973).

2. *Histological.* The eccrine secretory coil contains two types of secretory cells, the clear and dark cells, whereas apocrine secretory cells are of one cell type only. A classification based on these differences has been suggested but these differences occur only in primates (and perhaps the horse).

3. *Histochemical.* A classification based on the histochemical staining differences between apocrine and eccrine glands has been suggested, but there is a wide variety of histochemical characteristics of sweat glands in animals.

4. *Neural control.* The sudomotor mechanism is essentially cholinergic for eccrine glands and adrenergic for apocrine glands. It has been suggested that this is a satisfactory method for classifying sweat glands (Robertshaw, 1974).

ECCRINE SWEAT GLANDS

Function

The vast majority of sweat glands are eccrine and their function is mainly for temperature regulation. During prolonged fasting, the consumption of glucose for metabolic purposes decreases in the brain, kidney and muscle but sweat gland consumption of glucose decreases remarkably little. This suggests that sweat glands, because temperature control is so important must have a high priority during starvation, when carbohydrate supplies are limited (Benson et al, 1974). Disorders of sweat gland function may cause profound systemic effects.

Thermoregulation

Sweating occurs in response to heat stimulation either from rise in environmental temperature or endogenously from rise in body temperature due to exercise, infection, etc. Temperature change affects sweat glands via local and central mechanisms (Cooper, 1970; Myers, 1971).

LOCAL MECHANISMS

Nadel, Bullard and Stolwijk (1971) suggested that the release of transmitter substance (acetylcholine) from nerves supplying the sweat gland is directly temperature dependent. As skin temperature rises, more transmitter substance is released and sweating increases. Sato (1973b) finds direct cooling of sweat glands in vitro (to 4°C) abolishes sweating. Rising skin temperature increases the sensitivity of sweat glands, as shown by the fact that sweat produced by local injections of acetylcholine, is more easily triggered off when the skin temperature is raised (Ogawa, 1970): this effect is unchanged by nerve block.

CENTRAL MECHANISMS

Body temperature is controlled by centres in the hypothalamus (hypothalamic thermoregulation centre) where the 'thermostat setting' is regulated. Receptors in the hypothalamus which are temperature sensitive can alter the setting of the 'thermostat' (Benzinger, 1969). Sodium ions in the hypothalamus raise the 'set point' and calcium ions lower the 'set point' (Myers, 1971).

It has been suggested that circulating noradrenaline and 5-hydroxytryptamine might be important in hypothalamic tremperature regulation. In animal species, adrenaline and noradrenaline injected directly into cerebral ventricles lower body temperature (Handley and Spencer, 1972) while 5-hydroxytryptamine raises body temperature. Rise of body core temperature increases sweating, but skin temperature modifies this reaction possibly by setting the 'thermostat' in the hypothalamus at a different level. Cold receptors in the skin ensure that under normal circumstances one avoids extreme skin temperature changes by adjusting the amount of clothes worn, etc.

Emotional sweating

The palms and soles have been described as areas where eccrine sweating is triggered off by emotional stress rather than heat. Allen, Armstrong and Roddie (1973) have suggested that with emotional stimuli sweat glands in these areas behave in the same way as they do in the rest of the body, there are merely more of them. They found the sweat output from four different areas— hands and feet, head and neck, arms and legs, and the trunk, increased markedly with stress. The sweat output from each area was roughly proportional to the calculated number of sweat glands in that area. This confirms previous observations (Bettley and Grice, 1965). The density of sweat glands is highest on the sole, approximately $620/cm^2$, and lowest on the thigh $120/cm^2$ (Ellis, 1968).

Friction and grip

Sweat glands in the palms and soles are said to be analogous to those in the foot and toe pads of animals, the function of which is thought to be to help grip and prevent frictional damage (Weiner and Hellmann, 1960). Adams and Hunter (1969) have found at low sweat rates skin friction or grip is increased, due to elevation of the water content of the stratum corneum. This may be due to seepage of sweat through the walls of the duct as it corkscrews up in the stratum corneum. At higher sweat rates, however, even before microscopic sweat is seen on the surface, frictional resistance decreases. Ellis (1972) suggests that sweat needed to increase gripping power may be reinforced in other ways, as in the manual labourer who spits on his hands before grasping heavy loads or the South American roll-tail monkey who urinates on his hands and feet when frightened, possibly to ensure a speedy getaway.

The damage produced by friction can be judged by measuring the time a friction-producing machine takes to form a skin erosion (Comaish and Bottoms, 1971; Comaish, 1973). Glutaraldehyde, an antiperspirant, increases the time taken to produce skin damage by friction in normal subjects as well as in patients with epidermolysis bullosa, porphyria cutanea tarda and bullous pemphigoid. The effect of glutaraldehyde on friction may not be due solely to its antiperspirant effect as it is equally effective in vitro as well as in vivo. It was suggested that glutaraldehyde might be helpful in preventing blisters and indeed in epidermolysis bullosa this has been shown to be true.

Regional and individual variation in sweat production

The number of active and resting sweat glands at any one time varies not only in different regions but also in different individuals under identical conditions. Excluding the palm and sole the number of active glands is highest on the forehead (average $181/cm^2$, range 111–313) and lowest on the back (average $64/cm^2$, range 37–121). Sweat electrolyte content also varies. Sato and Dobson (1970a) thought the difference between people was largely due to a different capacity of the sweat gland both to secrete sweat in the secreting coil and also to reabsorb sodium in the duct. Some people's sweat glands are fired off more easily and at lower skin temperature, as happens with heat acclimatisation or sweat gland training. During acclimatisation, sweat sodium output is low only when there is a deficient sodium intake. When this is rectified sweat sodium concentration returns to normal (Smiles and Robinson, 1971).

The differences between various areas in the same person are thought to be due merely to a difference in the number of sweat glands present. An amusing method for studying regional variation in skin temperature is by Aga colour thermovision. A multicoloured man is shown on the screen, with different colours representing varying skin temperatures. When he starts running, the colours and patterns change dramatically (Clark, Mullan and Pugh, 1974).

Newborn infants

Hypothermia is common in the newborn; at birth sweating is deficient both in the premature and full-term infant (Hey and Katz, 1969). Very premature infants (less than 30 gestational weeks) are incapable of sweating at birth even though their rectal temperature be raised or acetylcholine injected (Foster, Hey and Katz, 1969). In less premature infants, at birth sweating is mainly confined to the face, and by 34 to 37 gestational weeks sweat appears on the limbs, spreading to the trunk later. By 7 to 14 days after birth sweat appears in all areas, palmar sweating usually being detected in normal newborn babies before or on the third day (Verbov and Baxter, 1974). Sweat glands in infants are less responsive to acetylcholine injection than are those of adults, maximum sweat rate being three times lower than that of adults, when tested 7 to 10 days after birth.

It seems that a fully functional sweat gland at birth depends on an intact central nervous system in utero, because infants with severe congenital brain defects (anencephalus, microencephalus, etc.) are incapable of sweating even though local pilocarpine be injected. At autopsy these infants show an apparently normal sympathetic system and normal sweat glands. Foster et al (1969) suggested that some of the fleeting rashes infants develop soon after birth may be due to miliaria.

Structure

The eccrine gland, a coiled blind tubule opening on to the skin surface, is usually divided into four segments for descriptive and functional purposes: the terminal secretory coil, the coiled duct, the straight duct, and the intra-epithelial duct (Ellis, 1968).

The secretory coil

Three cell types are surrounded by an amorphous basement membrane (Fig. 5.1).

Myoepithelial cells have ultrastructure reminiscent of muscle cells. Myofibrils nearly fill the cytoplasm and where there is contact between adjacent cells the bond is similar to that found between smooth muscle cells. Myoepithelial cells lie on the external basement membrane with some gaps between the cells. These gaps are filled by the clear cells and the heavily folded intercellular spaces or canaliculi. Myoepithelial cells may act as valves controlling the area of clear cells exposed to the basement membrane or extracellular fluid. They may also help expel sweat.

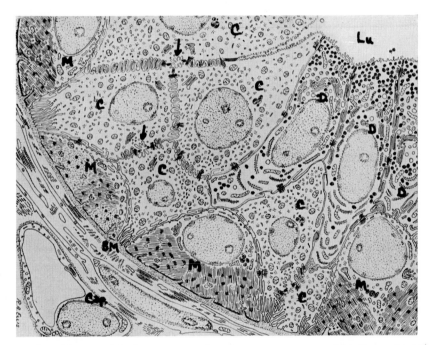

Figure 5.1 Diagram of the fine structure of eccrine sweat secretory coil kindly provided by Professor Ellis (Ellis, 1968). The pavement myoepithelium (M), clear cells (C), intercellular canaliculi (arrows), dark granular cells (D), capillary (cap), lumen (Lu), and basement membrane (BM)

Clear cells resemble the salt and water secreting epithelial cells from other parts of the body. They border on the intercellular spaces and have elaborately folded basal membranes. Extracellular fluid, from the capillary network surrounding the secretory coil, crosses the basement membrane filter, and enters the intercellular spaces. Fluid is absorbed into the clear cells where precursor sweat is formed and excreted into the lumen (Hashimoto, 1971).

Dark cells are smaller than clear cells. Their bases line the lumen with short microvilli, and their ultrastructure is that of a mucin-producing cell.

Basement membrane is a term applied to the extracellular tissue enveloping the secretory coil of the sweat gland as seen in light microscopy (Cotta-Pereira, Rodrigo and Bittencourt-Sampaio, 1975).

Electron microscopy has shown that the basement membrane consists of an inner layer formed by a dense filamentous sheet—the basal lamina—which is connected to the myoepithelial cells and clear cells by half desmosomes. Outside the basal lamina is an amorphous sheath surrounded by collagen fibres and two of the constituents of the elastic system—elaunin and oxytalan.

The pigment lipofuscin occurs in the secretory coil and is probably related to lysosomes. It has been known as the 'wear and tear' pigment as the number of granules in the secretory coil increases with age. The youngest child whose sweat glands showed pigment in one study was aged six years (Cawley et al, 1973).

Intradermal sweat duct (coiled and straight)

The duct is lined by two layers of cells, an outer ring of basal cells and an inner ring of cuticular cells.

Basal cells have ultrastructure similar to ion-secreting cells in the rest of the body. In the coiled duct the basal cells contain more mitochondria and have a more elaborate villous border than they do in the straight duct. This suggests the coiled duct is more active in sodium reabsorption than is the straight duct (Sato, Dobson and Mali, 1971). Mitotic activity is confined to the basal cells of the eccrine duct in mouse foot pads. An inhibitor of eccrine duct mitosis (sweat chalone) has been found in human sweat (Bullough and Deol, 1972).

Cuticular (superficial or luminal) cells line the lumen with short stumpy microvilli and a cuticular border formed by very fine fibrils. The cuticular border is more marked as it approaches the epidermis. The function of the cuticular border may be to impede absorption of ions. It has also been suggested that it strengthens and maintains the shape of the sweat duct. Cuticular cells have a great capacity for regeneration. After destruction of the intraepidermal sweat duct, cuticular cells of the straight duct migrate into the dermis in a tightly coiled spiral (Lobitz, Holyoke and Montagna, 1954).

Intraepidermal sweat duct

The inner sleeve of cells lining the lumen resemble the cuticular cells of the straight duct. The outer coats are formed by three or four layers of cells similar to epidermal cells. The coiling epidermal sweat duct unit also called the acrosyringium, projects down into the dermis. The duct coils two to three times in the epidermis before entering the stratum corneum where the duct then usually coils about six times (Christophers and Plewig, 1973).

The surface spirals of the sweat duct have been studied by microtopography (Sarkany, 1962; Sarkany, Shuster and Stammers, 1965). A mould is made of the skin surface. The impression thus made is coated and this replica of the skin surface which has been produced can be viewed by scanning electron microscopy (Johnson, Dawber and Shuster, 1970). Scanning electron micro-scopy has also been used on skin biopsies (Papa, 1972).

On the palms and soles the spirals of the sweat duct can be seen following the contours of the funnel-shaped sweat pore opening with a nipple-like projection in the centre (Fig. 5.2). Sweat pores on the palms, soles and dorsa of the distal phalanx and anterior surfaces of the wrist are pit-like and easily visible. Sweat pores from elsewhere are slit-like and difficult to see (Wolf,

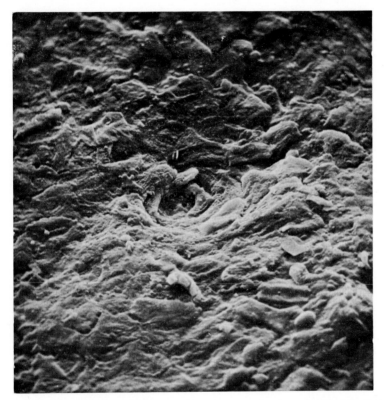

Figure 5.2   Palmar sweat pore. Imprint scanning electron microscopy. × 500. (Kindly lent by Dr R. Dawber)

1970). Johnson et al (1970) showed that on the forearms and trunk the terminal spiral was almost flush with the skin surface, occurring in elevations surrounded by fine skin creases so that even with electron microscopy orifices were easily missed.

On the palm, eccrine ducts open at the apices of ridges and only very rarely in the sulci or on ridge margins (Verbov, 1973). In the newborn infant there is no clear-cut relationship between ridge height and palmar sweating although marked ridge flattening is always associated with absence of sweating (Verbov, 1975).

Sweat Production

Discharge of sweat on to the skin surface depends upon the rate of sweat secretion into the secretory coil of sweat glands. The myoepithelial cells probably contract rhythmically, but seem likely to have little effect on the rate of sweat discharge in man (Bligh, 1967). Eccrine sweat is secreted through intact cellular membranes of the secreting cell and does not contain cytoplasmic material.

Secretory coil

Dark cells in the secretory coil produce mucin (a mucopolysaccharide) which is thought to line the sweat duct.

Clear cells produce aqueous sweat (Dobson and Sato, 1972). The fluid formed in the secretory coil is isotonic or slightly hypertonic to plasma. This has been shown by direct micropuncture of the sweat coil (Schulz et al, 1965; Schulz, 1969) and also by dissecting out the eccrine gland and collecting sweat in vitro by glass pipettes (Sato, 1973b).

The sweat precursor in the secretory coil is thought to be produced by active transport of sodium from the extracellular fluid, into the sweat coil, water then passively follows the sodium across. The sodium pump (or sodium transport system) is thought to be located in the clear cell intercanaliculi. It is suggested the sodium pump at the closed or distal end of the intercanaliculus, functions at low sweat rates. When sweating increases the pump starts functioning all along the canalicus (Slegers and Hof-Grootenboer, 1971; Dobson and Sato, 1972). The energy for the sodium pump involves the enzyme Na–K-sensitive ATPase and glucose (which is broken down to lactate or CO_2).

Sweat duct

The function of isolated sweat ducts has been studied in vitro by microanalytical methods (Mangos, 1973). The isotonic solution in the secretory coil passes into the coiled duct where more sodium than water is absorbed. Thus the hypotonic sweat solution is formed.

Reabsorption of water does not occur at high sweat rates, but with decreasing sweat rates, water reabsorption increases, but is still small. The net sodium reabsorption remains constant at different sweat flow rates. This can be explained by the fact that sodium is not only reabsorbed from the sweat, but is also excreted back into the lumen. This two-directional flow of sodium keeps the net sodium reabsorption constant. At high flow rates, less sodium is reabsorbed but more sodium diffuses back. Potassium is excreted into the sweat. Its passage across the duct wall is thus in the opposite direction to that of sodium. Sodium and potassium are thought to be actively transported through the duct by a mechanism involving Na–K-sensitive ATPase. The sweat coil and proximal duct contain 10 times more of this enzyme than does the distal tubule (Sato, Dobson and Mali, 1971).

From single human sweat gland studies, the sweat duct has been shown to take up bicarbonate and excrete hydrogen ions. The excretion is probably essential for sodium absorption and potassium excretion (Kaiser, Songo-Williams and Drack, 1974). The amount of sodium absorbed is much greater than the amount of potassium excreted. Hydrogen ions are probably exchanged with sodium. The hydrogen ion production is carbonic anhydrase dependent and acetazolamide (Diamox) sensitive. Lactate is excreted in high concentrations in sweat. It is known that as sweat rate increases, so also its sodium and chloride concentrations rise (Johnson, Morimoto and Robbins, 1969). This is what one would expect from the isotonic precursor fluid passing down the duct, and sodium being reabsorbed at a steady rate unrelated to the amount of sweat passing through the duct.

Prostaglandin E_2 has been found in human eccrine sweat (Frewin et al, 1973; Förström, Goldyne and Winkelmann, 1974) and it has been suggested its function might be to regulate sodium and water reabsorption in the sweat duct. In the kidney tubule and gut this is known to be one of their functions. In atopic eczema, psoriasis and hyperhidrosis, the prostaglandin activity in sweat is greater than normal.

Effect of aldosterone, hydrocortisone and antidiuretic hormone (ADH) in vivo. The rate of sweat flow is reduced, by local injection of D-aldosterone, but not by hydrocortisone. Both drugs increase the reabsorption of sodium by the duct and raise excretion of potassium (Sato and Dobson, 1970b). ADH increases both water and sodium reabsorption by the sweat duct (Fasciolo, Totel and Johnson, 1969). The concentration of sweat sodium chloride is increased in untreated adrenal insufficiency (Mearns, 1974).

Sweat compared with urine, saliva or other exocrine fluids. The sweat gland is often compared with the nephron. It has been pointed out, however, that although there are some similarities there are many differences. Urea clearance for example is similar in the nephron and sweat gland (sweat gland clearance being one fifth to one half of simultaneous renal clearance). The clearance of creatinine is quite different. Sweat gland clearance of creatinine is only 1/50 to 1/300 of that of the nephron (Johnson et al, 1969). These authors suggested the sweat gland should not be compared with the nephron or other exocrine glands as they all have different functions and different methods for producing their exocrine fluids.

Pharmacology of Eccrine Sweating

CHOLINERGIC CONTROL

As is well known, human eccrine sweat glands are innervated by sympathetic nerves transmitting cholinergic fibres. Electron microscopic studies suggest that the nerves may not supply the glands directly but supply the capillary plexus surrounding the glands (Jenkinson, 1973). Acetylcholine-induced sweating starts within a few seconds (5–15 s) of injection, is very protracted and the threshold dose is similar in all subjects ($10^{-3} \pm$ s.e. 10^{-4} μg/0.1 ml) (Foster, 1971).

ADRENERGIC CONTROL

The existence and importance of adrenergically controlled eccrine sweating in man has not yet been clarified. Eccrine sweat glands respond to intradermal, intravenous and intra-arterial adrenaline (Foster, Ginsburg and Weiner, 1970) but whether the response is merely a phylogenetic relic or whether it has functional importance is still unknown (Robertshaw, 1974).

Adrenaline-induced eccrine sweating is not blocked by atropine and is less than that produced by acetylcholine. The lower sweat output from adrenaline may be due to the concomitant vasoconstriction it produces, thus the dose of the drug reaching the sweat gland is less. Although eccrine sweat glands respond to adrenaline, no adrenergic fibres have been found in nerves supplying eccrine sweat glands. The catecholamines (adrenaline and noradrenaline) probably reach the eccrine glands via the circulation. The amount of catecholamines released into the blood stream by the adrenal medulla increases during asphyxia and exercise. In man the dose of intra-arterial adrenaline which induces eccrine sweating (4–10 μg/min) is probably higher than that ever reached during exercise or asphyxia but these levels are reached in the presence of pheochromocytoma (Foster, et al, 1970). Eccrine sweating induced by pheochromocytoma can, however, be blocked by atropine which suggests it is cholinergically controlled (Prout and Wardell, 1969).

Eccrine sweat glands possibly have both α-adrenocreceptors (Foster and Weiner, 1970) and β-adrenoreceptors (Allen and Roddie, 1972). In thyrotoxicosis the hyperhidrosis produced by circulating catecholamines from the adrenal medulla may be mediated via β-adrenoreceptors. The amount of sweat produced by adrenaline, whether in the palms or forearms, varies considerably in different individuals, is not abolished by atropine (Wolf and Maibach, 1974) and lasts for a short time (Warndorff and Neefs, 1971). Spontaneous palmar sweating is abolished by atropine.

The possible function that adrenaline may have on eccrine sweating has not been clarified. Contraction of eccrine myoepithelial cells may be under adrenergic control (Blight, 1967) but adrenaline may also affect sweat secretion. Sato (1973b) using the isolated sweat gland in vitro, found that acetylcholine and adrenaline produced a similar amount of sweat from the secretory coil and that the sweat sodium and potassium content was also similar. He suggested both drugs activate the sodium pump by increasing the rate of sodium passage from the extracellular fluid into the secretory cell. The adrenaline induced sweat response lasts for a much shorter time than does that produced by cholinergic stimulation. It was thought that the function of adrenaline might be similar to that found in the parotid and submandibular glands, i.e. to control various biochemical syntheses. β-adrenergic stimulation of eccrine sweat glands in vitro was found to stimulate glucose metabolism via the pentose cycle which is mediated by intracellular AMP (Sato, 1973a).

Excretion in Sweat

Non-electrolytes such as urea, are excreted in sweat. The main barrier to their passage from plasma to sweat is thought to be the basal membrane of the sweat gland secretory coil (Slegers, 1969).

Drugs

The sweat gland epithelium is more permeable to the unionised form of drugs (Schanker, 1964), the unionised molecule diffusing more readily through sweat gland epithelium.

Sulphonamide compounds which are completely unionised in plasma, appear in sweat in concentrations approaching that found in plasma, the more unionsed the compound the higher its relative concentration in sweat.

Antipyrine and aminopyrine are found in sweat at a concentration nearly as high as that in plasma (Brusilow and Gordes, 1966; Johnson and Maibach, 1971). These are lipid soluble drugs and dissolve in the lipid of the basement membrane as they diffuse through (Slegers, 1969). pH is important as it determines the fraction of drug present in the unionised lipid soluble state.

Ethyl alcohol. After absorption and equilibrium, ethyl alcohol is evenly distributed throughout total body-water, and its concentration in sweat and urine is the same (Pawan and Grice, 1968). Water-soluble drugs like ethyl alcohol probably pass through minute pores or channels in the sweat gland membrane. The concentration of drugs in sweat remains constant in spite of increasing sweat rate, produced by generalised heating (Johnson and Maibach, 1971) or localised pharmacological stimulation of sweat glands. Considering that the body can produce up to 12 litres of sweat per day, the amount of alcohol excreted in sweat can be very large and may explain the observation that tolerance to alcohol is higher in hot climates than in a more temperate one (Grice, J. W. H., personal communication).

Griseofulvin. Within 8 h of ingestion, griseofulvin appears in all layers of the stratum corneum (Knight, 1974). Its concentration is higher in the outermost layers of the stratum corneum. This concentration gradient disappears when sweat gland occlusion is produced by wearing a rubber glove. Griseofulvin has been found in sweat and it is suggested that the high surface content of the drug has been produced by deposition from surface sweat (Epstein, Shah and Riegelman, 1972; Shah, Epstein and Riegelman, 1974).

Bullous and necrotic lesions in drug-induced coma. Toxic skin lesions are found in 4 per cent of patients with barbiturate coma and in 40 per cent of those that die. The lesions consist of large bullae, vesicles or plaques followed by ulceration with a burn-like eschar (Almeyda and Levantine, 1972). The sites involved are pressure areas on the buttocks, posterior or lateral aspects of the thighs, and sides and dorsa of the fingers and toes. Beveridge (1970) suggests that barbiturates collect in sweat in large concentrations at sites where there is sweat duct blockage and skin maceration. Skin biopsy shows subepidermal bullae with barbiturates in the blister fluid, and necrosis of sweat gland and of periductal epithelium.

Similar lesions have been described in overdose due to imipramine, meprobamate, glutethimide, methadone, and nitrazepam (Ridley, 1971) and in carbon monoxide poisoning (Leavell, Farley and McIntyre, 1969).

Quinine (Comaish and Shelley, 1965) and *amphetamine* (Vree, Muskens and Van Rossum, 1972) have been found in sweat. Doping of athletes might be controlled by measuring sweat amphetamines.

Lead is excreted in sweat in a similar concentration to that found in urine (Allen, Moore and Hunter, 1975).

Drug eruptions. Skin eruptions due to drug sensitivity in some cases may be related to the fact that they are excreted in sweat (Johnson and Maibach, 1971).

Infections

Hepatitis. Hepatitis B antigen (HBAg) has been found in sweat (Telater et al, 1974) as well as in faeces, urine, saliva and semen (Heathcote, Cameron and Dane, 1974). Minute amounts of HBAg may be infectious, therefore with skin contaminated by sweat HBAg, direct contact with infectious hepatitis patients may be epidemiologically important.

Proteins. Amino acids and protein are excreted in sweat and it has been suggested that they may provide a medium for bacterial growth on the skin surface (Jenkinson, Mabon and Manson, 1974).

Immunoglobulins

IgG, IgA, IgD (Page and Remington, 1967) and IgE have been found in sweat (Förström, Goldyne and Winkelmann, 1975).

Hyperhidrosis

Excessive sweating occurs in a host of conditions such as hyperthyroidism, and hyperpituitarism. Recently some of the mechanisms involved have been clarified, new causes discovered and treatment improved.

Physiological

Acclimatisation, the menopause, gustatory sweating on the face after eating spicy food (and occasionally cheese and chocolate) can all produce profuse sweating. Sweat rate is usually the same on the two sides of the body (Gibiński et al, 1971) but differences can occur.

Neurological

'It has become apparent that defects in autonomic function occur commonly in many diseases and are more dangerous and disabling than was appreciated' (Johnson and Spalding, 1974). These authors pointed out that the site of damage to the sympathetic pathway can be investigated by the following simple tests:

INVESTIGATIONS

Total body heating. This will show up areas of hypohidrosis and hyperhidrosis. Legs or an arm placed in water at 42°C in a room temperature of 30°C produces copious sweating. Postganglionic fibres destined for sweat glands (sudomotor) are supplied by spinal cord segments: T2–T4 for the head and neck, T2–T8 for the upper limbs, T6–T10 for the trunk, and T11–L2 for the legs.

Ganglionic and postganglionic lesions. Sweat glands need an intact ganglionic and postganglionic nerve supply in order to respond to local injection of acetylcholine. Sweating and piloerection are produced by acetylcholine if the lesion is preganglionic, but not if the lesion is ganglionic or postganglionic.

Sweat gland. Pilocarpine acts directly on the sweat gland. Pilocarpine injection will produce sweat if there is a lesion in the sympathetic nerve but not if sweat glands are absent.

PERIPHERAL NERVE LESIONS AND CAUSALGIA

Causalgia, a painful condition caused by an incomplete lesion of a peripheral nerve, usually affects the sciatic or median nerve (Richards, 1967). Burning pain with partial sensory loss and hyperhidrosis results. A cervical rib can cause hyperhidrosis of the hand (Ellis, 1972).

SPINAL CORD LESIONS

These produce hyperhidrosis mostly at the border of the anaesthetic skin area. Sweating is thought to be an irritant phenomenon (Johnson and Prout, 1967).

PARKINSON'S DISEASE

Hyperhidrosis of the face may occur to compensate for anhidrosis of the limbs and trunk (Appenzeller and Goss, 1971).

PATHOLOGICAL GUSTATORY SWEATING

Pathological gustatory sweating occurs when parasympathetic nerves previously innervating a salivary gland or the stomach regenerate mistakenly along sympathetic nerves, innervating sweat glands.

Auriculo-temporal syndrome (Frey) occurs frequently after operations on the parotoid gland; the secreto-motor fibres of the parotoid growing into the auriculo-temporal branch of the trigeminal nerve. Unilateral facial sweating occurs after food. Various surgical techniques are used to interrupt the nerve pathways, e.g. the destruction of the nerve plexus around the middle ear (tympanic nerectomy) or the resection of the auriculo-temporal nerve or intracranial section of the glossopharyngeal nerve (Edison, 1974).

Cervical symapthetic plexus may be damaged at the thoracic inlet, for instance during operation for sympathectomy, and sweating then occurs when eating (Greenhalgh, Rosengarten and Martin, 1971).

Diabetes mellitus. Drenching bilateral facial sweating brought on by eating food, especially cheese, can spread to the neck, shoulder and upper chest (Watkins, 1973). Degeneration of the autonomic nervous system occurs in diabetes and it is suggested aberrant regeneration accounts for the gustatory sweating.

Idiopathic unilateral gustatory sweating has been described on the face, knee and wrist associated with enlarged sweat glands (Cunliffe, Johnson and Williamson, 1972).

Infections

During infections bacterial pyrogens are released in the blood and act directly on the hypothalamus to raise body temperature (by the release of 5-hydroxytryptamine from platelets and also by lowering the calcium concentration in the hypothalamus) (Myers, 1971).

Tetanus. Overactivity of sympathetic nerves comparable to the overactivity of motor nerves may produce hyperhidrosis in tetanus (Kerr et al, 1968).

Hirsutism

Burton et al (1972) studied 13 hirsute women and found significantly increased mean rates of sweat and sebum secretion and plasma testosterone concentration compared with control women. These writers suggested that the whole skin is virilised in hirsutism presumably due to androgenic stimulation.

Defects of neurohumoral transmitter

Shock, hypoglycaemia and pheochromocytoma. Profuse sweating and vaso-constriction in these conditions is possibly due to an increased amount of circulating noradrenaline and adrenaline (Foster, Ginsburg and Weiner, 1970). Hyperhidrosis induced by a pheochromocytoma can be inhibited by the cholinergic blocking agent hyoscine (Prout and Wardell, 1969).

Familial dysautonomia (Riley–Day syndrome) occurs in children and is characterised by drenching sweats, absence of tears ('crying without tears'), pain insensitivity and absence of fungiform papillae of the tongue. Many of the symptoms are due to autonomic nervous system disturbances. The blood vessel changes produce flushing with erythema in large blotches or in a pin-head sized pattern, oedema of the hands and face and labile hypertension (Brunt and McKusick, 1970). It is autosomal recessive and occurs only in Jewish children of Ashkenazi stock. The cause is unknown but there is

excessive sensitivity to acetylcholine and the excretion in urine of the metabolites of adrenaline and noradrenaline is abnormal—elevated excretion of
homovanillic acid (HVA) and decreased excretion of vanillylmandelic acid
(VMA) and 3-methoxy-4-hydroxyphenylethyleneglycol (HMPG). It has
been suggested that there is an abnormality in the synthesis of these catecholamines (Gitlow et al, 1970) which may be secondary to a neurological
defect.

Abnormalities in the central nervous system have been found and in the
peripheral nerves there is a paucity of unmyelinated nerves (Aguoyo, Nair and
Bray, 1971).

Idiopathic Hyperhidrosis

The aetiology of idiopathic hyperhidrosis is still unknown, but treatment
has improved.

BILATERAL HYPERHIDROSIS

Drenching sweats may be confined to the axillae, palms and soles or may be
widespread. Axillary hyperhidrosis, like that of the palms and soles, is due to
eccrine sweating. In a patient with idiopathic palmar hyperhidrosis, Allen,
Armstrong and Roddie (1974) studied the sweat rate from different areas
using various stimuli. The patient had a higher resting palmar sweat output
than did controls. Emotional stress produced excessive sweating from all
areas, but the effect of heat was the same as in controls. Blood flow in the
finger was increased in a patient with idopathic hyperhidrosis, when compared
with the other side which had been treated by sympathetomy: the capillaries
were dilated as shown by electron microscopy and there was an increased
bleeding time (Burch and Kones, 1973): The blood vessel changes could have
been secondary to vasodilator kinins excreted in sweat (Fox and Hilton,
1958).

UNILATERAL LOCALISED HYPERHIDROSIS

Unilateral hyperhidrosis of the scalp and forehead in the area of skin
supplied by the ophthalmic division of the trigeminal nerve was described by
Verbov (1974). Sweating was unrelated to food and was of recent origin.
Unilateral profuse sweating since infancy on the dorsum of the forearm was
investigated in two women by Cunliffe et al (1972). They found on the affected
side increased sweating was produced by heat and cholinergic stimuli, and the
sweat glands were enlarged. They suggested the hyperhidrosis could have been
due either to a congenital functional abnormality of sweat glands (functional
naevus) or to primary enlargement of the glands (anatomical naevus).

Treatment

Both medical and surgical treatment of hyperhidrosis has aroused a good
deal of interest (Frain-Bell, 1969; *Lancet*, 1974).

A. MEDICAL

The search continues for an effective, non-toxic antiperspirant for treating hyperhidrosis of the palms, soles and axillae. Sweating elsewhere can now be successfully treated.

1. *Anticholinergic compounds.* Frankland and Seville (1971) used propantheline (Probanthine) spray (1.8–3.6 mg dose) twice daily to the sole of the foot. Sweating diminishes and macerative keratolysis (keratolysis plantaris sulcatum) improves. Poldine methosulphate (Nacton) is a useful antiperspirant (Grice and Bettley, 1966). Topical application of poldine methosulphate (4–8 per cent) in methyl alcohol abolishes sweating for two to three days. Unfortunately like all antiperspirants it is less effective on the palms, soles and axillae especially in the presence of hyperhidrosis. The anhidrotic effect of the drug has been enhanced by polythene occlusion; in the axillae self-cling polythene (Cling-wrap) can be wrapped around the shoulders. For toe webs and groins 4 per cent poldine methosulphate in absorbable dusting powder (Boots K285) is useful. Side effects do not occur with low dosage, but when high concentrations are used on large areas, systemic effects such as a dry mouth, are produced.

Decrease of palmar sweating produced by poldine methosulphate under occlusion to one hand, may be associated with diminished sweating on the opposite untreated side. The mechanism of this contralateral sweat inhibition does not seem to depend always on systemic absorption. Thus, contralateral sweat inhibition was produced by applying unilaterally atropine sulphate or aluminium chloride to rat paws. The dose absorbed was too small to inhibit sweating and it was suggested the mechanism of contralateral sweat inhibition was neural in origin (Hitchens et al, 1972).

Mechanism of anhidrotic action. Anticholinergic compounds act directly on sweat glands. Scopolamine when applied topically to produce anhidrosis causes no blockage of the sweat duct at the level of the stratum corheum. This can be shown by the fact that the sweat rate is unaffected after the stratum corneum is stripped off.

2. *Aluminium and zirconium salts.* Aluminium chloride ($AlCl_3.6H_2O$) 25 per cent in distilled water is still thought to be the most effective axillary antiperspirant by Shelley and Hurley (1975). It is, however, only about 50 per cent effective. Polythene occlusion or dimethyl sulphoxide increases the penetration and hence the effectiveness of aluminium chloride (Kligman, 1965; Papa and Kligman, 1967). Thirty per cent aluminium chloride in distilled water applied to the feet decreases interdigital maceration, odour and pruritus (Leyden and Kligman, 1975). Aluminium chlorhydrate is commonly used in cosmetic preparations as it is less acid (pH 4.2–4.6) and therefore less irritating than aluminium chloride. It is, however, less effective as an antiperspirant but more effective as a deodorant as it kills off more bacteria.

Shelley and Hurley (1975) used anhydrous aluminium chloride. When applied to a dry axilla at night, 25 per cent $AlCl_3$ in absolute ethyl alcohol or zirconyl chloride in 20 per cent ethyl alcohol under polythene occlusion reduced sweating. Both solutions are highly irritating (pH less than 1) and contamination of the hands is avoided by using roll-on glass applicators; when applied to damp skin a primary irritant dermatitis occurs. Sneddon (personal communication) has found anhydrous aluminium chloride to be so effective for axillary hyperhidrosis that he has abandoned using surgery. Its preparation is, however, very time consuming for the pharmacy.

Mechanism of anhidrotic action. Aluminium anhidrosis is not produced by high level blockage of the sweat duct as stripping off the stratum corneum does not affect the sweat rate (Gordon and Maibach, 1968). Aluminium salts are thought to damage the sweat duct below the level of the stratum corneum, the periductal epidermis shows spongiosis, vesicles and rupture of the duct. There is also an upper dermal periductal inflammatory infiltrate (Papa and Kligman, 1967). Aluminium appears in the terminal sweat duct in rat foot pads after hypohidrotic doses of 25 per cent aluminium chloride is applied to their paws (Lansdown, 1973).

3. *Glutaraldehyde and methenamine.* Aqueous solutions of 10 per cent glutaraldehyde with 1.65 per cent sodium bicarbonate applied three times a week decreases hyperhidrosis of the feet. Concomitant bacterial and fungal infection also improves (Juhlin and Hansson, 1968). As brown staining occurs at a concentration above 2 per cent glutaraldehyde is not usually used in the axilla. Contact dermatitis (Sanderson and Cronin, 1968; Jordan, Dahl and Albert, 1972) and eye damage have been reported following the use of glutaraldehyde. Contact dermatitis may also result from the antibacterial agents used in deodorants: axillary dermatitis has been reported from a quarternary ammonium compound present in a roll-on deodorant (Schmunes and Levy, 1972).

In solution methenamine releases formaldehyde. For some years methanamine (Antihydral) in an ointment base has been on sale in Germany and Austria. Recently methenamine in a gel stick formulation has been found to decrease palmar and plantar sweating. It was said to be less likely than formalin to produce contact dermatitis (Cullen, 1975).

Mechanism of action. Formaldehyde causes anhidrosis by sweat duct plugging at the stratum corneum and probably also deeper in the epidermis (Gordon and Maibach, 1969). Scanning electron microscopy shows amorphous, non-cellular material in the sweat pore lumen during formalin anhidrosis (Papa, 1972).

INVESTIGATIONS ON ANTIPERSPIRANTS

Bakiewicz (1973) has reviewed the different methods used for testing antiperspirants. Using the rat foot pad as a model, Lansdown (1973) found 10 per cent formalin and 25 per cent aluminium chloride or aluminium chlorhydrate similarly effective as hypohidrotic agents. Tridihexethylchloride was found to be one of the more effective antiperspirants when tested on the foot pads of mice (Kaszynski and Frisch, 1974).

Goodall (1970) applied 41 cholinergic blocking agents as open patch tests to the palm and wrist. Trihexyphenidyl hydrochloride (Artane, Pipanol) and mannitol hexanitrate were found to be some of the more effective drugs. Diethylene glycol monomethyl ether was a better vehicle than propylene glycol or a cream base. Topically applied esters of scopolamine hydrobromide are effective antiperspirants (MacMillan, Reller and Synder, 1964) but there has been a reluctance to use them in view of their possible systemic effects and their instability. The levorotary isomer of hyoscine camphor sulphate is about 70 times more active than the dextrorotary isomer (Craig, 1970).

B. IONTOPHORESIS (ELECTROPHORESIS)

Hyperhidrosis of the palms and soles can be well controlled in some patients by iontophoresis. Levit (1968) used a simple apparatus providing a source of direct current of low voltage and low amperage. Tap water in contact with the palms and soles is used at the anode and cathode. Current ions flow into the sweat duct as at this site electrical resistance is lowest. Treatment given once or twice a week for six to eight weeks produces complete remission of symptoms in some patients for weeks or months (Grice, Satter and Baker, 1972; Abell and Morgan, 1974). The method is simple and safe, but is not sufficiently effective for severe hyperhidrosis. Iontophoresis of anticholinergic compounds is more effective but more difficlt to control in view of systemic absorption of the drugs. Poldine methosulphate (Grice et al, 1972) and the longer acting glycopyrronium bromide and hexopyrronium bromide (Abell and Morgan, 1974) suppress hyperhidrosis of the palms and soles for long periods but treatment may have to be abandoned owing to side effects. Gordon and Maibach (1969) showed anhidrosis produced by tap water iontophoresis results in sweat duct blockage.

C. SURGERY

As idiopathic hyperhidrosis of the palms, soles and axillae is self-limiting there is a reluctance to advocate surgery. Recently surgical treatment of axillary hyperhidrosis has been simplified and is relatively free of post-operative complications.

Axillary hyperhidrosis. Hurley and Shelley (1966) showed most axillary sweating is produced from a small area in the dome of the axilla. They found that removal of a small ellipse of skin (4–5 × 2.5 cm) gave good results. The sweating area may be mapped out with starch–iodine (Hurley and Shelley, 1966; Davis, 1971). An easy source of starch–iodine during operation is sterile povidine–iodine (Betadine) and sterile glove powder (Davis, 1971). Good results of surgery have been reported by Gillespie and Kane (1970), Weaver and Copeman (1971), Ellis (1972) and Munro et al (1974). Shaw (1974) suggests local anaesthesia should be used but if general anaesthesia is preferred care should be taken to see that the arm is not abducted at more than a right angle to the trunk because of the danger of compressing the nerves in the axilla by the head of the humerus which can result in muscle paralysis. Other complications of the axillary operation include postoperative infection, scarring and hidradenitis.

Hyperhidrosis of the hands. The results of bilateral cervical sympathectomy have been reviewed: Greenhalgh et al (1971) found 25 patients with hyperhidrosis of the hands were symptom free for two months to 10 years. Postoperative Horner's syndrome was the commonest complication but was permanent in only one case and pneumothorax and gustatory sweating were other complications. Ellis and Morgan (1971) advocated a transaxillary approach to reach the upper thoracic chain and thus avoided producing a Horner's syndrome.

Anhidrosis

Anhidrosis has been defined as the absence of sweating in spite of provocative testing by heat, exercise or local injection of cholinergic compounds. The patient may complain of pruritis and heat intolerance but neither he nor the clinician may notice he is unable to sweat (Kay and Maibach, 1969).

SYSTEMIC EFFECT OF SWEAT IMPAIRMENT

In hypohidrotic ectodermal dysplasia, where there is a diminution in the number of sweat glands, very little sweat is produced from the whole body. Rising environmental temperature causes hyperthermis, the central core temperature rises, heart rate and oxygen consumption increases; there is panting and marked distress (Total, 1974). However, in scarring produced by burns covering 50 per cent of the body surface, rising environmental temperature has little systemic effect. This occurs because there is compensatory hyperhidrosis in the rest of the undamaged skin. Anhidrosis is being found in a number of conditions.

Neurological

Interruption of the sympathetic pathways when it is complete results in anhidrosis (partial interruption produces hyperhidrosis) (Johnson and Spalding, 1974).

HOLMES–ADIE SYNDROME (ADIE SYNDROME)

Patients with Holmes–Adie syndrome may have a variety of autonomic disorders, the pupil changes being the best known. Impairment of sweating may occur (Johnson, McLellan and Love, 1971; Vanasse, Molina-Negro and Saint-Hilaire, 1974). Orthostatic hypotension results from a defect of reflex vasoconstriction in the upper and lower limbs. Impairment of sympathetic pathways may be central or peripheral.

HORNER'S SYNDROME

Anhidrosis of the forehead occurs in this syndrome.

MULTIPLE SCLEROSIS

Twenty-five out of 60 patients with multiple sclerosis had diminished or absent sweating (Noronha, Vas and Aziz, 1968).

QUADRIPLEGIA

In spite of quadriplegics having anhidrosis, these patients tolerate heat much better than do the patients with anhidrotic ectodermal dysplasia (Totel, 1974). This is said to be due to two factors:

(a) Patients with quadriplegia have skin receptors which are defective and and it is known that the 'hypothalamic thermostat' is affected by skin temperature receptors as well as by blood temperature;
(b) Sympathetic nervous control of blood vessels is impaired and peripheral vessels dilate. Blood pressure may thus be low and the distribution of heat by the circulation becomes impaired.

IDIOPATHIC ORTHOSTATIC HYPOTENSION

Segmental (Fisher and Maibach, 1970) or unilateral loss of sweating has been described with orthostatic hypotension and sexual impotence due to degeneration of sympathetic cells especially in the intermediolateral spinal columns (Johnson et al, 1966). The patients are usually middle-aged men and the autonomic failure may be associated with other primary neuronal degenerations such as olivoponto-cerebellar atrophy, Parkinsonism and motor neurone disease.

PERIPHERAL NERVE LESIONS

Sympathetic nerves supplying the distant parts of the limbs pass alongside peripheral nerves. Severe lesions of peripheral nerves produce anhidrosis and vasomotor changes in approximately the area of sensory loss. Polyarteritis nodosa and rheumatoid arthritis associated with mononeuritis multiplex may show anhidrosis (Yamamoto, 1967).

Hypohidrosis occurs in the hypopigmented lesions of leprosy. Sweat inhibition may occur before or at the same time as impairment of cutaneous sensation (Sehgal, 1974). After treatment sweating may return before cutaneous sensation improves (Willis, Harris and Moretz, 1973).

Chronic polyneuritis as occurs in chronic alcoholism may cause hypohidrosis. Failure of reflex vasoconstriction in the limbs may produce orthostatic hypotension. Anhidrosis and orthostatic hypertension has been reported in association with bronchogenic carcinoma (Ivy, 1961) and carcinoma of the pancreas (Thomas and Shields, 1970).

Lack of sweating may be very extensive in diabetic polyneuropathy or it may be patchy. Hyperhidrosis in the upper part of the body can occur as a compensatory mechanism during heating, when there is anhidrosis in the lower half of the body. It is not known if anhidrosis is produced by peripheral impairment of sympathetic pathways only or if there is also spinal cord damage (Goadby and Downman, 1973).

ANGIOKERATOMA CORPORIS DIFFUSUM (ANDERSON–FABRY DISEASE, AFD)

Wallace (1973) found that hypohidrosis commonly occurred in his 57 patients with AFD. The onset was usually during childhood or early adolescence. Other early symptoms are severe pain in the fingers and toes, and transient oedema in the ankles and sometimes in the face and hands. Fever, malaise, raised sedimentation rate and albuminuria also may occur. He suggests the diagnosis is often missed, as the characteristic angiectases may be minimal or may not become conspicuous until some years after the onset of the disease. Females usually remain symptom free and their skin eruption is minimal or absent. Men die at about the age of 42.

This sex-linked disorder of glycolipid metabolism results in an accumulation of trihexosyl ceramide (galactosylgalactosylglucosyl ceramide) and dihexosyl ceramide due to a deficiency of the lysosomal hydrolase γ-galactosidase (Kent and Carton, 1973). The storage of these catabolites throughout the body results in the typical skin lesions, cerebrovascular and cardiovascular disease, renal damage and ocular signs. Corneal dystrophy, fine curving lines seen with a slit lamp, is an early sign of AFD and is only very exceptionally absent in affected adults. The lipid catabolites are stored in lysosomes and produce the typical onion-skin occlusions (lamellar bodies) as seen by electron microscopy in many tissues including skin, renal biopsies and urine (Van Mullen, 1972). Gamma-galactosidase is decreased in plasma, leucocytes and fibroblasts, and urine contains excess trihexosyl ceramide. To prevent the disappearance of lipid from skin biopsies, the calcium formalin-fixed specimen should remain in 3 per cent potassium dichromate solution for a week, the solution being renewed every third day.

It seems AFD should be considered in any case of obscure heat intolerance. The cause of the hypohidrosis is presumably due to degeneration of sympathetic pathways. Lipid deposition causes gross changes in cerebral vessels, there is degeneration of peripheral autonomic nerves, and cellular degeneration in the hypothalamus and autonomic ganglia. Lipid deposition occurs in sweat glands.

Enzyme replacement by renal transplant is being investigated (Desnick et al, 1971). Renal transplant was rejected by a patient after two years but the rejected specimen showed no evidence of AFD (Wallace, 1973). Diphenylhydantoin may relieve the AFD crises (Kent and Carton, 1973).

COCKAYNE'S SYNDROME

Demyelinating peripheral neuropathy with hypohidrosis has been described in Cockayne's syndrome (Moosa and Dubowitz, 1970). Diminished lacrimation, intracranial calcification and nystagmus may be associated with the well-known progeria-like appearance and large Mickey Mouse-like feet, hands and ears. Photosensitivity and optic atrophy may also occur. It is said to be autosomal recessive and is one of the inborn errors of lipid metabolism.

Other disorders

Generalised anhidrosis has been reported as the presenting sign in multiple myeloma (Shelley and Lehman, 1961) and also may occur in Hodgkin's disease (English et al, 1963).

Sweat duct occlusion

PSORIASIS

Hypohidrosis occurs in psoriatic plaques and is thought to be due to sweat duct obstruction. Johnson and Shuster (1969) showed that less sweat is produced by local pharmacological stimulation of sweat glands in psoriatic skin, when compared with the normal adjacent skin. After stripping off the psoriatic stratum corneum, sweating increases, although the rate is still not as high as that in normal skin.

Neumann and Hard (1974) showed that the Munro microabscess and the spongiform pustule of Kogoj in psoriatic plaques and in generalised pustular psoriasis of Zumbusch are situated in the epidermal sweat duct unit. They suggested the epidermal cells surrounding the lining membrane of the sweat duct degenerate which not only causes the sweat duct to collapse, but also releases chemotactic substances which attract the invasion of leucocytes.

Accidental hypothermia with coma can occur in generalised psoriasis due to excessive skin heat loss from evaporation of the large transepidermal water loss and increased skin blood flow (Grice et al, 1968).

ERYTHRODERMA

Generalised hypohidrosis in erythroderma may cause hyperpyrexia (Shuster and Marks, 1970). Massive sweating occurs in normal subjects with the room temperature at 30°C and the legs in water at 42°C (Grice et al, 1975). Patients with erythroderma show under these conditions no visible sweating although some sweating does occur. They develop a rise in central core temperature, tachycardia, marked distress, faintness and hypotension (Grice, Sattar and Baker, unpublished data). Sweat glands in erythroderma due to psoriasis fail to respond to pharmacological stimulation (Suskind, 1954).

MILIARIA

It is known that miliaria is due to sweat duct blockage which occurs in hot humid conditions where sweat evaporation is at a disadvantage.

If water is applied for a short time to skin under occlusion, the stratum corneum absorbs water, swells and blocks the terminal sweat duct. Anhidrosis lasts for a short time after the occlusion is removed (Sarkany, Shuster and Stammers, 1965). Artificial miliaria rubra has been produced by covering about 70 per cent of the body surface with polythene for 48 h. If after removal of the occlusion the subjects are then exposed to heat, miliaria rubra and anhidrosis appear in 90 per cent of the area which has been occluded. After the miliaria clears clinically (only faint desquamation being seen) hypohidrosis persists and lasts for up to one to two weeks (Sulzberger and Griffin, 1969). The duration of the hypohidrosis is directly related to the severity of the miliaria. Occlusion for less than 48 h fails to produce miliaria. When the post-miliarial hypohidrosis is widespread (50–60 per cent of the body surface) incapacitating and dangerous heat exhaustion can occur.

Miliaria therefore seems to result from attempts at sweating through occluded sweat ducts. Stripping off the stratum corneum in most cases relieves the sweat obstruction (Sulzberger and Harris, 1972). In normal skin, stratum corneum stripping has no effect on sweat rate (Johnson and Shuster, 1970). Histological examination of polythene-induced miliaria rubra shows no abnormal plugs in the duct but there is damage to the sweat duct walls as shown by round-cell infiltration and spongiosis at the epidermodermal junction.

It has been suggested that bacterial infection may play some part in miliaria. Although the number of Gram-positive bacteria on the skin surface is increased in polythene-induced miliaria, the number of organisms bear no relationship to the severity of the miliaria rubra. The number of organisms varies enormously between individuals and the species of organisms, e.g. diphtheroids are not those found in normal skin (Henning, Griffin and Maibach, 1972).

Soaking the skin in water for three to six days produces subacute dermatitis but no anhidrosis. It is suggested prolonged soaking damages the stratum corneum barrier. The paddy foot seen in farmers working in rice paddy fields is the clinical manifestation of this (Willis, 1973).

Treatment. Measures to increase evaporation of sweat, such as air conditioning and appropriate clothes, help to prevent miliaria. Topical corticosteroid lotion reduces the skin eruptions. Oral ascorbic acid 1 g daily may decrease the duration of miliaria and anhidrosis (Hindson, 1968; Hindson and Worsley, 1969). High doses of ascorbic acid may be toxic however in some patients (Tan and Cunliffe, 1975). Pretreatment of the skin with anhydrous lanolin, topical neomycin or chloramphenicol, and acid buffers (aqueous solutions of 0.1 M citric acid and 0.1 M ascorbic acid), reduces experimental miliaria and hypohidrosis (Stillman, Hindson and Maibach, 1971).

ATOPIC ECZEMA

The function of sweat glands in atopic eczema has not yet been clarified. Some patients when exposed to heat in a sauna have no visible sweating (Warndorff, 1970) but attacks of hyperhidrosis may also occur. Injected acetycholine or isoprenaline (β-adrenergic-mimetic drug) produce more sweat in patients with atopic eczema than they do in normals (Warndorff and Hamer, 1974). It has been suggested that the increase in sweat sensitivity in atopic eczema may be related to the skin vascular hypersensitivity as shown by the well-known blanch phenomenon. Heating (and hence vasodilatation) has been shown to increase the sensitivity of receptor sites in sweat glands (Ogawa, 1970). Atopic sweat gland enzymes are normal (Cotton and Van Rossum, 1973).

Diminution in sweat gland population

Ectodermal dysplasia. To be classified as an ectodermal dysplasia a condition must show at least one of the following signs—trichodysplasia, abnormal dentition, onychodysplasia, dyshidrosis (hypo- or hyper-)—and at least one other sign (Freire-Maia, 1971).

ANHIDROTIC ECTODERMAL DYSPLASIA (AED) (Fig. 5.3)

The patients often show a similar facial appearance with the nose saddle-shaped with a depressed bridge, the chin small and pointed and the forehead bossed. Photophobia, absent lacrimation, corneal opacities, congenital cataracts or absence of the iris may occur. There may be absence of mucous glands in the pharynx, larynx, trachea, bronchus and oesophagus. The voice may be hoarse and respiratory infections common (Reed, Lopez, and Landing, 1970).

Sweat glands are diminished in number and total body sweating is slight (Totel, 1974). The anhidrotic heat syndrome or heat stroke may occur when there is a rise of body temperature due to exercise, infection or hot weather. The anhidrotic heat syndrome is characterised by lassitude, weakness, headache and mental confusion. The clinical implications of a tropical environment for AED have been studied in a Nigerian family (Familusi et al, 1975).

Scalp hair is short, fine and scanty and eyebrows and eyelashes sparse or absent. Atopic eczema may be present. Teeth may be absent or conical and the lower lip may pout. Males are more commonly and more severely affected and the classical severe AED is thought to be X-linked recessive. The evidence for an X-linked form fully expressed in males is beyond dispute (Kerr, Wells and Cooper, 1966) and female carriers may show some manifestations, i.e. they are manifesting heterozygotes. Dermatoglyphic patterns of palms and soles may be abnormal with ridge flattening and unilateral or bilateral distally situated axial triradii which are commonly associated with a high maximal atd angle. An increase in hypothenar pattern frequencies, as compared with the normal, is also common. Absent epidermal ridge pores have been shown (Frias and Smith, 1968; Verbov, 1970; Crump and Danks, 1971).

In a study of 53 members of 13 unrelated families with AED (Verbov, 1970; Verbov and Wells, 1972) a group of patients with a milder form of the disorder was distinguished. These patients showed, in addition to dental abnormalities, reasonable sweat gland function, both hypothenar pattern frequencies and atd angles were usually normal and hypotrichosis and nail abnormalities were sometimes found. It was suggested that this milder form of ectodermal dysplasia is inherited as an X-linked dominant form and should be termed hypohidrotic ectodermal dysplasia (HED) retaining the term an-hidrotic ectodermal dysplasia (AED) for the classical form. Treatment of AED consists of avoidance of heat and exercise beyond the patient's capacity. They tend to show an improved tolerance to environmental heat as they age.

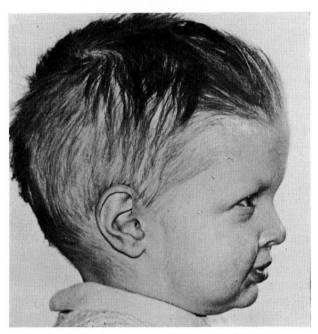

Figure 5.3 Classical type of anhidrotic ectodermal dysplasia at the age of 21 months, showing prominent forehead, sparse scalp hair and absent eyebrows

HYPODONTIA WITH NAIL DYSGENESIS (HND)

Hypodontia with nail dysgenesis is characterised by absence of some permanent teeth, koilonychia or absence of nails since birth, a pouting lower lip and occasionally some hypohidrosis (Hudson and Witkop, 1975). The disorder is transmitted as an autosomal dominant trait and affected individuals do not have the facial appearances characteristic of anhidrotic ectodermal dysplasia. Hudson and Witkop (1975) reported 29 cases of the disorder in six families.

A NEW SYNDROME

Freire-Maia et al (1975) described a new form of ectodermal dysplasia in a seven-year-old girl. Although the child had normal teeth, hypotrichosis, hypohidrosis, onychogryphosis, pigmentary disturbances and psychomotor and growth retardation were present in addition to other signs.

ICHTHYOSIS VULGARIS

Hypohidrosis of the trunk and limbs is described in the sex-linked and autosomal dominant varieties of ichthyosis vulgaris. Fewer sweat glands than normal were found in skin biopsies particularly from the sex-linked form, by Wells and Kerr (1966) but not by Feinstein, Ackerman and Ziprkowski (1970). Palmar sweating is only occasionally diminished (Grice and Bettley, 1967; Verbov, unpublished data).

Genetic Abnormalities of Sweat Gland Function

Cystic fibrosis

High sweat concentration of sodium, chloride, and to a lesser extent potassium, pancreatic deficiency, and chronic pulmonary disease are the salient feature of cystic fibrosis (CF). Excessive salt loss in sweat may cause low blood pressure (Lieberman and Rodbard, 1975).

Screening and diagnosis. The diagnosis of CF is usually made by finding sweat sodium levels above 60 to 70 mEq/litre (Mearns, 1974), although CF can exist with normal sweat electrolyte levels (Sarsfield and Davies, 1975). Screening for CF is useless under the age of one month (Steinrud, Winkel and Flensborg, 1974) as infants younger than one month may have high sweat electrolytes probably due to low sweat rates in the new born (Foster, Hay and Katz, 1969). The concentration of sweat chloride is 45 mEq/litre (range 8–100) before the age of one month, it then falls to about 20 mEq/litre (range 6–46) at which it remains during childhood. In females, CF sweat chlorides (mean 128 mEq/litre) are higher than in males (mean 112 mEq/litre).

Elliott (1974) suggested a simple new test for CF: soaking an infant's hand in tap water for 3 min causes wrinkling of CF skin due to high electrolyte content of the stratum corneum. Another screening test suggested is based on the finding that in CF the sodium, calcium and magnesium content of nails is raised (Leonard and Morris, 1972).

Immune complexes are found in many organs in CF, especially in the respiratory and intestinal tracts. Circulating immune complexes are present in serum and sputum (McFarlane et al, 1975). Serum α-fetoprotein levels (AFP) are raised (56–8825 µg/litre) in CF and in the parents and siblings of CF patients. AFP is a major component of normal fetal serum but falls after birth (normal range 5–25 µg/litre) (Chandra, Madhavankutty and Way, 1975).

Mechanism of sweat gland abnormality. The pathogenesis of CF is still unknown although various suggestions have been made. Mucin (mucus) is said to 'water-proof' membranes (Negus, 1967) and this inhibits the passive passage of water but not of ions through membranes. CF mucin is abnormally viscid with a raised calcium content. Gibson, Matthews and Minihan (1970) suggest CF mucin lining the sweat duct lets through too much water. As they point out, however, were more water than salt absorbed in the duct one would expect raised sweat concentrations of urea, lactic acid and creatinine in CF. In fact these concentrations are all normal. Dobson (1974) suggests CF mucin may bind more sodium, therefore hindering its reabsorption by the sweat duct. An inhibitor of sodium transport has been found in CF sweat (Kaiser, Drack and Rossi, 1970) but this is present in normal secretions and therefore is probably not of prime importance in CF (Gibson et al, 1970). Spock et al (1967) found an abnormal serum factor (ciliary dyskinetic factor) in CF which increases the permeability of rat intestine.

Mucopolysaccharidoses

The genetic mucopolysaccharidoses are characterised by hirsutism and skin thickening. Mucopolysaccharides are excreted in excess in the urine and deposited in various tissues (McKusick et al, 1965). Sweat sodium concentration is normal both in the type I (Hurler syndrome or gargoylism) and type II forms (Hunter syndrome). There is an increased deposition of mucopolysaccharides in all three cell types of the secretory sweat coil and also in the sweat duct (Belcher, 1973). There is relative sparing of the coiled duct which probably accounts for the normal sweat sodium concentration. The Hurler syndrome is inherited as an autosomal recessive trait whilst the Hunter syndrome is sex-linked recessive.

FUCOSIDOSIS (DEFICIENCY OF α-FUCOSIDASE)

In a new mucopolysaccharidosis (Durand et al, 1968; Loeb et al, 1969), fucosidosis, the sodium chloride concentration in sweat is even higher than that found in cystic fibrosis. Hyperhidrosis, skin thickening and mental degeneration also occur. Fucose is deposited in tissues as it accumulates due to absence of α-L-fucosidase in lysosomes. The rare disorder is transmitted as an autosomal recessive trait.

Glycogen storage disease (type I)

Sweat concentration of sodium chloride was increased in three boys with glucose-6-phosphatase deficiency (Harris and Cohen, 1963).

APOCRINE SWEAT GLANDS

Viscid apocrine sweat is said to be formed by breaking off the apical portion of the secretory cell. Schaumburg-Lever and Lever (1975) have shown by electron microscopy that this actually happens. They showed axillary apocrine secretion is formed by three mechanisms.

1. Apocrine secretion—true decapitation of the apical cap of the secretory cell occurs.

2. Merocrine secretion—vesicles form in the apical portion and discharge their granular contents into the lumen.
3. Holocrine secretion—whole secretory cells are detached from the basal lamina and are found lying free in the lumen (Braun-Falco and Rupec, 1968; Montagna and Parakkal, 1974).

The secretory coiled tubular apocrine gland consists of an inner layer of secretory cells and an outer layer of myoepithelial cells, surrounded by a thick basement membrane. Sweat expulsion may be mediated by the contractile myoepithelial cells (Jenkinson, 1973). Elongated balloon-like apocrine glands in the transparent bat's wing can be seen expelling sweat by contraction of ducts and gland (Cortese and Nicoll, 1970).

Axillary apocrine glands empty independently of one another, the rhythm in discharge is not regular and varies in different glands. There is a surge of activity in the morning which dies off during the evening (Fox, Mullen and Thornton, 1974). It is difficult to distinguish eccrine from apocrine sweat rhythm in the axilla as these glands occur in a 1:1 ratio (Montagna and Parakkal, 1974). Fox et al (1974) overcame this problem by using a plaster of paris disc in the axilla to absorb eccrine sweat. Apocrine sweat contaminated with sebum formed discrete spots on the disc which fluoresced with ultra-violet radiation.

Apocrine axillary secretion has been studied after injection of adrenaline (Bell, 1974). Electron microscopy shows that large secretory granules in the secretory cells of apocrine glands, discharge their contents into the surrounding cytoplasm. The granules contain particles, microfilaments and lipid droplets. Bell (1974) suggests during sweat secretion the particles land on the microfilaments which act as a springboard and possibly control the direction of the discharge of particles. 'Saltatory movement' of particles has been described in other cells. Two other types of granules are found in the secretory cells, one containing pigment (lipofuscin) and iron and the other is probably a precursor of the true secretory granule. Mitochondria may be large and are thought to be associated with energy producing processes.

Pharmacology of Apocrine Sweating

Apocrine sweating is essentially adrenergically controlled but there has been much controversy about the method by which adrenaline and noradrenaline reach the gland. In most animal species no nerves have been found close to the gland (Jenkinson, 1973). This is also true in the human axilla, although nerves have been found on a few occasions (Aoki, 1962; Montagna, 1964).

Two methods of adrenergic control are possibly employed.

1. Adrenergic sympathetic nerves may terminate on blood vessels close to the gland, and the final leg of transmission is vascular, i.e. there is a localised neurohumoral system for firing off apocrine sweating (Jenkin-

son, Sengupta and Blackburn, 1966). Sympathetic stimulation may either change the permeability of the vessel or release a transmitter substance (Jenkinson, 1973).

2. Circulating adrenaline from the adrenal medulla possibly supplements neural stimulation. This may occur in hypoglycaemia, asphyxia and exercise (Robertshaw, 1974).

Apocrine sweat glands of the human axilla are probably α-adrenergically controlled. Using excised skin, it seems in the horse and donkey, sweat secretion is under β-adrenergic control while sweat expulsion by the myo-epithelial cells is under α-adrenergic control. The cow's sweat secretion, on the other hand, seems to be α-adrenergically controlled (Johnson, 1975).

Human axillary apocrine sweat glands also respond to acetylcholine and where nerves have been found they are weakly cholinesterase reactive. This is said not necessarily to prove the cholinergic nature of the nerves as small amounts of the enzymes are also found in adrenergic nerves (Aoki and Hayashi, 1974).

Hidradenitis Suppurativa

Axillary apocrine glands are small and undifferentiated until about the age of seven and are probably not functioning fully until puberty. Hidradenitis suppurativa is, therefore, rare before puberty and disappears in old age (Shelley, 1972). Hidradenitis usually affects the axillae, groins, external genitalia and perianal region. It occurs less often in the submammary and periumbilical regions and in the areola of the breast (Letterman and Schurter, 1974).

Although it has been known for over 100 years that hidradenitis suppurativa is due to inflammation of apocrine sweat glands the pathogenesis is still little understood. Whereas in the past there was a tendency to soldier on with medical treatment, recently there is an increasing tendency to advocate earlier surgery. Hidradenitis suppurative has been classified into two stages.

EARLY (OR MEDICAL) STAGE

Tender inflammatory nodules at one or more apocrine sweat gland-bearing sites probably occur quite commonly and either clear spontaneously or can be treated successfully with short courses of systemic antibiotics. Similar lesions were produced experimentally in the axilla by Shelley (1972) using adhesive tape occlusion. This blocked apocrine sweat ducts and encouraged bacterial overgrowth.

The more recalcitrant cases have been successfully treated with oral contraceptives, intralesional or systemic corticosteroids and simple opening and drainage.

7

CHRONIC (OR SURGICAL) STAGE

Surgery is the treatment of choice where there are numerous interconnect-ing deep or tortuous sinus tracts, brawny induration, discharging sinuses and cord-like bands (Anderson and Perry, 1975). The following surgical procedures have been advocated.

1. Exteriorisation, curettage and electrocoagulation.
2. Complete excision of all the involved area and direct primary closure. This is possible where the disease is localised to a small preferably linear area (Ward, Washio and David, 1974) or in the axilla where a transverse primary closure has been used. Anderson and Perry (1975) advocate complete removal of hair-bearing skin in the axilla to decrease the risk of recurrence. They believe primary closure is the procedure of choice and showed it was unnecessary to postpone surgery until infection had cleared.
3. Excision and resurfacing with primary or delayed skin grafts.
4. Excision and closure by local flaps. Modified Z-plasty is used by Letterman and Schurter (1974).

SWEAT GLAND TUMOURS

There has been considerable controversy over the classification and histo-genesis of sweat gland tumours. Like Wilson-Jones (1971) one feels reluctant to plunge into the nosological jungle! Electron microscopy and histochemistry have helped in classification. Tumours derived from eccrine elements react with glycogen phosphorylase and branching enzymes. Tumours of apocrine origin react to acid phosphatase but glycogen phosphorylase is absent (Castro and Winkelmann, 1974).

Eccrine duct milium

Milia are small subepidermal keratin cysts that are formed usually from under-developed sebaceous glands. Milia that occur following subepidermal bullae, however, have been shown to arise in sweat ducts (Sanderson, 1972): the walls of the milium are formed by eccrine duct cells (Tsuji, Sugai and Suzuki, 1975) the sweat duct having been avulsed by the subepidermal blister.

Eccrine poroma

More than 100 eccrine poromas were observed in a patient aged 65 years. They were all on the palms and soles and had been present for 20 years. They were soft, red, sessile, nodules 1.5 to 3 cm in diameter which looked similar to the usual solitary lesion. Goldner (1970) suggested the term eccrine poromatosis for his unique case.

Pigmented nodular hidradenoma

Wilson-Jones (1971) described pigmentation in five tumours which otherwise were straightforward examples of benign sweat gland tumours in the 'nodular hidradenoma eccrine poroma spectrum'. One patient had a warty pigmented cellular-naevus-like lesion on the shoulder present since birth which recurred after excision. It had bled recently. Three other patients had tumours on the arms or scalp for three years. The tumour cells of the first case tended to be slightly larger and less regularly arranged than in the classical eccrine poroma. The other three tumours showed the usual characteristics of a nodular hidradenoma with eccrine poroma features. The other patient had a heel tumour which was clinically and histologically a typical eccrine poroma. The histochemical enzyme characteristics were those associated with an eccrine derivation. Extensive pigmentation with active melanogenesis was present in one tumour and patchy pigmentation, confined to the superficial layers, was present in the others. A mistaken histological diagnosis of seborrhoeic wart had been made in the first case.

Wilson-Jones (1971) wondered if the pigment in the sweat gland tumour was related to the fact that melanocytes are found in the sweat duct anlagen of the 14-week-old embryo, the melanocytes disappearing later.

Eccrine hidrocystoma (hidrocystoma)

Forty-five patients with eccrine hidrocystoma were reviewed by Smith and Chernosky (1973). The tumour is usually single (80 per cent of the cases), but multiple lesions can occur, one patient having over 200 lesions. The patients are usually female (3:2) aged around 50 years (range 35–75 years) and the duration of the tumour is from one month to five years. The lesions usually occur around the eye, sometimes on the lids or lid margin. The tumours are also found on the face, neck, trunk and leg. Hidrocystomas are small (0.1– 1.6 cm) smooth, shiny, dome-shaped, translucent and often bluish, the edges blending gradually into the surrounding normal skin. The fact that there is no telangiectasis, ulceration or haemorrhage helps to distinguish these lesions from basal cell carcinoma. The cyst contains a thin clear watery fluid. The clinical differentiation from apocrine hidrocystomas may be difficult, the latter do not usually occur around the eye except on the lid margin and their colour is often a deep bluish black.

Apocrine hidrocystoma (apocrine cystadenoma)

Forty-two patients with apocrine hidrocystomas were reviewed (Smith and Chernosky, 1974). The lesion is usually single (88 per cent), but up to four tumours can occur. Men and women are equally affected usually around the age of 55 years (range 35–79 years). The duration of the lesion varies from three days to 11 years and the tumour practically always occurs on the head and neck (96 per cent of the cases), often on the cheeks or lid margins. The glands of Moll are modified apocrine glands and retention cysts of these glands are said to be the same as apocrine hidrocystomas. The cysts are smooth, shiny, dome-shaped, devoid of hair or pores, the colour is translucent and clear in some, but most apocrine hidrocystomas are dark blue, often nearly black. The watery content of the cyst is often brownish or black; the colour is not due to melanin or haemosiderin but is probably due to pigment in the apocrine granules.

Hidradenoma papilliferum

This tumour, occurring in the anogenital region predominantly in females, was studied recently by electron microscopy (Hashimoto, 1973). It was confirmed that the papillary endothelium lining the ducts was composed of apocrine secretory cells and myoepithelial cells. There was an epithelial capsule, enclosing the apocrine gland elements, which it was suggested originated from the external hair sheath. Part of the capsule was keratinised but other areas of the capsule were less keratinised and resembled the wall of a steatocystoma multiplex or tricholemmal cyst.

Naevus sebaceus (organoid epidermal naevus)

Various types of sweat gland tumour can occur in a naevus sebaceus. Areas of syringocystadenoma papilliferum were found by Wilson-Jones and Heyl (1970) in 27 of their 140 cases of naevus sebaceus. The area of syringocystadenoma papilliferum was usually small but in some it formed a large part of the tumour. Most of the cases occurred on the scalp (17/27) but a few were found on the face, neck and trunk and none occurred behind the ear.

Apocrine naevus

Civatte, Tsoïtis and Préaux (1974) described two cases of a pure apocrine naevus. To their knowledge there had been only one previous case described. Both tumours had been present from birth, both appeared in the scalp as exudative tumours with alopecia. Histology showed numerous well-differentiated apocrine glands and absence of pilosebaceous units. There was basaloid proliferation of the overlying epidermis and possibly a basal cell carcinoma, as found in the naevus sebaceus.

Tubular apocrine adenoma

A woman aged 66 years with a red, slightly pedunculated verrucous lesion (2 cm in diameter) behind an ear was described by Landry and Winkelmann (1972). The tumour had been present since birth, but at the age of 51 years the lesion began to enlarge and continued to do so for five years, then further growth ceased. Histology showed a tumour consisting of widely dilated tubular structures, the walls being lined by two layers of epithelial cells which on histochemical and electron microscopic analysis showed it to be of apocrine origin. The overlying epidermis showed pseudoepitheliomatous hyperplasia with one area of basal cell carcinoma, similar to that found in a naevus sebaceus.

Dermal cylindroma (cylindroma, turban tumour)

Dermal cylindromas developed on the scalp of two patients with atrophic scarred alopecia following radiotherapy for tinea capitis. The tumours developed 30 and 39 years after radiotherapy and in one case the tumour was associated with two basal cell carcinomas (Black and Wilson-Jones, 1971).

Spiradenoma

In an effort to classify this tumour, Castro and Winkelmann (1974) studied two lesions. Both were movable, painful tumours which had been present for 15 to 20 years. One occurred on the chest and one on the wrist. The histological diagnosis was eccrine spiradenoma. Histochemistry and electron microscopy showed no evidence that this was a sweat gland tumour and the authors suggested that it originated from the basal cells of the epidermis.

Degos' acanthoma (clear cell acanthoma, acanthome à cellules claires)

The origin of this tumour is still unknown, it does not have the enzyme characteristics of a sweat gland tumour (Hu and Sisson, 1969). Lindgren and Neumann (1973) studied two patients with Degos' acanthoma, one had a scaling erythematous nodule of the leg and the other had a similar lesion on the back. The histology showed the typical acanthosis of the epidermis caused by pale enlarged glycogen-filled cells. In both cases the sheath cells of the intraepidermal sweat duct seemed to merge with the acanthoma and the authors suggested the origin of the tumour was from the epidermal-like cells of the intraepidermal sweat duct.

Eccrine gland tumour of clear cell origin

Rosen, Kim and Yermakov (1975) described a 47-year-old black man with a nodular indurated tumour involving the right eyelid. The tumour remained localised but recurred locally following attempts at complete or partial excision. On the basis of light and electron microscopic findings and the clinical behaviour of the lesion, the authors considered it to represent a hitherto undescribed low-grade malignant neoplasm of the clear cells of the secretory portion of the eccrine sweat gland.

Sweat-gland carcinoma (hidradenocarcinoma)

The histology and clinical features in 83 patents has recently been reviewed (El-Domeira et al, 1971). This rare tumour arises most commonly on the face, but can occur in all sites including the perineum. The commonest age at which diagnosis is made is between 50 and 70 years (range 7–86 years). It is slightly more common in females. The tumours are often painful and the clinical appearance varies between a tender bluish or red, smooth-surfaced nodule, to a large inflammatory-looking mass, which in one case was mistakenly thought to be an abscess and treated with antibiotics. The diameter of the tumour is usually under 5 cm but can be as much as 15 cm.

The tumours have often been present for some years. In over half the cases, the length of history is more than one year and in one patient it was 35 years. The prognosis is not affected by the length of history. After five years, 38 per cent of the patients who had received treatment to primary lesions were alive and well (26/68). The outlook is poor if the histology is anaplastic or there is lymph gland involvement.

The tumours are radio-resistant. Wide surgical excision is advised for more differentiated tumours. This should be combined with regional lymph gland dissection if the histology is anaplastic or highly undifferentiated, if there has been local skin recurrence after previous wide excision, or if there is clinical evidence of lymph gland involvement.

Single case reports of sweat gland carcinoma have also been described (Dave, 1972; Weiner, Richfield and Safdi, 1973; Fakhery and Fishman, 1974).

ACKNOWLEDGEMENT

We are most grateful to Dr D. McEwan Jenkinson for his help and advice, and we thank Dr K. V. Sanderson for his advice on sweat gland tumours.

REFERENCES

INTRODUCTION

Bligh, J. (1967) A thesis concerning the processes of secretion and discharge of sweat. *Environmental Research*, **1**, 28–45.

Ellis, R. A. (1968) Eccrine sweat glands. *Handbuch der Haut-und Geschlechtskrankheiten*, Vol. 1, Part 1, Jadassohn, J. Engänzungswerk, ed. Marchionini, A., pp. 224–260. Berlin: Springer-Verlag.

Jenkinson, D. McEwan (1969) Sweat gland function in domestic animals. In *The Exocrine Glands*, ed. Botelho, S. Y., Brooks, F. P. & Shelley, W. B., pp. 201–221. Philadelphia: University of Pennsylvania Press.

Jenkinson, D. McEwan (1973) Comparative physiology of sweating. *British Journal of Dermatology*, **88**, 397–406.

Robertshaw, D. (1974) Neural and humoral control of apocrine glands. *Journal of Investigative Dermatology*, **63**, 160–167.

Eccrine sweat glands

FUNCTION

Adams, T. & Hunter, W. S. (1969) Modification of skin mechanical properties by eccrine sweat gland activity. *Journal of Applied Physiology*, **26**, 417–419.

Allen, J. A., Armstrong, J. E. & Roddie, I. C. (1973) The regional distribution of emotional sweating in man. *Journal of Physiology*, **235**, 749–759.

Benson, J. W., Jr, Buja, M. L., Thompson, R. H. & Gordon, R. S., Jr (1974) Glucose utilisation by sweat glands during fasting in man. *Journal of Investative Dermatology*, **63**, 287–291.

Benzinger, T. H. (1969) Heat regulation: homeostasis of central temperature in man. *Physiological Reviews*, **49**, 671–759.

Bettley, F. R. & Grice, K. A. (1965) A method for measuring the transepidermal water loss and a means of inactivating sweat glands. *British Journal of Dermatology*, **77**, 627–638.

Clark, R. P., Mullan, B. J. & Pugh, L. G. C. E. (1974) Colour thermography in running. *Journal of Physiology*, **239**, 81–82P.

Comaish, S. (1973) Glutaraldehyde lowers skin friction and enhances skin resistance to acute friction injury. *Acta dermato-venereological (Stockholm)*, **53**, 455–460.

Comaish, J. S. & Bottoms, E. (1971) The skin and friction: deviations from Amonton's laws and the effects of hydration and lubrication. *British Journal of Dermatology*, **84**, 37–43.

Cooper, K. E. (1970) Studies of the human central warm receptor. In *Physiological and Behavioural Temperature Regulation*, ed. Hardy, J. D., Gagg, A. P. & Stolwijk, J. A. J., pp. 224–250. Springfield, Illinois: Charles C. Thomas.

Ellis, H. (1972) Hyperhidrosis. *British Journal of Hospital Medicine*, **7**, 641–644.

Ellis, R. A. (1968) Eccrine sweat glands. *Handbuch der Haut-und Geschlechtskrankheiten*, Vol. 1, Part 1, Jadassohn, J. Engänzungswerk, Ed. Marchionini, A., pp. 224–260. Berlin: Springer-Verlag.

Foster, K. G., Hey, E. N. & Katz, G. (1969) The response of the sweat glands of the new-born baby to thermal stimuli and to intradermal acetycholine. *Journal of Physiology*, **203**, 13–29.

Handley, S. L. & Spencer, P. S. J. (1972) Thermoregulatory effects of intraventricular injection of noradrenaline in the mouse and the influence of ambient temperature. *Journal of Physiology*, **223**, 619–631.

Hey, E. N. & Katz, G. (1969) Evaporative water loss in the new-born baby. *Journal of Physiology*, **200**, 605–619.

Myers, R. D. (1971) Hypothalamic mechanisms of pyrogen action in the cat and monkey. In *Pyrogens and Fever*, Ciba Foundation Symposium, ed. Wolstenholms, G. E. W. & Birch, J., pp. 131–153. London: Churchill Livingstone.

Nadel, E. R., Bullard, R. W. & Stolwijk, J. A. J. (1971) Importance of skin temperature in the regulation of sweating. *Journal of Applied Physiology*, **31**, 80–87.

Ogawa, T. (1970) Local effect of skin temperature on threshold concentration of sudorific agents. *Journal of Applied Physiology*, **28**, 18–22.

Sato, K. (1973b) Sweat induction from an isolated eccrine sweat gland. *American Journal of Physiology*, **225**, 1147–1152.

Sato, K. & Dobson, R. L. (1970a) Regional and individual variations in the function of the human eccrine sweat gland. *Journal of Investigative Dermatology*, **54**, 443–449.

Smiles, K. A. & Robinson, S. (1971) Sodium ion conservation during acclimatisation of men to work in the heat. *Journal of Applied Physiology*, **31**, 63–69.

Verbov, J. & Baxter, J. (1974) Onset of palmar sweating in newborn infants. *British Journal of Dermatology*, **90**, 269–276.

Weiner, J. S. & Hellmann, K. (1960) The sweat glands. *Biological Reviews of the Cambridge Philosophical Society*, **35**, 141–186.

STRUCTURE

Bullough, W. S. & Deol, J. U. R. (1972) Chalone control of mitotic activity in eccrine sweat glands. *British Journal of Dermatology*, **86**, 586–592.

Cawley, E. P., Hsu, Y. T., Sturgill, B. C. & Harman, L. E., Jr (1973) Lipofuscin ('wear and tear pigment') in human sweat glands. *Journal of Investigative Dermatology*, **61**, 105–107.

Christophers, E. & Plewig, G. (1973) Formation of the acrosyringium. *Archives of Dermatology*, **107**, 378–382.

Cotta-Pereira, G., Rodrigo, F. G. & Bittencourt-Sampaio, S. (1975) Ultrastructural study of elaunin fibres in the secretory coil of human eccrine sweat glands. *British Journal of Dermatology*, **93**, 623–629.

Ellis, R. A. (1968) Eccrine sweat glands. *Handbuch der Haut-und Geschlechtskrankheiten*, Vol. 1, Part 1, Jadassohn, J. Engänzungswerk, ed. Marchionini, A., pp. 224–260. Berlin: Springer-Verlag.

Hashimoto, K. (1971) Demonstration of the intercellular spaces of the human eccrine sweat gland by Lanthanum. 1. The secretory coil. *Journal of Ultrastructure Research*, **36**, 249–262.

Johnson, C., Dawber, R. & Shuster, S. (1970) Surface appearance of the eccrine sweat duct by scanning electron microscopy. *British Journal of Dermatology*, **83**, 655–660.

Lobitz, W. C., Holyoke, J. B. & Montagna, W. (1954) Responses of the human eccrine sweat duct to controlled injury. Growth centre of the 'epidermal sweat duct unit'. *Journal of Investigative Dermatology*, **23**, 329–344.

Papa, C. M. (1972) Mechanisms of eccrine anidrosis. III. Scanning electron microscopic study of poral occlusion. *Journal of Investigative Dermatology*, **59**, 295–298.

Sarkany, I. (1962) A method for studying the microtopography of the skin. *British Journal of Dermatology*, **74**, 254–259.

Sarkany, I., Shuster, S. & Stammers, M. C. (1965) Occlusion of the sweat pore by hydration. *British Journal of Dermatology*, **77**, 101–104.

Sato, K., Dobson, R. L. & Mali, J. W. H. (1971) Enzymatic basis for the active transport of sodium in the eccrine sweat gland. Localisation and characterisation of Na-K-adenosine triphosphatase. *Journal of Investigative Dermatology*, **57**, 10–16.

Verbov, J. (1973) Hypohidrotic ectodermal dysplasia: unusual palmprint in a heterozygote. *British Journal of Dermatology*, **88**, 92–93.

Verbov, J. (1975) Palmer ridge appearance in normal newborn infants and ridge appearance in relation to eccrine sweating. *British Journal of Dermatology*, **93**, 645–648.

Wolf, J. (1970) Configuration of orifices of the sweat ducts on the surface of the horny layer of the skin in man. *Folio morphologica (Prague)*, **18**, 14–20.

SWEAT PRODUCTION

Bligh, J. (1967) A thesis concurring the processes of secretion and discharge of sweat. *Environmental Research*, **1**, 28–45.

Dobson, R. L. & Sato, K. (1972) The secretion of salt and water by the eccrine sweat gland. *Archives of Dermatology*, **105**, 366–370.

Fasciolo, J. C., Totel, G. L. & Johnson, R. E. (1969) Antidiuretic hormone and human eccrine sweating. *Journal of Applied Physiology*, **27**, 303–307.

Förström, L., Goldyne, M. E. & Winkelmann, R. K. (1974) Prostaglandin activity in human eccrine sweat. *Prostaglandins*, **7**, 459–463.

Frewin, D. B., Eakins, K. E., Downey, J. E. & Bhattacherjee, P. (1973) Prostaglandin-like activity in human eccrine sweat. *Australian Journal of Experimental Biology and Medical Science*, **51**, 701–702.

Johnson, R. E., Morimoto, T. & Robbins, F. D. (1969) The excretion of solutes in human eccrine sweat. In *The Exocrine Glands*, ed. Botelho, S. Y., Brooks, F. P. & Shelley, W. B., pp. 105–129. Philadelphia: University of Pennsylvania Press.

Kaiser, D., Songo-Williams, R. & Drack, E. (1974) Hydrogen ion and electrolyte excretion of the single human sweat gland. *Pflügers Archiv. European Journal of Physiology*, **349**, 63–72.

Mangos, J. (1973) Transductal fluxes of Na, K and water in the human eccrine sweat gland. *American Journal of Physiology*, **224**, 1235–1240.

Mearns, M. B. (1974) Cystic fibrosis. *British Journal of Hospital Medicine*, **12**, 497–506.

Sato, K. (1973b) Sweat induction from an isolated eccrine sweat gland. *American Journal of Physiology*, **225**, 1147–1152.

Sato, K. & Dobson, R. L. (1970b) The effect of intracutaneous D-aldosterone and hydrocortisone on human eccrine sweat gland function. *Journal of Investigative Dermatology*, **54**, 450–462.

Sato, K., Dobson, R. L. & Mali, J. W. H. (1971) Enzymatic basis for the active transport of sodium in the eccrine sweat gland. Localisation and characterisation of Na-K-adenosine triphosphatase. *Journal of Investigative Dermatology*, **57**, 10–16.

Schultz, I. (1969) Site and mechanisms of the electrolyte transport of the sweat gland. *The Exocrine Gland*, ed. Botelho, S. Y., Brooks, F. P. & Shelley, W. B., pp. 126–128. Philadelphia: University of Pennsylvania Press.

Schultz, I., Ullrich, K. J., Frömter, E., Holzgreve, H., Frick, A. & Hegel, U. (1965) Mikropunktion und elektrische Potentialmessung an Schweissdrüsen des Menschen. *Pflügers Archiv. für die gesamte Physiologie des Menschen und der Tiere*, **284**, 360–372.

Slegers, J. F. G. & Hof-Grootenboer, A. E. van't (1971) The localisation of sodium transport sites in a forward pumping secretory system. *Pflügers Archiv. European Journal of Physiology*, **327**, 167–185.

PHARMACOLOGY OF ECCRINE SWEATING

Allen, J. A. & Roddie, I. C. (1972) The role of circulating catecholamines in sweat production in man. *Journal of Physiology*, **227**, 801–814.

Bligh, J. (1967) A thesis concurring the processes of secretion and discharge of sweat. *Environmental Research*, **1**, 28–45.

Foster, K. G. (1971) Factors affecting the quantitative response of human eccrine sweat glands to intradermal injections of acetylcholine and methacholine. *Journal of Physiology*, **213**, 277–290.

Foster, K. G., Ginsburg, J. & Weiner, J. S. (1970) Role of circulating catecholamines in human eccrine sweat gland control. *Clinical Science*, **39**, 823–832.

Foster, K. G. & Weiner, J. S. (1970) Effect of cholinergic and adrenergic blocking agents on the activity of the eccine sweat glands. *Journal of Physiology*, **210**, 883–895.

Jenkinson, D. McEwan (1973) Comparative physiology of sweating. *British Journal of Dermatology*, **88**, 397–406.

Prout, B. J. & Wardell, W. M. (1969) Sweating and peripheral blood flow in patients with phaeochromocytoma. *Clinical Science*, **36**, 109–117.

Robertshaw, D. (1974) Neural and humoral control of apocrine glands. *Journal of Investigative Dermatology*, **63**, 160–167.

Sato, K. (1973a) Stimulation of pentose cycle in the eccrine sweat gland by adrenergic drugs. *American Journal of Physiology*, **224**, 1149–1154.

Sato, K. (1973b) Sweat induction from an isolated eccrine sweat gland. *American Journal of Physiology*, **225**, 1147–1152.

Warndorff, J. A. & Neefs, J. (1971) A quantitative measurement of sweat production after local injection of adrenalin. *Journal of Investigative Dermatology*, **56**, 384–386.

Wolf, J. E. & Maibach, H. I. (1974) Palmar eccrine sweating—the role of adrenergic and cholinergic mediators. *British Journal of Dermatology*, **91**, 439–446.

EXCRETION IN SWEAT

Allen, B. R., Moore, M. R. & Hunter, J. A. A. (1975) Lead and the skin. *British Journal of Dermatology*, **92**, 715–719.

Almeyda, J. & Levantine, A. (1972) Drug reactions. XVII. Cutaneous reaction to barbiturates, chloral hydrate and its derivatives. *British Journal of Dermatology*, **86**, 313–316.

Beveridge, G. W. (1970) Sweat gland necrosis in barbiturate poisoning. *Archives of Dermatology*, **101**, 369.

Brusilow, S. W. & Gordes, E. H. (1966) The permeability of the sweat glands to non-electrolytes. *American Journal of Diseases of Children*, **112**, 328–333.

Comaish, J. S. & Shelley, W. B. (1965) Fluorimetric determination of quinine and fluorescein excretion in human sweat. *Journal of Investigative Dermatology*, **44**, 279–281.

Epstein, W. L., Shah, V. P. & Riegelman, S. (1972) Griseofulvin levels in stratum corneum. Study after oral administration in man. *Archives of Dermatology*, **106**, 344–348.

Förström, L., Goldyne, M. E. & Winkelmann, R. K. (1975) IgE in human eccrine sweat. *Journal of Investigative Dermatology*, **64**, 156–157.

Grice, J. W. H. Personal communication.

Heathcote, J., Cameron, C. H. & Dane, D. S. (1974) Hepatitis-B antigen in saliva and semen. *Lancet*, **1**, 71–73.

Jenkinson, D. McEwan, Mabon, R. M. & Manson, W. (1974) Sweat proteins. *British Journal of Dermatology*, **90**, 175–181.

Johnson, H. L. & Maibach, H. I. (1971) Drug excretion in human eccrine sweat. *Journal of Investigative Dermatology*, **56**, 182–188.

Knight, A. G. (1974) The activity of various topical griseofulvin preparations and the appearance of oral griseofulvin in the stratum corneum. *British Journal of Dermatology*, **91**, 49–55.

Leavell, U. W., Farley, C. H. & McIntyre, J. S. (1969) Cutaneous changes in a patient with carbon monoxide poisoning. *Archives of Dermatology*, **99**, 429–433.

Page, C. O'Neal, Jr & Remington, J. S. (1967) Immunologic studies in normal human sweat. *Journal of Laboratory and Clinical Medicine*, **69**, 634–650.

Pawan, G. L. S. & Grice, K. (1968) Distribution of alcohol in urine and sweat after drinking. *Lancet*, **2**, 1016.

Ridley, C. M. (1971) Bullous lesions in nitrazepam overdose. *British Medical Journal*, **3**, 28.

Schanker, L. S. (1964) Physiological transport of drugs. In *Advances in Drug Research*, Vol. 1, ed. Harper, N. J. & Simmonds, A. B., pp. 71–106. London: Academic Press.

Shah, V. P., Epstein, W. L. & Riegelman, S. (1974) Role of sweat in accumulation of orally administered griseofulvin in skin. *Journal of Clinical Investigation*, **53**, 1673–1678.
Slegers, J. F. G. (1969) Mechanisms of non-electrolyte transport through epithelial cells. In *The Exocrine Gland*, ed. Botelho, S. Y., Brooks, F.P. & Shelley, W. B., pp. 133–151. Philadelphia: University of Pennsylvania Press.
Telater, H., Keyhan, B., Kes, S. & Karacadağ, S. (1974) HBAg in sweat. *Lancet*, **2**, 461.
Vree, T. B. A., Muskens, Th. J. M. & Van Rossum, J. M. (1972) Excretion of amphetamines in human sweat. *Archives internationales de pharmacodynamie et de thérapie*, **199**, 311–317.

HYPERHIDROSIS
Abell, E. & Morgan, K. (1974) The treatment of idiopathic hyperhidrosis by glycopyrronium bromide and tap water iontophoresis. *British Journal of Dermatology*, **91**, 87–91.
Aguoyo, A. J., Nair, C. P. V. & Bray, G. M. (1971) Peripheral nerve abnormalities in the Riley–Day syndrome. *Archives of Neurology*, **24**, 106–116.
Allen, J. A., Armstrong, J. E. & Roddie, I. C. (1974) Sweat responses of a hyperhidrotic subject. *British Journal of Dermatology*, **90**, 277–281.
Appenzeller, O. & Goss, J. E. (1971) Autonomic deficits in Parkinson's syndrome. *Archives of Neurology*, **24**, 50–57.
Bakiewicz, T. A. (1973) A critical evaluation of the methods available for measurement of anti-perspirants. *Journal of the Society of Cosmetic Chemists*, **24**, 245–258.
Brunt, P. W. & McKusick, V. A. (1970) Familial dysautonomia. A report of genetic and clinical studies, with a review of the literature. *Medicine*, **49**, 343–374.
Burch, G. E. & Kones, R. J. (1973) Essential hyperhidrosis. Correlation of digital blood flow and capillary ultrastructure after unilateral sympathectomy. *American Journal of Medicine*, **54**, 378–389.
Burton, J. L., Johnson, C., Libman, L. & Shuster, S. (1972) Skin virilism in women with hirsutism. *Journal of Endocrinology*, **53**, 349–354.
Craig, F. N. (1970) Inhibition of sweating by salts of hyoscine and hyoscyamine. *Journal of Applied Physiology*, **28**, 779–783.
Cullen, S. I. (1975) Topical methenamine therapy for hyperhidrosis. *Archives of Dermatology*, **111**, 1158–1160.
Cunliffe, W. J., Johnson, C. E. & Williamson, D. M. (1972) Localised unilateral hyper-hidrosis—a clinical and laboratory study. *British Journal of Dermatology*, **86**, 374–378.
Davis, P. K. B. (1971) Surgical treatment of axillary hyperhidrosis. *British Journal of Plastic Surgery*, **24**, 99–100.
Edison, B. D. (1974) Frey's syndrome: diagnosis and treatment. *Eye, Ear, Nose and Throat*, **53**, 54–58.
Ellis, H. (1972) Hyperhidrosis. *British Journal of Hospital Medicine*, **7**, 641–644.
Ellis, H. & Morgan, M. W. (1971) Surgical treatment of severe hyperidrosis. *Proceedings of the Royal Society of Medicine*, **64**, 768–770.
Foster, K. G., Ginsburg, J. & Weiner, J. S. (1970) Role of circulating catecholamines in human eccrine sweat gland control. *Clinical Science*, **39**, 823–832.
Fox, R. H. & Hilton, S. M. (1958) Bradykinin formation in human skin as a factor in heat vasodilatation. *Journal of Physiology*, **142**, 219–232.
Frain-Bell, W. (1969) Anidrotics. *Practitioner*, **202**, 79–87.
Frankland, J. C. & Seville, R. H. (1971) The treatment of hyperhidrosis with topical propan-theline—a new technique. *British Journal of Dermatology*, **85**, 577–581.
Gibiński, K., Leszek, G., Zmudziński, J., Wacławczyk, J. & Dosiak, J. (1971) Body side related asymmetry in sweat gland function. *Journal of Investigative Dermatology*, **57**, 190–192.
Gillespie, J. A. & Kane, S. P. (1970) Evaluation of a simple surgical treatment of axillary hyperhidorisis. *British Journal of Dermatology*, **83**, 684–689.
Gitlow, S. E., Bertani, L. M., Wilk, E., Li, B. L. & Dziedzic, B. S. (1970) Excretion of cate-cholamine metabolites by children with familial dysautonomia. *Pediatrics*, **46**, 513–522.
Goodall, Mc. C. (1970) Innervation and inhibition of eccrine and apocrine sweating in man. *Journal of Clinical Pharmacology and Journal of New Drugs*, **10**, 235–246.
Gordon, B. I. & Maibach, H. I. (1968) Studies on the mechanism of aluminium anhidrosis. *Journal of Investigative Dermatology*, **50**, 411–413.

Gordon, B. I. & Maibach, H. I. (1969) Eccrine anhidrosis due to glutaraldehyde, formaldehyde and iontophoresis. *Journal of Investigative Dermatology*, **53**, 436–439.
Greenhalgh, R. M., Rosengarten, D. S. & Martin, P. (1971) Role of sympathectomy for
hyperhidrosis. *British Medical Journal*, **1**, 332–334.
Grice, K. A. & Bettley, F. R. (1966) Inhibition of sweating by poldine methosulphate (Nacton). Its use for measuring insensible respiration. *British Journal of Dermatology*, **78**, 458–
464.
Grice, K., Sattar, H. & Baker, H. (1972) Treatment of idiopathic hyperhidrosis with iontophoresis of tap water and poldine methosulphate. *British Journal of Dermatology*, **86**,
72–78.
Hitchens, J. T., Gomez, L., Goldstein, S. & Shemano, I. (1972) Contralateral inhibition of
eccrine sweating in rats after topical application of drugs. *Journal of Pharmacology and
Experimental Therapeutics*, **183**, 385–392.
Hurley, H. J. & Shelley, W. B. (1966) Axillary hyperhidrosis. Clinical features and local
surgical management. *British Journal of Dermatology*, **78**, 127–140.
Johnson, R. H. & Prout, B. J. (1967) Dissociation of some sympathetic nervous functions.
Bibliotheca anatomica (Basel) **9**, 349–354.
Johnson, R. H. & Spalding, J. M. K. (1974) Sweating. *Disorders of the Autonomic Nervous
System*, 1st edn, Ch. 10, pp. 179–198. Oxford: Blackwell.
Jordan, W. P., Jr, Dahl, M. V. & Albert, H L. (1972) Contact dermatitis from glutaraldehyde.
Archives of Dermatology, **105**, 94–95.
Juhlin, L. & Hansson, H. (1968) Topical glutaraldehyde for plantar hyperhidrosis. *Archives
of Dermatology*, **97**, 327–330.
Kaszynski, E. & Frisch, S. B. (1974) Mouse foot screen for the inhibition of sweating by anti-
cholinergic drugs. *Journal of Investigative Dermatology*, **62**, 510–513.
Kerr, J. H., Corbett, J. L., Prys-Roberts, C., Crampton Smith, A. & Spalding, J. M. K. (1968)
Involvement of the sympathetic nervous system in tetanus. Studies on 82 cases. *Lancet*,
2, 236–241.
Kligman, A. M. (1965) Topical pharmacology and toxicology of dimethyl sulfoxide—Part 1.
Journal of the American Medical Association, **193**, 796–804.
Lancet (1974) A prescription for perspiration. *Lancet*, **2**, 90–91.
Lansdown, A. B. G. (1973) The rat foot pad as a model for examining antiperspirants. *Journal
of the Society of Cosmetic Chemists*, **24**, 677–684.
Levit, F. (1968) Simple device for treatment of hyperhidrosis by iontophoresis. *Archives of
Dermatology*, **98**, 505–507.
Leyden, J. J. & Kligman, A. M. (1975) Aluminium chloride in the treatment of symptomatic
athlete's foot. *Archives of Dermatology*, **111**, 1004–1010.
MacMillan, F. S. K., Reller, H. H. & Synder, F. H. (1964) The antiperspirant action of
topically applied anticholinergics. *Journal of Investigative Dermatology*, **43**, 363–377.
Munro, D. D., Verbov, J. L., O'Gorman, D. J. & du Vivier, A. (1974) Axillary hyperhidrosis.
Its quantification and surgical treatment. *British Journal of Dermatology*, **90**, 325–329.
Myers, R. D. (1971) Hypothalamic mechanisms of pyrogen action in the cat and monkey. In
Pyrogens and Fever, Ciba Foundation Symposium, ed. Wolstenholme, G. E. W. &
Birch, J., pp. 131–153. London: Churchill Livingstone.
Papa, C. N. (1972) Mechanisms of eccrine anidrosis. III. Scanning electron microscopic study
of poral occlusion. *Journal of Investigative Dermatology*, **59**, 295–298.
Papa, C. M. & Kligman, A. M. (1967) Mechanisms of eccrine anhidrosis. II. The anti-
perspirant effect of aluminium salts. *Journal of Investigative Dermatology*, **49**, 139–145.
Prout, B. J. & Wardell, W. M. (1969) Sweating and peripheral blood flow in patients with
phaeochromocytoma. *Clinical Science*, **36**, 109–117.
Richards, R. L. (1967) Causalgia. A centennial review. *Archives of Neurology*, **16**, 339–350.
Sanderson, K. V. & Cronin, E. (1968) Glutaraldehyde and contact dermatitis. *British Medical
Journal*, **3**, 802.
Schmunes, E. & Levy, E. J. (1972) Quarternary ammonium compound contact dermatitis
from a deodorant. *Archives of Dermatology*, **105**, 91–93.
Shaw, M. H. (1974) A serious complication of an operation for axillary hyperhidrosis. *British
Journal of Plastic Surgery*, **27**, 196–197.
Shelley, W. B. & Hurley, H. J., Jr (1975) Studies on topical antiperspirants control of axillary
hyperhidrosis. *Acta dermato-venereologica (Stockholm)*, **55**, 241–260.

Verbov, J. (1974) Unilateral localised hyperhidrosis over face and scalp. *British Journal of Dermatology*, **90**, 470.

Warndorff, J. A. (1971) The response of the sweat glands to β-adrenergic stimulation. *British Journal of Dermatology*, **86**, 282–285.

Watkins, P. J. (1973) Facial sweating after food: a new sign of dibetic autonomic neuropathy. *British Medical Journal*, **1**, 583–587.

Weaver, P. C. & Copeman, P. W. M. (1971) Simple surgery for axillary hyperhidrosis (two cases). *Proceedings of the Royal Society of Medicine*, **64**, 607–608.

ANHIDROSIS

Cotton, D. W. K. & Van Rossum, E. (1973) Hexokinase, glucose-6-phosphate dehydrogenase and malate dehydrogenase in the isolated sweat glands of normal and atopic subjects. *British Journal of Dermatology*, **89**, 459–465.

Crump, I. A. & Danks, D. M. (1971) Hypohidrotic ectodermal dysplasia. A study of sweat pores in the X-linked form and in a family with probable autosomal recessive inheritance. *Journal of Pediatrics*, **78**, 466–473.

Desnick, R. J., Allen, K. Y., Simmons, R. L., Najarian, J. S. & Krivit, W. (1971) Treatment of Fabry's disease: correction of the enzymatic deficiency by renal transplantation. *Journal of Laboratory and Clinical Medicine*, **78**, 989–990.

English, R. S., Hurley, H. J., Witkowski, J. S. & Sanders, S. (1963) Generalised anhidrosis associated with Hodgkin's disease and acquired ichthyosis. *Annals of Internal Medicine*, **58**, 676–681.

Familusi, J. B., Jaiyesimi, F., Ojo, C. O. & Attah, Ed.'B. (1975) Hereditary anhidrotic ecto-dermal dysplasia. Studies in a Nigerian family. *Archives of Disease in Childhood*, **50**, 642–647.

Feinstein, A., Ackerman, A. B. & Ziprkowski, L. (1970) Histology of autosomal dominant ichthyosis vulgaris and X-linked ichthyosis. *Archives of Dermatology*, **101**, 524–527.

Fisher, D. A. & Maibach, H. I. (1970) Postural hypotension and anhidrosis. The autonomic insufficiency syndrome. *Archives of Dermatology*, **102**, 527–531.

Freire-Maia, N. (1971) Ectodermal dysplasias. *Human Heredity*, **21**, 309–312.

Freire-Maia, N., Fortes, V. A., Pereira, L. C., Opitz, J. M., Marcallo, F. A. & Cavalli, I. J. (1975) A syndrome of hypohidrotic ectodermal dysplasia with normal teeth, peculiar facies, pigmentary disturbances, psychomotor and growth retardation, bilateral nuclear cataract, and other signs. *Journal of Medical Genetics*, **12**, 308–310.

Frias, J. L. & Smith, D. W. (1968) Diminished sweat pores in hypohidrotic ectodermal dysplasia: a new method for assessment. *Journal of Pediatrics*, **72**, 606–610.

Goadby, H. K. & Downman, C. B. B. (1973) Peripheral vascular and sweat-gland reflexes in diabetic neuropathy. *Clinical Science and Molecular Medicine*, **45**, 281–289.

Grice, K. A. & Bettley, F. R. (1967) Skin water loss and accidental hypothermia in psoriasis, ichthyosis and erythroderma. *British Medical Journal*, **4**, 195–198.

Grice, K., Blendis, L. M., Keir, M. I. & Harvey, R. T. (1968) Accidental hypothermia in erythroderma from generalised psoriasis. *Archives of Dermatology*, **98**, 263–267.

Grice, K., Sattar, H. & Baker, H. Unpublished data.

Grice, K., Sattar, H., Casey, T. & Baker, H. (1975) An evaluation of Na^+, Cl^- and pH ion-specific electrodes in the study of the electrolyte contents of epidermal transudate and sweat. *British Journal of Dermatology*, **92**, 511–518.

Henning, D. R., Griffin, T. B. & Maibach, H. I. (1972) Studies on changes in skin surface bacteria in induced miliaria and associated hypohidrosis. *Acta dermato-venereologica (Stockholm)*, **52**, 371–375.

Hindson, T. C. (1968) Ascorbic acid for prickly heat. *Lancet*, **1**, 1347–1348.

Hindson, T. C. & Worsley, D. E. (1969) The effects of administration of ascorbic acid in experimentally induced miliaria and hypohidrosis in volunteers. *British Journal of Dermatology*, **81**, 226–227.

Hudson, C. D. & Witkop, C. J. (1975) Autosomal dominant hypodontia with nail dysgenesis. *Oral Surgery, Oral Medicin and Oral Pathology*, **39**, 409–423.

Ivy, H. K. (1961) Renal sodium loss and bronchogenic carcinoma. Associated autonomic neutophy. *Archives of Internal Medicine*, **108**, 47–55.

Johnson, C. & Shuster, S. (1969) Eccrine sweating in psoriasis. *British Journal of Dermatology*, **81**, 119–124.

Johnson, C. & Shuster, S. (1970) The patency of sweat ducts in normal-looking skin. *British Journal of Dermatology*, **83**, 367–370.

Johnson, R. H., Lee, G. de J., Oppenheimer, D. R. & Spalding, J. M. K. (1966) Autonomic failure with orthostatic hypotension due to intermediolateral column degeneration. *Quarterly Journal of Medicine*, **35**, 276–292.

Johnson, R. H., McLellan, D. L. & Love, D. R. (1971) Orthostatic hypotension and the Holmes–Adie syndrome: a study of two patients with afferent baroreceptor block. *Journal of Neurology, Neurosurgery and Psychiatry*, **34**, 562–570.

Johnson, R. H. & Spalding, J. M. K. (1974) Sweating. *Disorders of the Autonomic Nervous System*, 1st edn, Ch. 10, pp. 179–198. Oxford: Blackwell.

Kay, D. M. & Maibach, H. I. (1969) Pruritus and acquired anhidrosis. Two unusual cases. *Archives of Dermatology*, **100**, 291–293.

Kent, J. A. & Carton, D. (1973) In *Fabry's Diseases, Lysosomes and Storage Diseases*, ed. Hers, H. G. & Van Hoff, F., pp. 357–381. New York: Academic Press.

Kerr, C. B., Wells, R. S. & Cooper, K. E. (1966) Gene effect in carriers of anhidrotic ectodermal dysplasia. *Journal of Medical Genetics*, **3**, 169–176.

Moosa, A. & Dubowitz, V. (1970) Peipheral neuropathy in Cockayne's syndrome. *Archives of Disease in Childhood*, **45**, 674–677.

Neumann, E. & Hard, S. (1974) The significance of the epidermal sweat duct unit in the genesis of pustular psoriasis (Zumbusch) and the microabscess of Munro–Sabouraud. *Acta dermato-venereologica (Stockholm)*, **54**, 141–146.

Noronha, M. J., Vas, C. J. & Aziz, H. (1968) Autonomic dysfunction (sweating responses) in multiple sclerosis. *Journal of Neurology, Neurosurgery and Psychiatry*, **31**, 19–22.

Ogawa, T. (1970) Local effect of skin temperature on threshold concentration of sudorific agents. *Journal of Applied Physiology*, **28**, 18–22.

Papa, C. M. (1972) Mechanisms of eccrine anidrosis. III. Scanning electron microscopic study of poral occlusion. *Journal of Investigative Dermatology*, **59**, 295–298.

Reed, W. B., Lopez, D. A. & Landing, B. (1970) Clinical spectrum of anhidrotic ectodermal dysplasia. *Archives of Dermatology*, **102**, 134–143.

Sarkany, I., Shuster, S. & Stammers, M. C. (1965) Occlusion of the sweat pores by hydration. *British Journal of Dermatology*, **77**, 101–104.

Sehgal, V. N. (1974) Significance of the local sweat response in the diagnosis of leprosy. *Dermatologica*, **148**, 217–223.

Shelley, W. B. & Lehman, J. M. (1961) Generalised anhidrosis associated with multiple myeloma. *Archives of Dermatology*, **83**, 903–909.

Shuster, S. & Marks, J. (1970) In *Systemic Effects of Skin Disease*. London: Heinemann.

Stillman, M. A., Hindson, T. C. & Maibach, H. I. (1971) The effect of pretreatment of skin on artificially induced miliaria rubra and hypohidrosis. *British Journal of Dermatology*, **84**, 110–116.

Sulzberger, M. B. & Griffin, T. B. (1969) Induced miliaria, postmiliarial hypohidrosis, and some potential sequelae. *Archives of Dermatology*, **99**, 145–151.

Sulzberger, M. B. & Harris, D. R. (1972) Miliaria and anhidrosis. III. Multiple small patches and the effects of different periods of occlusion. *Archives of Dermatology*, **105**, 845–850.

Suskind, R. R. (1954) Eccrine function in psoriasis. *Journal of Investigative Dermatology*, **23**, 345–357.

Tan, S. G. & Cunliffe, W. J. (1975) High doses of ascorbic acid. *British Journal of Dermatology*, **93**, 731.

Thomas, J. P. & Shields, R. (1970) Associated autonomic dysfunction and carcinoma of the pancreas. *British Medical Journal*, **4**, 32.

Totel, G. L. (1974) Physiological responses to heat of resting man with impaired sweating capacity. *Journal of Applied Physiology*, **37**, 346–352.

Vanasse, M., Molina-Negro, P. & Saint-Hilaire, J. M. (1974) Syndrome d'Adie associé à une hypohidrose segmentaire. Étude clinique et neurophysiologique. *Revue Neurologique*, **130**, 237–244.

Van Mullem, P. J. (1972) Ultrastructure of lipid bodies and lysosomes in the skin in Fabry's disease. *Archives belges de dermatologie et de syphiligraphie*, **28**, 41–49.

Verbov, J. (1970) Hypohidrotic (or anhidrotic) ectodermal dysplasia—an appraisal of diagnostic methods. *British Journal of Dermatology*, **83**, 341–348.

Verbov, J. Unpublished data.

Verbov, J. & Wells, R. S. (1972) Hypohidrotic ectodermal dysplasia. Paper (unpublished) read at the British Association of Dermatology, Summer meeting, 6th July, 1972, London.

Wallace, H. J. (1973) Anderson–Fabry disease. *British Journal of Dermatology*, **88**, 1–23.

Warndorff, J. A. (1970) The response of the sweat gland to acetylcholine in atopic subjects. *British Journal of Dermatology*, **83**, 306–311.

Warndorff, J. A. & Hamer, M. (1974) The response of the sweat glands to β-adrenergic stimulation with isoprenaline. *British Journal of Dermatology*, **90**, 263–268.

Wells, R. S. & Kerr, C. B. (1966) The histology of ichthyosis. *Journal of Investigative Dermatology*, **46**, 530–535.

Willis, I. (1973) The effects of prolonged water exposure on human skin. *Journal of Investigative Dermatology*, **60**, 166–171.

Willis, I., Harris, D. R. & Moretz, W. (1973) Normal and abnormal variations in eccrine sweat gland distribution. *Journal of Investigative Dermatology*, **60**, 98–103.

Yamamoto, K. (1967) Autonomic involvement in polyneuritis and its related disorders. *Brain Nerve (Tokyo)*, **19**, 1199–1208.

GENETIC ABNORMALITIES OF SWEAT GLAND FUNCTION

Belcher, R. W. (1973) Ultrastructure and function of eccrine glands in the mucopolysaccharidoses. *Archives of Pathology*, **96**, 339–341.

Chandra, R. K., Madhavankutty, K. & Way, R. C. (1975) Serum α-fetoprotein levels in patients with cystic fibrosis and their patents and siblings. *British Medical Journal*, **1**, 714–716.

Dobson, R. L. (1974) The normal eccrine sweat gland. In *Clinical Dermatology*, ed. Demis, D. J., Crounse, R. G., Dobson, R. L. & McGuire, J., Vol. 2, Section 9A-1. Maryland: Harper and Row.

Durand, P., Borrone, C., Della Cella, G. & Philippart, M. (1968) Fucosidosis. *Lancet*, **1**, 1198.

Elliott, R. B. (1974) Wrinkling of skin in cystic fibrosis. *Lancet*, **2**, 108.

Foster, K. G., Hey, E. N. & Katz, G. (1969) The response of the sweat glands of the newborn baby to thermal stimuli and to intradermal acetycholine. *Journal of Physiology*, **203**, 13–29.

Gibson, L. E., Matthews, W. J., Jr & Minihan, P. T. (1970) Hyperpermeable mucus in cystic fibrosis. *Lancet*, **2**, 189–191.

Harris, R. C. & Cohen, H. I. (1963) Seat electrolytes in glycogen storage disease, Type I. *Pediatrics*, **31**, 1044–1046.

Kaiser, D., Drack, E. & Rossi, E. (1970) Effects of cystic fibrosis sweat on sodium reabsorption by the normal sweat gland. *Lancet*, **1**, 1003.

Leonard, P. J. & Morris, W. P. (1972) Sodium, calcium, and magnesium levels in nails of children with cystic fibrosis of the pancreas. *Archives of Disease in Childhood*, **47**, 495–498.

Liberman, J. & Rodbard, S. (1975) Low blood pressure in young adults with cystic fibrosis. An effect of chronic salt loss in sweat? *Annals of Internal Medicine*, **82**, 806–808.

Loeb, H., Tondeur, M., Toppet, M. & Cremer, N. (1969) Clinical, biochemical and ultrastructural studies of an atypical form of mucopolysaccharidosis. *Acta paediatrica scandinavica*, **58**, 220–228.

McFarlane, H., Holzel, A., Brenchley, P., Allen, J. D., Wallwork, J. C., Singer, B. E. & Worsley, B. (1975) Immune complexes in cystic fibrosis. *British Medical Journal*, **1**, 423–428.

McKusick, V. A., Kaplan, D., Wise, D., Hanley, W. B., Suddarth, S. B., Sevick, M. E. & Maumanee, A. E. (1965) The genetic mucopolysaccharidoses. *Medicine*, **44**, 445–483.

Mearns, M. B. (1974) Cystic fibrosis. *British Journal of Hospital Medicine*, **12**, 497–506.

Negus, V. (1967) The function of mucus: a hypothesis. *Proceedings of the Royal Society of Medicine*, **60**, 75–77.

Sarsfield, J. K. & Davies, J. M. (1975) Negative sweat tests and cystic fibrosis. *Archives of Disease in Childhood*, **50**, 463–466.

Spock, A., Heick, H. M. C., Cress, H. & Logan, W. S. (1967) Abnormal serum factor in patients with cystic fibrosis of pancreas. *Pediatric Research*, **1**, 173–177.

Steinrud, J., Winkel, S. & Flensborg, E. W. (1974) Screening for cystic fibrosis with chloride electrode. *Danish Medical Bulletin*, **21**, 251–255.

Apocrine Sweat Glands

Bell, M. (1974) The ultrastructure of human axillary apocrine glands after epinephrine injection. *Journal of Investigative Dermatology*, **63**, 147–159.

Braun-Falco, I. & Rupec, M. (1968) Apokrine schweissdrüsen. *Handbuch der Haut-und Geschlechtskrankheiten*, Vol. 1, Part 1, Jadassohn, J. Ergänzungswerk, ed. Marchionini, A., pp. 267–338. Berlin: Springer-Verlag.

Cortese, T. A., Jr & Nicoll, P. A. (1970) In vivo observations of skin appendages in the bag wing. *Journal of Investigative Dermatology*, **54**, 1–10.

Fox, R. H., Mullen, B. J. & Thornton, C. (1974) A technique for studying apocrine gland function in man. *Journal of Physiology*, **239**, 75–76 p.

Jenkinson, D. McEwan (1973) Comparative physiology of sweating. *British Journal of Dermatology*, **88**, 397–406.

Montagna, W. & Parakkal, P. F. (1974) Apocrine glands. *The Structure and Function of the Skin*, 3rd edn, Ch. 11, pp. 332–365. New York: Academic Press.

Schaumburg-Lever, G. & Lever, W. F. (1975) Secretion from human apocrine glands: an electron microscopic study. *Journal of Investigative Dermatology*, **64**, 38–41.

PHARMACOLOGY OF APOCRINE SWEATING

Aoki, T. (1962) Stimulation of human axillary apocrine sweat glands by cholinergic agents. *Journal of Investigative Dermatology*, **38**, 41–44.

Aoki, T. & Hayashi, H. (1974) Some morphologic and pharmacologic observations on the apocrine glands in the tail of the goat. *Journal of Investigative Dermatology*, **63**, 168–173.

Jenkinson, D. McEwan (1973) Comparative physiology of sweating. *British Journal of Dermatology*, **88**, 397–406.

Jenkinson, D. McEwan, Sengupta, B. P. & Blackburn, P. S. (1966) The distribution of nerves, monoamine oxidase and cholinesterase in the skin of cattle. *Journal of Anatomy*, **100**, 593–613.

Johnson, K. G. (1975) Sweat gland function in isolated perfused skin. *Journal of Physiology*, **250**, 633–649.

Montagna, W. (1964) Histology and cytochemistry of human skin. XXIV. Further observations on the axillary organ. *Journal of Investigative Dermatology*, **42**, 119–129.

Robertshaw, D. (1974) Neural and humoral control of apocrine glands. *Journal of Investigative Dermatology*, **63**, 160–167.

HIDRADENITIS SUPPURATIVA

Anderson, D. K. & Perry, A. W. (1975) Axillary hidradenitis. *Archives of Surgery*, **110**, 69–72.

Letterman, G. & Schurter, M. (1974) Surgical treatment of hyperhidrosis and chronic hidradenitis suppurativa. *Journal of Investigative Dermatology*, **63**, 174–182.

Montagna, W. (1959) Histology and cytochemistry of human skin. XIX. The development and fate of the axillary organ. *Journal of Investigative Dermatology*, **33**, 151–161.

Montes, L. F., Baker, B. L. & Curtis, A. C. (1960) The cytology of the large axillary sweat glands in man. *Journal of Investigative Dermatology*, **35**, 273–283.

Shelley, W. B. (1972) Hidradenitis suppurative. In *Consultations in Dermatology*, pp. 74–79. Philadelphia: W. B. Saunders, Co.

Ward, J. N., Washio, H. & David, H. S. (1974) Hidradenitis suppurativa of scrotum and perimeum. *Urology*, **4**, 463–466.

Sweat Gland Tumours

Black, M. & Wilson-Jones, E. (1971) Dermal cylindroma following x-ray epilation of the scalp. *British Journal of Dermatology*, **85**, 70–72.

Castro, C. & Winkelmann, R. K. (1974) Spiradenoma. Histochemical and electron microscopic study. *Archives of Dermatology*, **109**, 40–48.

Civatte, J., Tsoïtis, G. & Préaux, J. (1974) Le naevus apocrine. Étude de 2 cas. *Annales de Dermatologie et Syphiligraphie*, **101**, 251–261.

Dave, V. K. (1972) Eccrine sweat gland carcinoma with metastases. *British Journal of Dermatology*, **86**, 95–97.

El-Domeira, A. A., Brasfield, R. D., Huvos, A. G. & Strong, E. W. (1971) Sweat gland carcinoma: a clinico-pathologic study of 83 patients. *Annals of Surgery*, **173**, 270–274.

Fakhery, B. & Fishman, L. N. (1974) Sweat gland carcinoma. Report of a case in an usual location and review of the literature. *Journal of the Maine Medical Association*, **65**, 80–87.

Goldern, R. (1970) Eccrine poromatosis. *Archives of Dermatology*, **101**, 606–608.

Hashimoto, K. (1973) Hidradenoma papilliferum. An electron microscopic study. *Acta dermato-venereologica (Stockholm)*, **53**, 22–30.

Hu, F. & Sisson, J. K. (1969) The ultrastructure of the pale cell acanthoma. *Journal of Investigative Dermatology*, **52**, 185–188.

Landry, M. & Winkelmann, R. K. (1972) An unusual tubular apocrine adenoma. Histo-chemical and ultrastructural study. *Archives of Dermatology*, **105**, 869–879.

Lindgren, A. G. H. & Neumann, E. (1973) Some evidence concerning the sweat duct origin of clear cell acanthoma. *Acta dermato-venereologica (Stockholm)*, **53**, 511–514.

Rosen, Y., Kim, B. & Yermakov, V. A. (1975) Eccrine sweat duct tumour of clear cell origin involving the eyelids. *Cancer*, **36**, 1034–1041.

Sanderson, K. V. (1972) Tumours of the skin. In *Textbook of Dermatology*, 2nd edn, ed. Rook, A., Wilkinson, D. S. & Ebling, F. J. G., Vol. 2, Ch. 66, pp. 1911–2007. Oxford: Blackwell.

Smith, J. D. & Chernosky, M. E. (1973) Hidrocystomas. *Archives of Dermatology*, **108**, 676–679.

Smith, J. D. & Chernosky, M. E. (1974) Apocrine hydrocystoma (cystadenoma). *Archives of Dermatology*, **109**, 700–702.

Tsuji, T., Sugai, T. & Suzuki, S. (1975) The mode of growth of milia. *Journal of Investigative Dermatology*, **65**, 388–393.

Weiner, A. L., Richfield, D. F. & Safdi, S. A. (1973) Sweat gland carcinoma: a little known and treacherous neoplasm. *Cutis*, **11**, 179–182.

Wilson-Jones, E. & Heyl, T. (1970) Naevus sebaceus. A report of 140 cases with special regard to the development of secondary malignant tumours. *British Journal of Dermatology*, **82**, 99–117.

Wilson-Jones, E. (1971) Pigmented nodular hidradenoma. *Archives of Dermatology*, **104**, 117–123.

6
LEG ULCERS

Robin D. G. Peachey

Leg ulcers may be associated with a large number of medical and dermatological conditions (Table 6.1), and their origin is often multifactorial (Ryan and Wilkinson, 1972). In a single chapter it is impossible to deal with all types of ulceration, and for this reason certain topics only have been singled out for discussion. Much of the following discussion is particularly related to venous leg ulceration, as this is the major cause of leg ulceration in most populations.

Incidence

The prevalence of a condition within a community may be affected by many factors, such as the genetic constitution of its members, nutritional status, environmental factors, customs and occupations. Accurate data concerning the incidence of a non-fatal disease are difficult to obtain, and statistics are usually drived from hospital attendance records or general practice surveys. Particularly in underdeveloped countries the incidence of a particular condition may be greatly underestimated, and apparent differences between populations may be affected by differences in age structure.

Even in the best centres it is difficult to provide an aetiological diagnosis for every patient with a leg ulcer, and it is not surprising that in most surveys of the incidence of skin diseases no attempt has been made to subdivide 'leg ulcers' into aetiological groups. Indeed, in many surveys leg ulcers as a group are not mentioned at all.

Population studies are few, and no adequate survey of the incidence of leg ulcers has been carried out in the United Kingdom. In Europe, the Basle study of 4422 healthy working adults aged 20 to 70 years, detected chronic venous insffiuciency in 19 per cent of men and in 25 per cent of women, while the severer forms with ulceration were present in 1.1 and 1.4 per cent respectively (Da Silva et al, 1974). Figures from American and other European series are similar (Borschberg, 1967), and all surveys confirm the increased incidence of ulceration in females, who usually outnumber males by 2–4 to 1.

In Britain the incidence of leg ulcers seen in dermatological outpatients varies. In central London, leg ulcer patients comprised 0.4 per cent of new patients attending St John's Hospital for Diseases of the Skin between 1952 and 1963 (Neves, 1966). Of these patients, 0.3 per cent had venous ulcers while

Table 6.1 Causes of leg ulceration

Trauma	
External	Injuries, burns, chemicals, trophic ulceration
Self-inflicted	Artefacts
Infections	
Acute	Pyococcal
Chronic	Mycobacterial, syphilis, yaws
Mycotic	
Leishmaniasis	
Miscellaneous	'Desert sore', accidental infections
Phagedenic	Meleney's ulcer, tropical ulcer
Infestations and bites	Guinea worm, spider bites, etc.
Pyoderma gangrenosum	
Venous	
Primary and post-thrombotic	
Atrophie blanche	
Cutaneous vasculitis	
Small vessel	Allergic vasculitis, Schönlein–Henoch purpura
Nodular forms	Erythema induratum, nodular vasculitis, nodular erythrocyanosis, polyarteritis nodosa
Erythrocyanoid	Livedo with ulceration
Necrobiotic	Necrobiosis lipoidica
Granulomatous	
Neoplastic	
Skin neoplasms	
Reticuloses	
Leukaemia	
Arteriovenous aneurysm	
Congenital	
Acquired	Especially post-traumatic
Ischaemia (arterial)	
Extramural	Strangulation by scar tissue, fibrosis, radiodermatitis
Mural	Thickening of vessel wall with thrombosis or reduced flow
Intramural	Thrombosis, embolism, coagulation disorders, blood dyscrasias, dysglobulinaemias, sludging of red cells
Miscellaneous	Chronic haemolytic anaemias, ulceration of rheumatoid nodules, Paget's disease, systemic sclerosis, Werner's syndrome, Jaffe–Lichtenstein disease, associated with calcinosis, Drugs, e.g. Warfarin

Modified from: Ryan, T. J. & Wilkinson, D. S. (1972) Diseases of the veins: leg ulcers. In *Textbook of Dermatology*, 2nd edn, ed. Rook, A., Wilkinson, D. S. & Ebling, F. J. G., Vol. 1, Ch. 33, Tab. 33.3. Oxford: Blackwell.

0.004 per cent had arteriosclerotic ulcers, and 0.1 per cent were unspecified. Warin (1965) reported that leg ulcers made up about 2 per cent of new dermatological outpatient attendances in Bristol, and figures for 1974 show this incidence to be virtually unchanged. Comparable figures have been reported from other centres (Rook and Wilkinson, 1972).

Information from parts of the world other than Europe and America is sparse, but it is generally held that ulceration due to venous insufficiency is less common in African natives. Schulz, Finlay and Scott (1962), in the Transvaal, found that 0.1 per cent of 2000 consecutive Bantu patients attending dermatological outpatients had venous leg ulcers, but do not give figures for the incidence of non-venous leg ulcers, while Dogliotti (1970), in Johannesburg, found the incidence of leg ulcers (unspecified) in Bantu patients referred to hospital to be 1.75 per cent. Finlay and Park (1969) compared the incidence of varicose eczema in their middle-aged Indian patients (7 per cent) with that in comparable 'white' patients (3 per cent) and Bantu (1 per cent), but give no figures for the incidence of venous ulceration. In Nigeria, Shrank and Harman (1966) found no varicose ulcers among 1156 Nigerian outpatients, but noted tropical ulcers in 1.1 per cent. Hill (1968) reported that 0.5 per cent of patients referred to dermatological outpatients in Hong Kong had varicose ulcers, compared with an incidence of 0.6 per cent in New Zealand.

Circulatory Factors

Arteries

The arterial supply to the lower third of the leg is relatively poor, and there has been some discussion concerning the part that arterial changes might play in leg ulceration. Anning (1952) noted 'arterial' ulcers in 1.8 per cent of 715 patients with leg ulcers, while Haeger (1965) stated that about 90 per cent of leg ulcers were venous in origin, 4 to 5 per cent were due to ischaemia without venous stasis, and that about 4 per cent were venous ulcers with superadded and important arterial ischaemia. Weidmann (1954) considered that arterial disease played a significant role in many patients with venous ulcers, while Wittels and Zuchristian (1967) observed arterial circulatory changes in 50 per cent of post-thrombotic cases.

More recent work by Thune (1972), using piezoelectric and photoplethysmographic pulse curve recordings, has shown that—with the exception of some areas of atrophie blanche and dermatosclerosis—the arterial cutaneous blood supply in 35 patients with venous leg ulcers was not significantly reduced. A zone of vasodilatation and decreased vascular reactivity was present around the ulcer. Fäs et al (1973) also were unable to find any evidence in men that severe venous insufficiency was associated with an increased incidence of arterial disease or vice versa.

Welbourn (1967), using arteriography, studied 51 patients with leg ulcers, varicose veins, or both. Twenty-three patients showed arteriovenous shunts at or near the ulcer site, or in relation to the varicosities. Some also showed concomitant arterial disease and/or an inflammatory circulation at the ulcer site. A further 23 patients had no evidence of arteriovenous shunts, but had other significant abnormalities—arterial disease (7), inflammatory circulation at the ulcer site (7), deep vein thrombosis (3), congenital abnormality (6), arterial hypoplasia (5), and the Klippel Trenauney syndrome (1). Five patients had no arterial abnormality.

Veins

In the lower leg the deep and superficial venous systems are connected by a limited number of thin, barely visible perforating veins. These short, horizontally running vessels are of two types. Direct perforators—about 40 in each lower limb—form a direct link between the main superficial and deep veins. Each perforates the deep fascia as a single channel, and then usually divides into three or four branches which enter the deep veins separately. Indirect perforators—160 to 200 in each lower limb—connect a main superficial vein to an intramuscular vein and then to a main deep vein. Most of the perforating veins are very small, inconstant in site, and valveless, but Linton (1938) and Dodd and Cockett (1956) pointed out that the perforators that most frequently became incompetent were larger and more constant vessels above the ankle, where the results of venous insufficiency are most obvious. In this region there are two to four direct perforators on the lateral side, and three to five on the medial side which do have valves and which direct blood from the superficial to the deep system.

If both saphenous veins are removed, the blood in the superficial system still finds its way into the deep veins without any apparent difficulty, and without any obvious change in pressure gradient. Daintree Johnson and Pflug (1975) consider that only a fraction of this blood could pass through the 200 to 300 thin perforating veins, and suggest that most of the blood must pass through the 'microscopic veins' which they consider in normal people to be of more importance in venous return than the perforating veins.

In the normal leg the pressure of blood in a superficial vein on the foot, with the patient standing and at rest, is equivalent to a pressure of 85 to 90 mmHg (Dodd and Cockett, 1956). As soon as the calf muscles are exercised, this pressure drops to 0 to 30 mmHg due to blood flowing from the superficial to the deep venous system, and on cessation of exercise, slowly rises to its previous level in about 31 s. In patients with incompetent superficial varicose veins the pressure falls to about 45 to 60 mmHg rising, within a few seconds, to the initial figure on cessation of exercise. In patients who have had a deep vein thrombosis with loss of valves in the deep venous system, there may be dilatation and incompetence or loss of valves in the ankle perforating veins, and in these cases, following exercise, there is either no fall at all or only a slight fall in pressure in the superficial veins, with an immediate return to the pre-exercise level on cessation of exercise.

Microvasculature

The common vascular pattern in adult skin is based on a characteristic micro-anatomy, and has been summarised by Ryan (1973). An artery of about 100 μm in diameter enters the lower dermis, and divides once or twice to give vertical or obliquely running branches which divide again in the mid and upper dermis to produce a 'candelabra' pattern of vertically orientated arterioles. The calibre of these vessels is reduced to about 15 μm by the time they reach the upper dermis, lose their muscle coats and become capillaries. Branching of capillaries gives rise to a network of capillaries lying horizontal to the surface, and above this may be found individual vertical terminal capillaries which arise from arterioles, and loop up into the dermal papillae. These capillaries empty into the horizontal subpapillary venous plexus. Venules in the upper and mid-dermis are, for the most part, horizontally disposed and are more numerous than arterioles.

In recent years it has become clear that blood vessel permeability is closely related to venular function. Venoconstriction may cause increased intra-capillary pressure, and thus increased capillary permeability (Haddy, 1960). It has been shown (Majno, Palade and Schoefl, 1961) that venules are them-selves permeable, and that permeability is greatest at the venular end of the capillary (Wiederhielm, 1966).

With increasing age the horizontal subpapillary venous plexus in the lower leg tends to become dilated, and leashes of arborising horizontal venules may be seen around the ankles. Blood flow in these vessels is slow with consequent cooling and increase in viscosity, and the overlying skin is often thin and atrophic (Ryan, 1969). Although these changes may be marked, they usually give rise to little pathology. More of a problem are changes in the papillary vessels. Allen (1972) has shown that dilatation of the papillary capillaries and the subpapillary venous plexus occurs in normal subjects when they are tilted from the horizontal to the vertical. The degree of filling noted is proportional to the hydrostatic pressure of the blood. Muscular exercise results in emptying of the skin capillaries and subpapillary venous plexus. In patients with varicose veins and the post-thrombotic syndrome, there is an over-all reduction in the number of papillary vessels, and the capillary loops are elongated and tortuous. In such cases capillary microscopy reveals a single arteriole dividing into one or more loosely coiled capillaries, which drain into a single venule (Ryan, 1973). These vessels are highly permeable, leading to local haemoconcentration, and often become blocked and throm-bosed or bleed, with resultant purpura and haemosiderin pigmentation. The abnormal vessel morphology, which occurs as a result of venous insufficiency, tends to lead to microvascular stasis and it is believed (Ryan, 1973) that some aspects of inflammation are enhanced in distorted vessels.

There is evidence (Piulachs and Vidal-Barraquer, 1953; Haeger and Bergman, 1963) that in patients with venous insuffiicency, small and normally non-functioning shunts may open up between arteries and veins. These shunt vessels are very small, and therefore difficult to demonstrate. Following femoral angiography (Haimovici, Steinman and Caplan, 1966) premature opacification of veins, indicating arteriovenous anastomoses, occurred first in the pedal vessels in patients with varicose veins and around the ankle in patients with the postphlebitic syndrome. Evidence of shunting could also be shown in patients with occlusive arterial disease and in those with ischaemic manifestations in the absence of organic occlusive disease.

When shunting occurs in patients with venous stasis, there is likely to be a further decrease in capillary blood flow, which will exacerbate the effects of stasis in the papillary vessels. Flow is most impaired in dilated capillaries because large red cell aggregates may obstruct them. Narrow capillaries are not easily obstructed by the normal flow of plasma and single red cells (Ryan, 1973).

The histology of veins in the lower leg reflects the pressures these vessels have to withstand. The muscle layer in the wall of these veins may be twice as thick as elsewhere and even capillaries have a thickened basement membrane (Kügelgen, 1955).

Atrophie blanche

Atrophie blanche consists typically of small plaques of white scar tissue, spotted with residual and greatly dilated papillary vessels. It is often seen on the feet and lower legs in patients with venous stasis, but may occur in association with other disorders. Stevanović (1974) has reported atrophie blanche in essential cryoglobulinaemia, systemic lupus erythematosus, scleroderma, and within a tumour plaque in a patient with lymphoma. Histologically, there are ischaemic zones in which there is total loss of papillary vessels and a thin, atrophic epidermis overlies a band of acellular collagen which separates the horizontal plexus from the surface of the skin. Some mid-dermal blood vessels show pronounced endothelial proliferation, with the deposition of fibrinoid material within the lumen and resulting partial or complete occlusion. The area of atrophy is surrounded and frequently pierced by residual, grossly dilated capillaries (Ryan, 1969). These vessels have broken or survived the barrier of scar tissue separating the epidermis from its blood supply, and can be shown to be excessively permeable and fragile.

Copeman and Ryan (1971) consider that atrophie blanche represents the end result of various pathological processes. They believe that blood stasis in the dermal vessels must be sufficiently prolonged to cause clotting and atrophy of the capillary-venule with subsequent ischaemic scarring. Predisposing factors are haemodynamic back pressure due to venous stasis, cold, altered blood viscosity and damage by immune phenomena.

Types of Leg Ulceration

Skin ulceration in the lower leg usually results from physical or chemical trauma, infection in various forms or occurs as a result of ischaemia. Frequently more than one factor is present.

Venous ulceration

Venous ulceration occurs as an end result of venous incompetence and is usually seen in association with oedema, purpura, pigmentation and fibrosis. Eczema may also be present.

Anning (1952) showed that 80 per cent of his cases of leg ulceration had a history of a previous deep vein thrombosis, while 7 per cent were associated with varicose veins and 10 per cent were due to venous insufficiency of doubtful cause.

Bauer (1942) followed 100 patients who had had a major deep vein thrombosis, and showed that all patients had some permanent residual oedema of the affected lower leg. After an interval of five years, 45 per cent of his patients had developed induration of the skin around the ankle and 20 per cent had developed ulceration. After 10 years these figures had increased to 72 and 52 per cent respectively.

Most authors now agree that primary saphenous insufficiency accounts for a relatively small proportion of venous ulcers, and it is largely accepted that the majority are associated with perforator vein incompetence, most commonly due to a preceding deep venous thrombosis (Anderson and McDonald, 1963). In some cases, however, venous incompetence may be produced in other ways such as by trauma, or by a superficial thrombosis which extends into a perforating vein. Sarjeant (1964) believes that in some patients a process which he calls phlebosclerosis, causes a contracture of the valve cusps rendering them incompetent. A number of workers (Sarjeant, 1964; Arnoldi, 1966, 1967; Haeger, 1966) believe that incompetent perforating veins are to be found in association with every venous ulcer, and that even when an ulcer is associated with gross incompetence of the superficial venous system, there is likely to be incompetence of one or more perforating veins in addition.

Although the importance of recognising and locating incompetent perforating veins in patients with leg ulcers is well established (Cockett and Elgan Jones, 1953; Sherman, 1964; Arnoldi, 1967), clinical examination alone will only detect up to 60 per cent and they may be difficult to localise. In recent years various tests have been devised to localise these veins more accurately.

Operative phlebography using intraosseous injection of contrast medium into the medial malleolus has an accuracy of 92 per cent (Townsend, Jones and Williams, 1967), but the technique is painful and requires a general anaesthetic, and in the presence of leg ulceration may cause osteomyelitis. It is usually performed immediately prior to surgery. A simplified technique of phlebography for preoperative use was described by Lea Thomas et al (1972), and was reported to be 81 per cent accurate in localising incompetent perforating veins. Several groups of workers have compared the accuracy of preoperative clinical assessment with phlebography and other techniques such as thermography and the fluorescein test, in the diagnosis of incompetent perforating veins, and have related their results to the localisation of incompetent veins found at surgery. Callum, Gray and Lea Thomas (1973) found clinical assessment to be 48 per cent accurate, the fluorescein test 39 per cent accurate, and phlebography 69 per cent accurate. Thermography is said to have an accuracy of between 94 per cent (Patil, Williams and Lloyd Williams, 1970) and 62 per cent (Noble and Gunn, 1972), but the necessary apparatus is expensive and not generally available in most hospitals. Miller and Foote (1974) reported a success rate of 82 per cent in detecting incompetent perforating veins using an ultrasonic scanning technique. Callum et al (1973) consider that phlebography is the best method of preoperative detection of incompetent perforating veins at present available, but feel that it is not sufficiently accurate to replace an adequate surgical exploration.

Associated abnormalities

Investigations have shown (Butcher and Hoover, 1955) that the superficial lymphatics are absent in and around venous ulcers, and there is evidence to suggest that obliteration or distortion of lymphatics may contribute to hyperkeratosis and dermal fibrosis.

Subcutaneous ossification in the legs was noted on radiological examination in 10 per cent of 600 patients with chronic venous insufficiency, examined by Lippmann and Goldin (1960). The calcified deposits, which may be widespread, are easily distinguished from phleboliths and arteriosclerotic calcification, and have been shown to occur in areas of fat necrosis and fibrosis (Sarkany and Kreel, 1966). In occasional cases subcutaneous ossification may be a cause of delayed healing of an ulcer.

Periostitis with new bone formation may be present beneath a chronic ulcer.

Non-venous ulceration

Lack of space precludes any detailed account of current views in most types of non-venous ulceration and only vasculitis, the hereditary haemolytic anaemias and hypertensive ischaemic ulceration will be singled out for brief discussion here.

Vasculitis. In this group of conditions the primary pathological event is an alteration in or around the vessel wall. Due to a failure of repair mechanisms a chain of events occurs which may present clinically in the skin as urticaria, purpura, blistering, infarction, or necrosis and ulceration. In cutaneous vasculitis the precipitating factors are thought to be immunological. Work in this field has been reviewed by a number of authors including Cream and Turk (1971) and Asghar and Cormane (1974), and will not be discussed further.

It has been shown (Cliff, 1966) that antigen–antibody complexes produce their damaging effects chiefly at the venular end of the microvascular tree. Stasis of blood and increased permeability in the venules allow irritant substances to lodge, causing subsequent damage. This is especially likely to occur in the legs, where blood flow in the skin is slow due to haemodynamic back pressure, skin papillary vessels may be tortuous, coiled, and distorted, and where cooling of blood is also a factor. Stasis encourages fibrin deposition and platelet aggregation, and is particularly likely to occur in grossly coiled vessels (Copeman and Ryan, 1970). When the microvascular system is blocked by fibrin or platelets, the lesion produced may be predominantly haemorrhagic or ischaemic. Studies of the Schwartzman phenomenon by Illig, Schneider and Winkelmann (1969) have indicated that haemorrhage and vessel block are two separate phenomena influenced by the degree of fibrinolytic activity.

The hereditary haemolytic anaemias. Chronic leg ulcers are a poorly under-stood complication of chronic haemolytic disease. They are particularly characteristic of sickle-cell anaemia and hereditary spherocytosis, but may also occur in association with other haemolytic disorders. Interruption of the haemolytic process, for example by splenectomy in hereditary spherocytosis, is followed by healing of the ulcers. Afifi et al (1975) have reported increased healing of leg ulcers in β-thalassaemia major, in eight patients who were treated with 3 g of ascorbic acid daily in a controlled, double-blind cross-over study.

In homozygous sickle-cell anaemia (Hb SS) the incidence of chronic leg ulcers in older children and adults is about 75 per cent in the United States of America and 50 per cent in Jamaica. The incidence in patients with combina-tion haemoglobinopathies is lower. Occasional patients with the sickle-cell trait (Hb As) may develop similar ulceration if there is associated systemic disease, such as pneumonia (Wolfort and Krizek, 1969). Serjeant and Gueri (1970) noted the sickle-cell trait in 49 of 250 patients attending a leg ulcer clinic in Jamaica, while the incidence of the trait in the Negro population was 10.8 per cent. This difference was statistically significant, and they concluded that there was a relationship between the two conditions.

Ulcers in sickle-cell anaemia are situated on the lower third of the leg, and are often on the lateral or medial side of the ankle. There is a tendency for ulcers to heal with age, and the incidence of active ulceration decreases in the older age-groups. The ulcer may start as a result of local trauma or an insect bite, or may occur without obvious cause. Current pathophysiological concepts have been recently reviewed by Gabuzda (1975). It seems likely that a reduction of local oxygen tension in an area of poor vascularity causes sickling of red cells, increased viscosity, thrombosis, and ischaemia, leading to tissue break-down and ulceration. If blood flow through the capillary bed is suffic-iently rapid, the time of exposure of the erythrocyte to hypoxia may be too short to allow sickling to occur. However, in capillary beds subjected to venous stasis the time factor adds to the detriment of the erythrocyte. There is evid-ence that a low Hb F, thought to be associated with greater sickling and an increased thrombotic tendency, is significantly more common in patients with spontaneous ulcers than in those with a history of preceding trauma (Serjeant, 1974).

Hypertensive ischaemic ulcers. Martorell (1945) described four female patients with hypertensive ischaemic ulcers and later (Martorell, 1950) included the following criteria for diagnosis—hypertension, palpable pulses in the legs, absence of disturbance in the venous circulation, and a superficial ulcer on the anterolateral aspect of the leg at the junction of the lower and middle thirds.

Hines and Farber (1946) reported 11 similar cases but with some variation in the site of the ulceration. The lesions originated as painful red-blue, or purpuric plaques which broke down to give a painful superficial ulcer. The ulcer often enlarged by extension of the purpuric and haemorrhagic area of skin, and subsequent break-down. Fully developed lesions varied from 1 to 11 cm in diameter. Histological examination showed thickening of arteriolar walls in the area of the ulcer, with considerable narrowing—and occasionally complete occlusion of the lumen. It was concluded that these ulcers were ischaemic in nature.

In 1966 Schnier, Sheps and Juergens reviewed 40 patients seen at the Mayo Clinic with ulcers that were considered, on clinical grounds, to be typical hypertensive ischaemic ulcers. Most patients were female and over 60 years of age. In this group of patients, atherosclerosis obliterans was present in 19, venous insufficiency in 16, and diabetes mellitus in 9. All except four patients were hypertensive, but only 14 patients had hypertension with no other vascular disease.

It seems clear that local ischaemia may play some part in the causation of leg ulceration in patients who are hypertensive, even though they may have normally palpable arterial pulses.

Microbiology

Leg ulcers may support a varied bacterial flora, most having a mixed flora of common pathogens. There is still dispute as to the significance of these organisms, some workers believing that they exacerbate and worsen the ulcer, while others believe that they are just colonizing a suitable site.

Friedman and Gladstone (1969), in a survey of 40 patients with untreated arterial or venous leg ulcers, found *Staphylococcus aureus* and the Entero-bacteriaceae to be most common in ulcers which appeared to be inflamed on clinical examination, while non-inflamed ulcers tended to have less virilent organisms. Perera (1970) on the other hand, could find no link between degree of inflammation and the type of organism present, and work by Somerville et al (as yet unpublished) and quoted by Noble and Somerville (1974) apparently supports this latter finding. Somerville et al did, however, find that an inflamed ulcer was more likely to be colonised by three or more pathogenic organisms, and also noted that *Staph. aureus* was more common in dry ulcers, and coliforms, particularly *Pseudomonas aeruginosa*, in moist ones. Mitchell, Pettigrew and MacGilvray (1970) have shown that varicose ulcers may act as reservoirs for hospital strains of *Staph. aureus* and *Ps. aeruginosa*, and that a high incidence of cross-infection may occur among patients attending a leg ulcer clinic.

Although clinical observation suggests that the bacterial flora is often of little importance, there is no doubt that ulcers may, on occasion, enlarge and become much more exudative as a result of frank bacterial infection. Van Duyn (1967) has suggested that particularly destructive, deep, and punched out ulcers may occur if staphylococci and *Proteus bacilli* occur together and act synergistically. There is some experimental evidence in mice to show that a potentiating substance produced by *Staph. aureus* may increase the pathogenicity of *Proteus vulgaris* and a wide variety of other microorganisms (Arndt, Young and Ritts, 1963). Little research has been carried out on the pathogenic capacity of mixed infections in leg ulcers, but in view of the previously mentioned finding of Somerville et al, this might be of considerable interest.

English, Smith and Harman (1971) studied the fungal flora of the legs of patients with venous ulcers. *Candida parapsilosis, Fusarium oxysporum,* and *F. solani* were commonly found in the moist skin surrounding the ulcer, rather than in the ulcer itself. The two *Fusarium* species were found only in legs with severe moist ulcers. It was thought that the presence of *C. parapsilosis* had little effect on ulcer healing, but no firm conclusion could be reached as to the effect of the *Fusarium* species. *Candida albicans* was isolated from only one patient in this investigation, but others have isolated it frequently from leg ulcers (Orbach, 1965; Simonart, 1968).

Phagedenic ulcers, which occur usually on the lower leg in young adults and children in hot, humid forest regions, are thought by most authors to be caused by an association of fusiform bacilli with spirochaetes, but fusiform bacilli may be present alone (Basset, 1969).

Treatment

The majority of leg ulcers will respond satisfactorily to treatment with suitable non-sensitising topical therapy and adequate elastic supportive bandaging or bed rest. Improvement is often particularly noticeable when the medical and nursing teams take a special interest in the condition and are willing to supervise therapy on a long-term basis. Treatment of any associated condition such as hypothyroidism, anaemia, cardiac failure, arthritis or diabetes is of great importance.

Although there have been a number of reports in recent years of new and beneficial treatments—often topical—for leg ulcers, few of these have been subjected to an adequately controlled trial, and most have failed to live up to the enthusiastic claims made for them. In the following account discussion has been limited to a number of general topics, and no attempt has been made to review in detail the field of topical therapy.

Control of oedema

It is generally held that venous leg ulcers heal best if oedema can be removed or prevented. Oedema is a consequence of venous hypertension, and methods of successful oedema control such as bandaging and posture (Bourne, 1974) exert a similar effect on the venous stasis so that it may be difficult to know whether the beneficial response is due to control of oedema alone, or to control of venous hypertension. Haeger (1964), in a controlled trial of diuretic treatment in patients with stasis oedema, showed that oedema improved and that the speed of ulcer healing increased. Myers and Cherry (1971), however, reported that the rate of healing of ulcers was related to the elimination of stasis, but was not directly related to the amount of oedema present. In their series of conservatively treated outpatients, no topical or systemic agent was as effective in healing leg ulcers as firm external elastic support. The fastest rates of ulcer healing were produced by treatment with bed rest.

Hyperbaric oxygen treatment

The application of topical oxygen at ambient pressure to leg ulcers is generally considered to be of little benefit, but hyperbaric oxygen has been shown to cause rapid healing in patients with venous ulceration. Fisher (1969), using pure oxygen applied continuously at a pressure of 22 mmHg for 4 to 12 h a day, noted complete healing in 16 patients with leg ulcers after 3 to 24 days. Oxygen was applied by means of a vinyl chamber with a self-sealing device and automatic relief valve, which enveloped the leg from the knee downwards. Three patients with bilateral ulcers showed rapid healing of the treated leg, while the untreated leg showed no improvement. Similar good results have been reported by Bass (1970) using the Vicker's 'Lotus' hyperbaric bed. In patients with arterial insufficiency or arterial ulceration healing was not promoted. The use of hyperbaric oxygen necessitates the availability of suitable equipment for the administration of oxygen under pressure, and requires stringent fire precautions.

Troxerutin

Troxerutin (trihydroxyethylrutoside) is a semisynthetic derivative of rutin, and has been shown, on oral administration, to diminish capillary permeability, reduce oedema, enhance capillary resistance, and augment venous return, when used in patients with venous insufficiency.

McEwan and McArdle (1971) found that oxygen levels in blood from varicose leg veins were significantly lower than those in blood from normal leg veins taken from the same site on the limb under the same conditions. Treatment with hydroxyethylrutosides significantly increased the oxygen levels in blood from varicose veins, and this was associated with an improvement in leg symptoms attributable to venous insufficiency. FirtzGerald (1967), Allen (1970), Rose (1970) and Van Cauwenberge (1972) have all noted improvement in symptoms such as night cramps, aching or 'heavy' legs, and ankle oedema in patients with varicose veins treated with Troxerutin, while Allen (1970) also noted accelerated healing of leg ulcers. Personal experience of this drug, in the treatment of a small number of recalcitrant venous leg ulcers, has not suggested that it speeds healing, but no properly controlled trials of its effects on leg ulcer healing have, as yet, been carried out.

Zinc

Zinc is believed to be essential for normal growth in plants, animals and man, and its relationship to the skin and skin disease has been recently reviewed by Goolamali and Comaish (1975). Zinc deficiency in rats impairs wound healing, while zinc supplementation is said to accelerate wound repair. Savlov, Strain and Huegin (1962) showed that zinc is preferentially accumulated at the wound site—especially in the first few days after injury, and have suggested that it is incorporated into enzyme systems. Pories et al (1967) have reported accelerated wound healing in man following zinc supplementation.

Greaves and Boyde (1967) reported low plasma zinc levels in patients with venous leg ulceration, and similar low levels have been found in patients with bed sores (Abbott et al, 1968), ulceration due to vascular insufficiency (Halsted and Smith, 1970), and sickle cell ulcers (Serjeant, Galloway and Gueri, 1970). Oon et al (1974) have reported low serum zinc levels in patients with leprosy—with or without trophic ulceration.

Accelerated healing of venous leg ulcers in patients treated with oral zinc sulphate was reported by Husain (1969) and by Hallböök and Lanner (1972), who also noted that healing was slower in untreated patients with low serum zinc levels. Serjeant et al (1970) reported accelerated healing of sickle cell ulceration following oral zinc sulphate and, more recently, Gueri et al (1975) have reported improved healing in non-sickle cell ulcers in the West Indies. Greaves and Skillen (1970), in an uncontrolled trial of zinc sulphate in the treatment of venous leg ulcers, thought that this treatment caused accelerated healing, but in a further double blind trial Greaves and Ive (1972) were unable to show a significantly increased rate of healing in the zinc treated group. Myers and Cherry (1970) were also unable to show any acceleration of healing in patients treated with oral zinc therapy.

Goolamali and Comaish (1975) point out that serum zinc levels have not always been monitored in the various conflicting studies, and it is clear that further investigation of tissue distribution and metabolism of zinc in patients with leg ulceration is overdue.

Local treatment

The local treatment of venous ulceration has been accorded exaggerated importance in the past, but there is little evidence to show that topical therapy is of great importance in most patients. Local antibiotics are almost certainly over-prescribed, and in an area of skin where allergic contact sensitisation may all too easily occur, it is important that any local treatment should be, as far as possible, harmless.

Perera (1970), working in London, performed routine patch tests on 37 patients with leg ulcers, and found positive results in 30 patients. The most common positive reactions were to neomycin and lanolin, followed by vioform, colophony, parabens, balsam of Peru, CTAB, Dettol, Eurax, and Viscopaste. The majority of patients had multiple sensitivities, but only two patients had positive responses to substances other than medicaments. Malten and Kuiper (1974) have shown that the incidence of contact allergy in leg ulcer patients is about five times that in patients with eczema due to non-venous causes. Positive reactions in this Dutch series were produced by para-phenylenediamine, para-amino-azobenzene, pellilol, benzocaine, diamino-diphenylmethane, coal tar, and sesame oil, as well as by lanolin, neomycin, and other substances already noted to be frequent sensitisers by Perera (1970). Angelini, Rantuccio and Meneghini (1975) have reported similar results from Italy—the main sensitisers being neomycin, sulphonamide, promethazine, parabens, lanolin, and benzoyl peroxide. The pattern of sensitivity clearly varies from country to country depending on prevailing customs in the local treatment of leg ulcers.

A few cases have been reported of anaphylactic reactions following topical treatment of leg ulcers with antibiotics (Pippen, 1966; Comaish and Cunliffe, 1967).

Harman (1974) has pointed out that the misguided application of topical steroids to leg ulcers, may delay healing and cause even deeper ulceration, with secondary infection and a possible risk of haemorrhage. In 1971 there were 23 deaths in England and Wales due to spontaneous haemorrhage from varicose veins (Evans et al, 1973), and in 10 of 18 cases haemorrhage occurred from a chronic large ulcer.

Surgical treatment

There is still controversy concerning the place of surgery in venous leg ulceration and this stems, in part, from dispute as to the relative importance of deep and superficial venous incompetence. Although a few surgeons believe that venous ulcers are usually due to 'varicose veins' (Rivlin, 1970), most authorities now consider that deep venous incompetence or incompetent perforating veins around the ankle are present in the majority, if not in all patients with venous ulceration.

Any assessment of the merits of surgery is made difficult because of the lack of adequately controlled trials. In addition, it has been pointed out that surgical results may be influenced by factors such as the length of follow-up, the effect of elastic support given at the same time, the period of bed rest in hospital, and any change of occupation (Dodd and Cockett, 1956).

Anning (1956) followed up 100 patients, whose venous leg ulcers had been healed by compression bandaging alone and who had been advised to continue elastic support. During a follow-up period of $2\frac{1}{2}$ to $7\frac{1}{2}$ years, 59 patients had recurrences of ulceration. Most surgical series have reported better results than this, but may not be comparable because of selection. Lofgren, Lauvstad and Bonnemaison (1965), at the Mayo Clinic, reviewed 129 patients with leg ulcers who had been healed following treatment with split-skin grafts in 1951 to 1960. Incompetent superficial veins had been stripped, but deep venous incompetence was controlled by elastic support, and no patients had had ligation of incompetent perforating veins. Follow-up showed that 30 per cent of ulcers recurred. Fegan (1970), treating leg ulcers by compression sclerotherapy, also reported a 30 per cent recurrence rate over a 5 to 10 year period. Linn (1972), treating his patients by subfascial ligation of incompetent perforators, noticed a recurrence rate of 40 per cent. In this series, significantly better results were obtained in patients who had three or more perforators ligated, good arterial pulses, and other correctable venous problems. Surprisingly, factors such as the duration of the ulcer, obesity, bilateral leg involvement, and smoking did not adversely affect the surgical outcome.

Surgical techniques vary, but the majority of surgeons now favour either surgical ligation or compression sclerotherapy (Fegan, 1967) for patients who have incompetent deep perforators, while saphenofemoral incompetence, when present, is probably best treated by surgery—most surgeons agreeing that sclerotherapy is unsatisfactory when used at or above knee level (*Lancet*, 1975). Unfortunately, as already discussed, many incompetent perforating veins are easily missed—particularly if the surgeon relies heavily on clinical examination, and in these cases recurrence of ulceration may be expected. Leigh (1970) pointed out that in occasional patients there may be a wide communication between the long and short superficial venous collecting systems in the lower leg, and that in cases in which there is a persisting medial venous ulcer, in spite of long saphenous vein stripping and perforator ligation, dissection of the popliteal fossa with stripping of the short saphenous system may be a worth-while procedure.

In recurrent ulceration, Silver et al (1971) have advocated radical surgery consisting of resection of the ulcer, the underlying subcutaneous tissue, and deep fascia, ligation of all perforating veins at their point of origin, and delayed split-skin grafting of the ulcer bed.

Skin grafting

In 1964 Battle noted that small pinch grafts, taken with a needle and scalpel, took well on a clean ulcer base, and in 1969 Chilvers and Freeman reported good results with an outpatient skin grafting technique whereby split-skin grafts, taken under local anaesthesia, were cut into 1 cm squares and seeded on to the base of the ulcer. Although many dermatologists have a clinical impression that pinch grafts speed healing, there has been no controlled trial to show that this is really so.

Hackett (1975) has advocated the use of lyophilised homograft in venous ulceration. This is human freeze-dried skin which is dead, but which when reconstituted in normal saline acts as a superior biological dressing. This offers the advantages of rapid relief of pain, promotion of healing, and preparation of full thickness defects for autograft acceptance if necessary. Similar benefits may be obtained by the use of lyophilised xenograft, in the form of irradiation-sterilised porcine skin, which is now being produced commercially (Elliott and Hoehn, 1973). Granulation tissue and epithelial growth is stimulated by the graft, which is changed every four days so that it does not become firmly bonded to the ulcer base.

Prevention of the Postphlebitic Syndrome

Venous ulceration is frequently a sequel to an earlier episode of deep-vein thrombosis, and any measures which decrease the incidence of deep-vein thrombosis should eventually also reduce the prevalence of venous ulceration.

Deep vein thrombosis may follow child-birth and surgical operations, or may occur as the result of injury. Some cases occur during the course of medical illnesses, prolonged recumbency from any cause, or the use of sclerosants in the treatment of varicose veins. Less common causes are thrombophlebitis, burns, blood dyscrasias and intravenous infusions. 'Silent' or undetected thrombosis of perforating veins may occur more frequently than is generally recognised (Cockett and Elgan Jones, 1953).

Browse and Negus (1970) have shown that about 70 per cent of cases of postoperative venous thrombosis occur during the first three days after operation, and the remaining 30 per cent between the fourth and sixth days. It has been suggested that there is a primary phase when thrombi tend to be initiated by venous stasis and a second phase initiated by increased platelet adhesiveness, which has been shown to reach a maximum on the third day (Dhall, Bennett and Matheson, 1967).

Earlier mobilisation and active leg exercises have probably reduced the incidence of massive deep vein thrombosis in postoperative patients and in women after child-birth in the last two decades, but thrombosis is still common and may be missed if dignosis rests only on clinical symptoms and signs.

Flanc, Kakker and Clarke (1968), using the ^{125}I-labelled fibrinogen test, showed that in patients aged 40 and over, venous thrombosis developed after operation in 35 per cent, and that in half of these the thrombosis first developed during the operation itself. In this study only 50 per cent of patients with proven thrombosis had clinical signs. Isotopically detected thrombi are often small and of little clinical significance, in that they are unlikely to generate emboli of sufficient size to cause symptoms, and do not damage veins to the extent of producing post-thrombotic swelling or ulceration. Their danger, however, lies in the fact that they may propagate to form clinically significant or major thrombi.

Sharnoff and De Blasio (1970) showed that small doses of heparin injected subcutaneously in patients undergoing surgery, would effectively reduce the incidence of postoperative venous thrombosis. This work has been confirmed in a large clinical multicentre trial by Kakkar et al (1975), who have shown that surgical patients on a low-dose heparin regime have an incidence of isotopically detected deep vein thrombosis of 7.7 per cent, compared with 24.6 per cent in controls. The incidence of fatal pulmonary emboli in this trial was reduced from 0.7 per cent in the controls to 0.09 per cent in the treated group.

Kline, Hughes and Campbell (1974) have shown that Dextran 70, given during operation, will reduce the incidence of postoperative pulmonary emboli, but in this trial the incidence of deep-vein thrombosis detected clinically and by ^{125}I fibrinogen was similar in the two groups. Calf muscle stimulation (Browse and Negus, 1970) and intermittent calf compression (Hills et al, 1972) effectively reduce the incidence of isotopically detected thrombi, but have not been subjected to large-scale trial.

In recent years there have been a number of papers detailing the use of the plasminogen activator—streptokinase—in the treatment of venous thrombosis. Unfortunately streptokinase is extremely expensive, and may cause complications such as bleeding or allergic manifestations. Kakkar et al (1969a), in a comparative study of the treatment of deep-vein thrombosis with streptokinase, heparin, and Arvin, showed that streptokinase, given for five days by intravenous infusion, caused complete lysis of thrombi in six of nine patients with extensive thrombosis of less than four days' duration. In a further paper (Kakkar et al, 1969b) the treated patients were reassessed 6 to 12 months later by ascending functional cinephlebography. Seven streptokinase-treated patients were available for review. Of five patients who had had complete clearance of thrombi after the initial treatment, four were found to have normal valve function, while in one valvular function was poor. In two patients who had not attained complete thrombolysis at the time of the original treatment, recanalisation of veins was complete in one, and incomplete in the other. No patient in the Arvin-treated group of seven patients, and only one of the heparin-treated group of eight patients had normal valve function 6 to 12 months after the original deep vein thrombosis. The authors concluded that treatment at an early stage with streptokinase produced lysis of thrombi, and the preservation of valvular function. A more recent trial by Duckert et al (1975) in acute or subacute deep-vein thrombosis, monitored by phlebography, showed that streptokinase produced complete clearing of occluded veins in 42 per cent, and partial clearing in 25 per cent of affected patients. Comparable figures for treatment with heparin were 0 and 10 per cent. Streptokinase was more effective when the thrombus was in the proximal rather than the calf veins, and the authors commented that, not only early thrombi, but those that had been present for 6 to 15 days were readily lysed. There are, as yet, no reports of prolonged follow-up of patients treated

8

with streptokinase, to show whether the late complications of chronic venous insufficiency are prevented.

REFERENCES

INTRODUCTION

Ryan, T. J. & Wilkinson, D. S. (1972) Diseases of the veins: leg ulcers. In *Textbook of Dermatology*, 2nd edn, ed. Rook, A., Wilkinson, D. S. & Ebling, F. J. G., Vol. 1, Ch. 33. Oxford: Blackwell.

INCIDENCE

Borschberg, E. (1967) *The Prevalence of Varicose Veins of the Lower Extremities*. Basle: Karger.

Da Silva, A., Widmer, L. K., Martin, H., Mall, T., Glaus, L. & Schneider, M. (1974) Varicose veins and chronic venous insufficiency: prevalence and risk factors in 4376 subjects of the Basle Study II. *Vasa*, **3**, 118–125.

Dogliotti, M. (1970) Skin disorders in the Bantu: a survey of 2000 cases from Baragwaneth Hospital. *South African Medical Journal*, **44**, 670–672.

Finlay, G. H. & Park, R. G. (1969) Common skin diseases in the Transvaal: an analysis of 22 000 dermatological outpatient cases. *South African Medical Journal*, **43**, 590–595.

Hill, B. H. R. (1968) The incidence and comparison of skin diseases in Hong Kong and New Zealand. *Australian Journal of Dermatology*, **9**, 248–255.

Neves, H. (1966) Incidence of skin diseases 1952–1965. *Transactions of the St John's Hospital Dermatological Society*, **52**, 255–271.

Rook, A. & Wilkinson, D. S. (1972) The prevalence, incidence and ecology of diseases of the skin. In *Textbook of Dermatology*, 2nd edn, ed. Rook, A., Wilkinson, D. S. & Ebling, F. J. G., Vol. I, Ch. 3, Oxford: Blackwell.

Schulz, E. J., Finlay, G. H. & Scott, F. P. (1962) Skin disease in the Bantu. *South African Medical Journal*, **36**, 199–202.

Shrank, A. B. & Harman, R. R. M. (1966) The incidence of skin disease in a Nigerian Teaching Hospital Dermatological Clinic. *British Journal of Dermatology*, **78**, 235–241.

Warin, R. P. (1965) The incidence of skin disease in man. In *The Comparative Physiology and Pathology of the Skin*, ed. Rook, A. J. & Walton, G. S., pp. 21–31. Oxford: Blackwell.

Circulatory Factors

ARTERIES

Anning, S. T. (1952) The cause and treatment of leg ulcers. *Lancet*, **2**, 789–794.

Fäs, J., Widmer, L. K., Da Silva, M. A. & Glaus, L. (1973) Zur Frage der arteriosklerotischen Venopathie. *Schweizerische medizinische Wochenschrift*, **103**, 1189–1191.

Haeger, K. (1965) Ischaemic ulcers of the lower limb. A comparison of general and local methods of treatment. *Acta chirurgica scandinavica*, **130**, 584–592.

Thune, P. (1972) Plethysmographic recordings of skin pulses. V. Piezoelectric and photoelectric measurements in venous leg ulcers. *Acta dermato-venereologica (Stockholm)*, **52**, 24–30.

Weidmann, A. (1954) Die arterielle Genese des Ulcus cruris 'Varicosum'. *Hautarzt*, **5**, 85–91.

Welbourn, E. (1967) The value of radiological investigation of chronic stasis ulcers of the leg. *Clinical Radiology*, **18**, 372–378.

Wittels, W. & Zuchristian, G. (1967) Verlauf und Prognose des post-thrombotische Syndroms. *Medizinische Welt*, **18**, 648–650.

VEINS

Daintree Johnson, H. & Pflug, J. (1975) *The Swollen Leg: Causes and Treatment*, pp. 27–28. London: Heinemann.

Dodd, H. & Cockett, F. B. (1956) *The Pathology and Surgery of the Veins of the Lower Limb*. London: Livingstone.

Linton, R. R. (1938) A new surgical technique for the treatment of postphlebitic varicose ulcers of the lower leg: a preliminary report. *New England Journal of Medicine*, **219**, 367–373.

MICROVASCULATURE

Allen, J. C. (1972) The microcirculation of the skin of the normal leg, in varicose veins and in the post-thrombotic syndrome. *South African Journal of Surgery*, **10**, 29–40.

Haddy, F. J. (1960) Effect of histamine on small and large vessel pressures in the dog forelimb. *American Journal of Physiology*, **198**, 161–168.

Haeger, K. H. M. & Bergman, L. (1963) Skin temperature of normal and varicose legs and some reflections on the aetiology of varicose veins. *Angiology*, **14**, 473–479.

Haimovici, H., Steinman, C. & Caplan, L. H. (1966) Role of arteriovenous anastomoses in vascular diseases of the lower extremity. *Annals of Surgery*, **164**, 990–1002.

Kügelgen, A. V. (1955) Uber das Verhältnis von Ringmuskulatur und innendruck in Menschlichen Grossen Venen. *Zeitschrift für Zellforschung*, **43**, 168–183.

Majno, G., Palade, G. E. & Schoefl, G. I. (1961) Studies on inflammation. II. The site of action of histamine and serotonin along the vascular tree: a topographic study. *Journal of Biophysical and Biochemical Cytology*, **11**, 607–628.

Piulachs, P. & Vidal-Barraquer, F. (1953) Pathogenic study of varicose veins. *Angiology*, **4**, 59–100.

Ryan, T. J. (1969) The epidermis and its blood supply in venous disorders of the leg. *Transactions of the St John's Hospital Dermatological Society*, **55**, 51–63.

Ryan, T. J. (1973) Structure, pattern and shape of the blood vessels of the skin. In *The Physiology and Pathophysiology of the Skin*, ed. Jarrett, A., Vol. 2, Ch. 16. London: Academic Press.

Weiderhielm, C. A. (1966) Transcapillary and interstitial transport phenomena in the mesentery. *Federation Proceedings. Federation of American Societies for Experimental Biology*, **25**, 1789–1798.

ATROPHIE BLANCHE

Copeman, P. W. M. & Ryan, T. J. (1971) Cutaneous antiitis. Patterns of rashes explained by (1) flow properties of blood; (2) anatomical disposition of vessels. *British Journal of Dermatology*, **85**, 205–214.

Ryan, T. J. (1969) The epidermis and its blood supply in venous disorders of the leg. *Transactions of the St John's Hospital Dermatological Society*, **55**, 51–63.

Stevanović, D. V. (1974) Atrophie blanche: a sign of dermal blood occlusion. *Archives of Dermatology*, **109**, 858–862.

Types of Ulceration

VENOUS ULCERATION

Anderson, M. N. & McDonald, K. E. (1963) Results of surgical therapy of severe stasis ulceration of the legs. *Annals of Surgery*, **157**, 281–286.

Anning, S. T. (1952) The cause and treatment of leg ulcers. *Lancet*, **2**, 789–794.

Arnoldi, C. C. (1966) Venous pressure in patients with valvular incompetence of the veins of the lower limb. *Acta chirurgica scandinavica*, **132**, 628–645.

Arnoldi, C. C. (1967) Venous leg ulcers. *Vascular Diseases*, **4**, 309–319.

Bauer, G. (1942) A roentgenological and clinical study of the sequels of thrombosis. *Acta chirurgica scandinavica*, **86**, Suppl. 74, 5–116.

Butcher, H. R. & Hoover, A. L. (1955) Abnormalities of human superficial cutaneous lymphatics associated with stasis ulcers, lymphoedema, scars and cutaneous autografts. *Annals of Surgery*, **142**, 633–653.

Callum, K. G., Gray, L. J. & Lea Thomas, M. (1973) An evaluation of the fluorescein test and phlebography in the detection of incompetent perforating veins. *British Journal of Surgery*, **60**, 699–702.

Cockett, F. B. & Elgan Jones, D. E. (1953) The ankle blow-out syndrome: a new approach to the varicose ulcer problem. *Lancet*, **1**, 17–23.

Haeger, K. (1966) Three- to six-year results with standardised surgical therapy of venous ulcers. *Vascular Diseases*, **3**, 106–108.

Lea Thomas, M., McAllister, V., Rose, D. H. & Tonge, K. (1972) A simplified technique of phlebography for the localisation of incompetent perforating veins of the legs. *Clinical Radiology*, **23**, 486–491.

Lippmann, H. I. & Goldin, R. R. (1960) Subcutaneous ossification of the legs. *Radiology*, **74** 279–288.
Miller, S. S. & Foote, A. V. (1974) The ultrasonic detection of incompetent perforating veins. *British Journal of Surgery*, **61**, 653–656.
Noble, J. & Gunn, A. A. (1972) The detection of incompetent perforating veins. *British Journal of Surgery*, **59**, 304.
Patil, K. D., Williams, J. R. & Lloyd Williams, K. (1970) Thermographic localisation of incompetent perforating veins in the leg. *British Medical Journal*, **1**, 195–197.
Sarjeant, T. R. (1964) Surgical anatomy in the treatment of venous stasis. *Surgical Clinics of North America*, **44**, 1383–1402.
Sarkany, I. & Kreel, L. (1966) Subcutaneous ossification of the legs in chronic venous stasis. *British Medical Journal*, **2**, 27–28.
Sherman, R. S. (1964) Varicose veins: anatomy, re-evaluation of Trendelenburg tests, and an operative procedure. *Surgical Clinics of North America*, **44**, 1369–1381.
Townsend, J., Jones, H. & Williams, J. E. (1967) Detection of incompetent perforating veins by venography at operation. *British Medical Journal*, **3**, 583–585.

NON-VENOUS ULCERATION

(a) Vasculitis

Asghar, S. S. & Cormane, R. H. (1974) Vasculitis. In *Immunological Aspects of Skin Diseases*, ed. Fry, L. & Seah, P. P., Ch. 5. Lancaster: Medical and Technical Publishing Co. Ltd.
Cliff, W. J. (1966) The acute inflammatory reaction in the rabbit ear chamber with particular reference to the phenomenon of leukocytic migration. *Journal of Experimental Medicine*, **124**, 543–556.
Copeman, P. W. M. & Ryan, T. J. (1970) The problems of classification of cutaneous angiitis with reference to histopathology and pathogenesis. *British Journal of Dermatology*, **82**, Suppl. 5, 2–14.
Cream, J. J. & Turk, J. L. (1971) A review of the evidence for immune-complex deposition as a cause of skin disease in man. *Clinical Allergy*, **1**, 235–247.
Illig, L., Schneider, K. & Winkelmann, R. K. (1969) Modification of local Schwartzman reaction by drug-induced fibrinolysis. *Biblio anatomica*, **10**, 464–468.

(b) Hereditary haemolytic anaemias

Afifi, A. M., Ellis, L., Huntsman, R. G. & Said, M. I. (1975) High dose ascorbic acid in the management of thalassaemia leg ulcers—a pilot study. *British Journal of Dermatology*, **92**, 339–341.
Gabuzda, T. G. (1975) Sickle cell leg ulcers. *International Journal of Dermatology*, **14**, 322–325.
Serjeant, G. & Gueri, M. (1970) Sickle cell trait and leg ulceration. *British Medical Journal*, **1**, 820.
Serjeant, G. R. (1974) The clinical features of sickle cell disease. In *Clinical Studies*, ed. Bearn, A. G., Black, D. A. K. & Hiatt, H. H., Vol. 4. Amsterdam: North-Holland Publishing Company.
Wolfort, F. G. & Krizek, T. J. (1969) Skin ulceration in sickle cell anaemia. *Plastic and Reconstructive Surgery*, **43**, 71–77.

(c) Hypertensive ischaemic ulcers

Hines, E. A. & Farber, E. M. (1946) Ulcer of the leg due to arteriolosclerosis and ischemia, occurring in the presence of hypertensive disease (hypertensive-ischemic ulcers): a preliminary report. *Proceedings of the Staff Meetings of the Mayo Clinic*, **21**, 337–346.
Martorell, F. (1945) Las úlcera supramaleolares por arteriolitis de las grandes hipertensas. *Actas de las reuniones científicas del cuerpo facultativo del Instituto Policlínico de Barcelona*, **1**, 6–9.
Martorell, F. (1950) Hypertensive ulcer of the leg. *Angiology*, **1**, 133–140.
Schnier, B. R., Sheps, S. G. & Juergens, J. L. (1966) Hypertensive ischaemic ulcer: a review of 40 cases. *American Journal of Cardiology*, **17**, 560–565.

Microbiology

Arndt, W. F., Young, E. J. & Ritts, R. E. (1963) Staphylococcal enhancement of susceptibility to bacterial infections in the mouse. *Journal of Infectious Diseases*, **112**, 255–263.

Basset, A. (1969) Tropical phagedenic ulcer. In *Essays on Tropical Dermatology*, ed. Simons, R. D. G. Ph. & Marshall, J., Vol. 1, pp. 25–33. Amsterdam: Excerpta Medica Foundation.

English, M. P., Smith, R. J. & Harman, R. R. M. (1971) The fungal flora of ulcerated legs. *British Journal of Dermatology*, **84**, 567–581.

Friedman, S. A. & Gladstone, J. L. (1969) The bacterial flora of peripheral vascular ulcers. *Archives of Dermatology*, **100**, 29–32.

Mitchell, A. A. B., Pettigrew, J. B. & MacGilvray, D. (1970) Varicose ulcers are reservoirs of hospital strains of *Staph. aureus* and *Pseudomonas pyocyanea*. *British Journal of Clinical Practice*, **24**, 223–226.

Noble, W. C. & Somerville, D. A. (1974) Microbiology of human skin. In *Major Problems in Dermatology*, ed. Rook, A., Vol. 2, pp. 260–261. London: Saunders.

Orbach, E. J. (1965) *Candida albicans*, a contributing cause of torpid vascular ulcers of the lower extremity. *Angiology*, **16**, 664–672.

Perera, P. (1970) An investigation of varicose ulcers. *Transactions of the St John's Hospital Dermatological Society*, **56**, 175–177.

Simonart, J. M. (1968) L'ulcere de jambe et le *Candida albicans*. *Archives Belges de dermatologie et de syphiligraphie*, **24**, 49–54.

Somerville, D. A., Smith, R. J., English, M. P. & Thorne, N. (in preparation) The microbial flora of stasis ulcers and its relationship to healing.

Van Duyn, J. (1967) *Proteus–Staphylococcus* synergism in punched out ulcers. *Plastic and Reconstructive Surgery*, **40**, 86–88.

Treatment

CONTROL OF OEDEMA

Bourne, I. H. J. (1974) Vertical leg drainage of oedema in treatment of leg ulcers. *British Medical Journal*, **2**, 581–583.

Haeger, K. (1964) Further observations on the effect of diuretics on stasis oedema of the leg. *Angiology*, **15**, 417–423.

Myers, M. B. & Cherry, G. (1971) Pathophysiology and treatment of stasis ulcers of the leg. *American Surgeon*, **37**, 167–174.

HYPERBARIC OXYGEN TREATMENT

Bass, B. H. (1970) The treatment of varicose leg ulcers by hyperbaric oxygen. *Postgraduate Medical Journal*, **46**, 407–408.

Fisher, B. H. (1969) Topical hyperbaric oxygen treatment of pressure sores and skin ulcers. *Lancet*, **2**, 405–409.

TROXERUTIN

Allen, S. (1970) The treatment of chronic venous disorder of the leg. *Practitioner*, **205**, 221–224.

Fitzgerald, D. E. (1967) A clinical trial of Troxerutin in venous insufficiency of the lower limb. *Practitioner*, **198**, 406–407.

McEwan, A. J. & McArdle, C. S. (1971) Effect of hydroxyethylrutosides on blood oxygen levels and venous insufficiency symptoms in varicose veins. *British Medical Journal*, **2**, 138–141.

Rose, S. S. (1970) A report on the use of an hydroxyethylrutoside in symptoms due to venous back pressure and allied conditions in the lower limbs. *British Journal of Clinical Practice*, **24**, 161–164.

Van Cauwenberge, H. (1972) Double-blind study of the efficacy of a soluble rutoside derivative in the treatment of venous disease. *Archives internationales de pharmacodynamie et de thérapie*, Suppl. 196, 122–125.

ZINC

Abbott, D. F., Exton-Smith, A. N., Millard, P. H. & Temperley, J. M. (1968) Zinc sulphate and bed sores. *British Medical Journal*, **2**, 763.

Goolamali, S. K. & Comaish, J. S. (1975) Zinc and the skin. *International Journal of Dermatology*, **14**, 182–187.

Greaves, M. & Boyde, T. R. C. (1967) Plasma-zinc concentrations in patients with psoriasis, other dermatoses, and venous leg ulceration. *Lancet*, **2**, 1019–1020.

Greaves, M. W. & Ive, F. A. (1972) Double-blind trial of zinc sulphate in the treatment of chronic venous leg ulceration. *British Journal of Dermatology*, **87**, 632–634.

Greaves, M. W. & Skillen, A. W. (1970) Effects of long-continued ingestion of zinc sulphate in patients with venous leg ulceration. *Lancet*, **2**, 889–891.

Gueri, M., Van Devanter, S., Serjeant, B. E. & Serjeant, G. R. (1975) Zinc sulphate treatment of non-sickle cell ulcers. *West Indian Medical Journal*, **24**, 26–29.

Hallböök, T. & Lanner, E. (1972) Serum-zinc and healing of venous leg ulcers. *Lancet*, **2**, 780–782.

Halsted, J. A. & Smith, J. C., Jr (1970) Plasma-zinc in health and disease. *Lancet*, **1**, 322–324.

Husain, S. L. (1969) Oral zinc sulphate in leg ulcers. *Lancet*, **1**, 1069–1071.

Myers, M. B. & Cherry, G. (1970) Zinc and the healing of chronic leg ulcers. *American Journal of Surgery*, **120**, 77–81.

Oon, B. B., Khong, K. Y., Greaves, M. W. & Plummer, V. M. (1974) Trophic skin ulceration of leprosy: skin and serum zinc concentrations. *British Medical Journal*, **2**, 531–533.

Pories, W. J., Henzel, J. H., Rob, C. G. & Strain, W. H. (1967) Acceleration of wound healing in man with zinc sulphate given by mouth. *Lancet*, **1**, 121–124.

Savlov, E. D., Strain, W. H. & Huegin, F. (1962) Radiozinc studies in experimental wound healing. *Journal of Surgical Research*, **2**, 209–212.

Serjeant, G. R., Galloway, R. E. & Gueri, M. C. (1970) Oral zinc sulphate in sickle-cell ulcers. *Lancet*, **2**, 891–892.

LOCAL TREATMENT

Angelini, G., Rantuccio, F. & Meneghini, C. L. (1975) Contact dermatitis in patients with leg ulcers. *Contact Dermatitis*, **1**, 81–87.

Comaish, J. S. & Cunliffe, W. J. (1967) Absorption of drugs from varicose ulcers: a cause of anaphylaxis. *British Journal of Clinical Practice*, **21**, 97–98.

Evans, G. A., Evans, D. M. D., Seal, R. M. E. & Craven, J. L. (1973) Spontaneous fatal haemorrhage caused by varicose veins. *Lancet*, **2**, 1359–1362.

Harman, R. R. M. (1974) Haemorrhage from varicose veins. *Lancet*, **1**, 363.

Malten, K. E. & Kuiper, J. P. (1974) Skin contact allergy in 100 cases of varicose ulcer. *Phlebologie*, **27**, 417–420.

Perera, P. (1970) An investigation of varicose ulcers. *Transactions of the St John's Hospital Dermatological Society*, **56**, 175–177.

Pippen, R. (1966) Anaphylactoid reaction after Chymacort ointment. *British Medical Journal*, **1**, 1172.

SURGICAL TREATMENT

Anning, S. T. (1956) Leg ulcers—the results of treatment. *Angiology*, **7**, 505–516.

Dodd, H. & Cockett, F. B. (1956) *The Pathology and Surgery of the Veins of the Lower Limb*. London: Livingstone.

Fegan, G. (1967) *Varicose Veins: Compression Sclerotherapy*. London: Heinemann.

Fegan, G. (1970) Skin-grafting and leg ulcers. *Lancet*, **1**, 416.

Lancet (1975) The treatment of varicose veins. *Lancet*, **2**, 311–312.

Leigh, B. (1970) Venous ulceration: a further factor. *Medical Journal of Australia*, **2**, 1030–1031.

Linn, B. S. (1972) Subfascial ligation of incompetent perforating veins: a rational therapy to prevent recurrence of venous stasis ulcers. *Southern Medical Journal*, **65**, 1063–1066.

Lofgren, K. A., Lauvstad, W. A. & Bonnemaison, M. F. (1965) Surgical treatment of large statis ulcer—review of 129 cases. *Proceedings of the Staff Meetings of the Mayo Clinic*, **40**, 560–563.

Rivlin, S. (1970) Skin-grafting leg ulcers. *Lancet*, **1**, 247–248.

Silver, D., Gleysteen, J. J., Rhodes, G. R., Georgiade, N. G. & Anlyan, W. G. (1971) Surgical treatment of the refractory postphlebitic ulcer. *Archives of Surgery*, **103**, 554–560.

SKIN GRAFTING

Battle, R. J. V. (1964) *Plastic Surgery*. London: Butterworth.

Cilvers, A. S. & Freeman, G. K. (1969) Out-patient skin grafting of venous ulcers. *Lancet*, **2**, 1087–1088.

Elliott, R. A. & Hoehn, J. G. (1973) Use of commercial porcine skin for wound dressings. *Plastic and Reconstructive Surgery*, **52**, 401–405.

Hackett, M. E. J. (1975) Preparation, storage and use of homograft. *British Journal of Hospital Medicine*, **13**, 272–284.

Prevention of Postphlebitic Syndrome

Browse, N. L. & Negus, D. (1970) Prevention of post-operative leg vein thrombosis by electrical muscle stimulation: an evaluation with ^{125}I-labelled fibrinogen. *British Medical Journal*, **3**, 615–618.

Cockett, F. B. & Elgan Jones, D. E. (1953) The ankle blow-out syndrome: a new approach to the varicose ulcer problem. *Lancet*, **1**, 17–23.

Dhall, D. P., Bennett, P. N. & Matheson, N. A. (1967) Effect of Dextran on platelet behaviour after abdominal operation. *Acta chirurgica scandinavica*, Suppl. 387, 75–79.

Duckert, F., Müller, G., Nyman, D., Benz, A., Prisender, S., Madar, G., Da Silva, M. A., Widmer, L. K. & Schmitt, H. E. (1975) Treatment of deep vein thrombosis with streptokinase. *British Medical Journal*, **1**, 479–481.

Flanc, C., Kakkar, V. V. & Clarke, M. B. (1968) The detection of venous thrombosis of the legs using ^{125}I-labelled fibrinogen. *British Journal of Surgery*, **55**, 742–747.

Hills, N. H., Pflug, J. J., Jeyasingh, K., Boardman, L. & Calnan, J. S. (1972) Prevention of deep vein thrombosis by intermittent compression of calf. *British Medical Journal*, **1**, 131–135.

Kakkar, V. V., Flanc, C., Howe, C. T., O'Shea, M. & Flute, P. T. (1969a) Treatment of deep vein thrombosis. A trial of heparin, streptokinase and Arvin. *British Medical Journal*, **1**, 806–810.

Kakkar, V. V., Howe, C. T., Laws, J. W. & Flanc, C. (1969b) Late results of treatment of deep vein thrombosis. *British Medical Journal*, **1**, 810–811.

Kakkar, V. V., Corrigan, T. P., Fossard, D. P., Sutherland, I., Shelton, M. G., Thirlwall, J. & others (1975) Prevention of fatal post-operative pulmonary embolism by low doses of heparin. An international multicentre trial. *Lancet*, **2**, 45–51.

Kline, A. L., Hughes, L. E. & Campbell, H. (1974) Dextran prophylaxis of deep vein thrombosis: organisation of a clinical trial. *British Journal of Surgery*, **61**, 332.

Sharnoff, J. G. & De Blasio, G. (1970) Prevention of fatal post-operative thromboembolism by heparin prophylaxis. *Lancet*, **2**, 1006–1007.

7

COMMON BALDNESS AND ALOPECIA AREATA

Arthur Rook

The inadequacy of undergraduate teaching in dermatology in the great majority of medical schools is readily admitted by most doctors after even a few months' experience of general practice. Diseases of the hair occupy such an insignificant fraction of the very limited time allowed for the systematic teaching of dermatology that many doctors do not know how to approach the investigation of hair disorders, and find their therapeutic repertoire confined to sympathy and a placebo. Yet the advances of the past two decades have provided steadily increasing evidence that most disorders of hair growth are caused by or associated with changes in other organs; the main exceptions are chemical or physical damage to the hair inflicted on cosmetic or supposedly therapeutic grounds. Many disorders of hair growth are manifestations of systemic disease and a patient's complaint that she is losing her hair is an indication for a history as detailed and an investigation as thorough as would be instituted if she had complained of cough, headache or any other symptom.

Of the many advances in our knowledge of the hair only a small number can be covered in this chapter. Two clinical situations have been selected, because they are frequently encountered. Common baldness—the term male-pattern alopecia is often inaccurate and misleading—is often misdiagnosed, misunderstood and overtreated. Alopecia areata remains an enigma, but many aspects of its natural history have been profitably explored and many misconceptions have been eliminated.

COMMON BALDNESS

The term male-pattern baldness is very commonly applied in many countries to that pattern of frontovertical baldness which is a physiological concomitant of maturation in the genetically predisposed. The term is perhaps misleading since the pattern of hair loss in the mildly affected female is not necessarily identical to that seen in the male.

Some textbooks of the last 50 years are monuments to human credulity in their uncritical endorsement of aetiological hypotheses ranging from tight hats and reflex interference with hair growth in cerebral congestion in brain workers, to a wide range of unconvincing microorganisms. Hamilton's (1942) now classic paper established the role of androgens in inducing common baldness; his work has received such unequivocal confirmation that it is surprising that the older myths have not yet been completely extinguished.

Phylogeny of baldness

Several primate species other than man also develop baldness as a natural phenomenon associated with sexual maturity (Montagna and Uno, 1968). In the chimpanzee, frontal baldness begins at adolescence and becomes conspicuous in adult life. A smaller monkey, more cheaply and conveniently handled in the laboratory, is the stump-tailed macaque, *Macaca speciosa*, in which also baldness develops from adolescence onwards. Detailed investigations have shown that this baldness is in every way comparable to the process as it occurs in man. The importance of this work lies not only in its direct contribution to our knowledge of the mechanism by which baldness is produced, but also in the irrefutable confirmation which it provides for the physiological nature of human baldness, which in the male and in the endocrinologically normal female must no longer be regarded as a disease. Under the influence of androgens, terminal follicles are progressively transformed into 'vellus' follicles, which differ from primary vellus follicles in that they may still have attached to them the remnants of fibres of the arrector pili muscles.

Prevalence and genetics

The prevalence of common baldness in any population has not been accurately recorded, but it may be true that, at least in the Caucasoid races it approximates to 100 per cent, for the replacement of some terminal follicles by vellus type follicles from puberty onwards is a universal phenomenon. Making assessments at the clinical level of evident sparsity of terminal hair a number of investigations have been carried out, but few of them have made any real attempt at quantification. An exception is that of Hamilton (1951) of New York who examined 312 white males and 214 white females aged 20 to 89 and proposed a system of grading baldness, which remains valuable.

Type   I   Full hair
Type   II   Bitemporal recession ⎫ Scalps not bald
Type   III   Borderline ⎭
Type   IV   Deep frontotemporal recession. Usually also some mid-frontal recession. In older subjects this degree of frontotemporal loss may be associated with some vertical thinning
Type   V   Increased frontotemporal recession and marked denudation of vertex
Type   VI   Increased loss from both areas, which are becoming confluent
Type   VII   Enlarged frontotemporal and vertical areas surpassed only by band of sparse hair
Type   VIII   Complete confluence of both areas

Type I was the normal scalp in both sexes before puberty, when it was replaced by Type II in 96 per cent of men and 79 per cent of women. Of men aged 50 or more, 58 per cent had scalps of Types V to VIII, and the extent of baldness tended to increase to the age of 70. About 25 per cent of women developed Type IV scalps by the age of 50, after which there was no further increase. Indeed after 50 some women who have developed Type II at puberty may revert to Type I. Types V to VIII were not found in any woman.

Type I scalp was retained after puberty by most Chinese. Baldness is uncommon, mild and of late onset.

Other statistics, much less accurately recorded, tend to group together what Hamilton has classified as Types II, III and IV, and are therefore of interest only in confirming the great frequency of common baldness in other populations of Caucasoids. For example, Buschke and Grenepert (1926) in Germany found bitemporal recession in 62.5 per cent of men aged 20 to 40. Beek (1946) in Holland found baldness in 27 per cent of women aged 35 to 40 and 64 per cent of those aged 40 to 70. Figures from Italy (Binazzi and Wierolis, 1962) also serve to emphasise the frequency of baldness in women of Caucasoid descent.

The incidence and patterns of baldness in American whites and Negroes have been compared (Setty, 1970). The more severe degrees of alopecia were more common in whites; and, taking all age groups together, a full head of hair—Hamilton Type I—was four times more frequent in Negroes than in whites.

This very frequency of common baldness has complicated the many attempts to establish its mode of inheritance. Moreover it is by no means clear that common baldness is genetically homogeneous, and some authorities differentiate between baldness of early onset (before 30 in men) and the same pattern of baldness becoming evident 20 years later.

Osborne (1916) thought that baldness was determined by a single pair of sex-influenced factors and Snyder and Yingling (1935) considered that both gene frequency studies and family histories supported this hypothesis. According to this theory both men and women of genotype BB are bald, and so are men but not women of genotype Bb. The genotype bb does not predispose to baldness in either sex.

Harris (1946) insisted that early baldness must be distinguished from late baldness, and that the former is transmitted by a single autosomal dominant gene. He assumed that the heterozygous female was normally not affected, but was uncertain about the homozygous female.

A clinical study (Smith and Wells, 1964) of the first degree relatives of 56 women with ordinary baldness, showed that of those who were 30 or over, 54 per cent of the males and 23 per cent of the females were similarly affected. These authors considered on the basis of their material that baldness could apparently develop in the heterozygous female and they postulated either dominant inheritance with increased penetrance in the male, or multifactorial inheritance. The probability of multifactorial inheritance was supported also by Salamon (1968). However, the question remains open. It is still uncertain whether early and late onset baldness are separately inherited. It is nevertheless certain that both are inherited and that both depend upon androgenic stimulation of susceptible follicles.

The association of baldness with susceptibility or resistance to certain diseases has been claimed, but the evidence is unsatisfactory; for example, an increased incidence of coronary artery disease, but a four-fold decrease in the incidence of carcinoma of the bronchus has been claimed for bald men as compared with non-bald controls (Bruchner, Brown and Tretsea, 1964).

The claim that baldness in men was associated with increased fertility could not be confirmed (Damon, Burr and Gerson, 1965).

Pathology

The combination of changes seen in common baldness is distinctive. The earliest change detected is focal perivascular basophilic degeneration in the lower third of the connective tissue sheath of otherwise apparently normal anagen follicles. The affected follicles become progressively smaller over a succession of hair cycles. Beneath the shrinking follicle can at first be seen the basophilic sclerotic remains of the connective tissue sheath, but eventually this too disappears. The arrector pili muscle decreases in size but its atrophy lags behind that of the follicle (Maguire and Kligman, 1962; Lettenand and Johnson, 1975). In any area of balding scalp, follicles at all stages can be found. In the scalp which appears totally bald almost all follicles are short and small and producing at best only tiny vellus hairs. However, even in such scalps there is usually a number of quiescent terminal follicles which may sometimes be stimulated into growth to raise false hopes of 'a cure' for baldness (Montagna and Parakkal, 1974). Careful studies of the differences between bald and non-bald scalp at various ages have been published by Goerttler (1965).

As the balding scalp loses its protective covering of hair so solar degenerative changes may be added to those described above (Singh and McKenzie, 1961; Allegra, 1968).

Soft tissue x-ray showed no correlation between the thickness of the scalp and the development of baldness (Garn, Selby and Young, 1954), and the reduction of blood supply has been shown to follow, not precede, the baldness (Cormia and Ernyey, 1961), though the degree of degenerative change in arterioles and capillaries may eventually be considerable (Allegra, 1968). When the follicles become small or disappear, their now unsupported nerve networks coil and twist and come to resemble encapsulated end-organs (Giacometti and Montagna, 1968).

The statement has often been made that the sebaceous glands of the scalp are enlarged and overactive in common baldness, but planimetric studies

(Rampini, Bertammo and Moretti, 1968) have shown that during the course of baldness the total number of sebaceous glands decreases significantly.

The development of baldness is associated with shortening of the anagen phase of the hair cycle and consequently with an increase in the proportion of telogen hairs, which may be detected in trichograms of the frontovertical region before evident baldness is present (Rassner, Zaun and Braun-Falco, 1963; Braun-Falco and Christophers, 1968). This is no doubt the explanation of the recorded differences in the force required to extract hairs from various regions of the adult male scalp (Light, 1951).

The reduction in the size of the affected follicles, which is the essential feature of ordinary baldness, necessarily results in a reduction in the diameter of the hairs they produce. This reduction is said to be greater in women than in men (Silvestri, 1967). The shaft diameter was found to be reduced in women with ordinary baldness also by Jackson, Church and Ebling (1972). Normal subjects showed a symmetrical distribution of shaft diameters with a peak at 0.08 mm; the patients showed a wide spread of shaft diameters with peaks at 0.04 and 0.06 mm.

The studies of the shaft in common baldness show no abnormality on electron microscopy (Puccinelli, Caputo and Casinelli, 1968) and preliminary studies show no abnormality in its chemical composition (Salamon, 1971).

Pathogenesis

Hypotheses formerly accepted by some scientists, but now abandoned since they lack any support from irrefutable evidence, have been mentioned above. Our knowledge of the pathogenesis of ordinary baldness is still incomplete but reliable facts are steadily accumulating and a working hypothesis can be proposed with some confidence. It must be remembered that any hypothesis put forward to explain human baldness must also be applicable to the identical condition occurring in other primates.

Hamilton's (1942) classic investigation showed that no baldness developed in 10 eunuchoids, 10 men castrated before puberty and in 34 men who had undergone orchidectomy during adolescence. The expected incidence of baldness in these 54 adult men was about 40 per cent. Common baldness developed in those individuals who were genetically so predisposed when testosterone was administered; when testosterone was discontinued the baldness did not progress but it was not reversed. Certain aspects of this work were confirmed in later publications (Hamilton, 1948, 1960). No subsequent investigator has been able to challenge Hamilton's findings; indeed much work in man and other primates has established beyond doubt that ordinary baldness is androgen-dependent.

The possibility that men who developed baldness might produce an excess of androgen was studied, but there is no evidence of increased output of testicular or of adrenal androgen in bald men as compared with control subjects matched for age and race. Studies in women with ordinary baldness have given conflicting results, but as technical procedures have improved and as more women have been adequately studied, it has become apparent that whilst a mild degree of baldness (Types II–IV) may occur in women with normal systemic androgen metabolism, more extensive baldness is usually (Apostolakis, Ludwig and Voigt, 1965; Binazzi and Calandra, 1968; Ludwig, 1968; Kuhn, 1972), probably always, associated with an increased output of ovarian or adrenal androgens, or of both. Normal male levels of androgen are sufficient to make manifest the degree of baldness genetically determined for the individual. Normal female levels of androgen can induce baldness only in women who are heavily genetically predisposed. In a larger proportion in whom the genetic predisposition is less strong, baldness is manifest only when androgen production is increased, and the severity of the baldness is related to the degree to which the androgen output is raised. In this group of patients hirsutism and acne may also develop, but in the lower abnormal range the genotype influences the degree and pattern of hirsutism and at all levels the genotype determines the presence or absence of acne. In a third group of women even grossly abnormal levels of androgen cause no clinically significant baldness, although all such patients are necessarily hirsute. There is no evidence that the non-sexual hormones are in any way involved in causing ordinary baldness (Stüttgen and Goerz, 1968), but the changes resulting from such states as hypothyroidism may of course occur in chance association with ordinary baldness.

Accepting that androgens are the initiating factor in ordinary baldness, it remains to consider by what mechanism they induce it.

The significance of sebum.   During the early decades of the present century the observed association of the presence of sebum with common baldness prompted many speculations and some uncritical experimental work on the relationship between the two phenomena. For many years microorganisms were held responsible for both, and when the role of such organisms was no longer accepted, the seborrhoea was considered to cause the loss of hair and the use of the term seborrhoeic alopecia as a synonym for common baldness emphasizes the widespread acceptance of this concept. The association of seborrhoea with baldness is of course a valid observation because both are androgen-dependent. In both sexes the bald scalp appears more greasy than the fully haired scalp. However, gravimetric studies of the casual levels of sebum and the hourly production of sebum in the bald scalp and hairy scalp of balding men and of the scalp of fully haired controls showed no differences between these groups (Maibach et al, 1968). Their subjects were all male. No similar investigation appears to have been carried out in females, but it is probable that some balding women will show greater sebum output than non-bald controls, as an inevitable result of their raised androgen levels. However, it is clear that increased sebum output does not in itself result in hair loss, but is an associated androgen-dependent phenomenon.

As early as 1926 Eliassow suggested an abnormality in the composition of sebum might influence hair growth. Later workers (Bloom, Woods and Nicolaides, 1955) could find no abnormality in the content of squalene or of free or esterified fatty acids in the sebum of balding subjects. More recently a number of investigators, e.g. Kuchinska (1973), reviewed by Thiele (1975), have suggested that the autoxidation of hair lipids gives rise to substances which have depilatory activity. The evidence that such substances play any part in ordinary baldness is unconvincing. Kuchinska's (1967) observation that washing the hair appears to reduce the rate of hair loss for the subsequent 24 h is readily explained by the fact that washing the hair removes club hairs nearing the end of normal telogen, and thus temporarily changes the tricho-gram and reduces physiological hair-fall for a few days. Moreover, if auto-oxidation products are depilatory why do they act only on certain follicles?

The metabolism of the hair follicles.   The weight of evidence strongly supports the opinion that the essential inherited factor responsible for ordinary baldness concerns the manner in which certain follicles in the frontovertical region of the scalp respond to androgens. However, regional variations in the metabolism of testosterone by hair follicles do not adequately explain observed differences in androgen-mediated hair growth (Schwiekert and Wilson, 1974). Reviewing the now very extensive literature on this subject Montagna and Parakkal (1974) suggest that the initial stage in the process of balding is probably the accumulation in the condemned follicles of 5α-dihydrotestosterone. This is the tissue-active androgen which activates sebaceous glands but inhibits the metabolism of hair follicles (Adachi, 1973). The conversion of testosterone to dihydrotestosterone (DHT) is catalysed by 5α-reductase but Adachi has shown that it is not this enzyme which controls the conversion. What factors exert this control, and what mechanisms are involved after the accumulation of DHT, remains to be established. The findings of published investigations offer abundant material for speculation, but are to some extent contradictory (Allegra et al, 1970; Fazekas and Sandor, 1973; Crovato, Moretti and Butamino, 1973).

Clinical features

Until further genetic studies have clarified the situation, ordinary baldness of early and of late onset are regarded as variants of a single clinical syndrome. The very high incidence of some degree of common baldness, and the great frequency of many disorders of hair growth, in particular the temporary and reversible disturbances of the hair cycle, inevitably results in the frequent fortuitous association of one or more disorders with common baldness.

The essential clinical feature of common baldness in both sexes is the replacement of terminal hairs by progressively finer hairs, which are even-tually very short and virtually unpigmented. This process may begin at any age after puberty and may become clinically apparent by the age of 17 in the normal male and by 25 to 30 in the endocrinologically normal female. The reduction in the size of the follicles is accompanied by shortening of anagen and therefore necessarily by increased shedding of telogen hairs. This shedding often attracts the patient's attention and induces him or her to seek advice. The replacement of terminal by smaller hairs occurs characteristically in a distinctive pattern, which spares the posterior and lateral scalp margins, even in the most advanced cases, and even in old age. The sequence of patterns in the male has been well described by Hamilton (page 224). Bitemporal recession is followed by balding of the vertex. Eventually more uniform frontal recession joins the bald areas and the entire frontovertical region bears only inconspicuous secondary vellus hair, which may also finally be lost. Variations in the pattern are governed at least in part by genetic factors, as can be confirmed in any collection of family portraits. The rate of progression too is probably determined largely by heredity; however, in the absence of evidence it would be wrong to exclude the possible influence of other factors.

The use of the term 'male-pattern alopecia' must be held partly responsible for the frequent failure to appreciate that in its earlier stages common baldness in women does not conform to the 'male pattern'. As in the male increased shedding of telogen hairs accompanies the reduction of shaft diameter, but the follicles first affected are more widely distributed over the frontovertical region. As a result many secondary vellus hairs are interspersed with hairs still normal, and others only slightly reduced in diameter. Partial baldness is sometimes first apparent on the vertex, but is more commonly diffusely distributed over the frontovertical region. Hair loss in this pattern has been regarded as a distinct entity (Guy and Edmundson, 1960) often known as 'chronic diffuse alopecia'. We entirely agree with those authors (Maguire and Kligman, 1963; Ludwig, 1964; Vadasz and Debreczeni, 1967) who claim that the most frequent presentation of common baldness in women is as a diffuse alopecia.

In women who are endocrinologically normal the rate of progression of common baldness is usually very slow, but nevertheless a severe degree of baldness, though still 'diffuse' may be present by the seventh decade. However, many women with ordinary baldness, particularly if it is of early onset, produce an excess of testosterone (Pierard, Kint and Backer, 1968). According to their genetic constitution this may give rise to hirsutism and/or recurrence or aggravation of existing acne or to no detectable abnormality other than the baldness. The entire clinical spectrum is seen according to the degree of androgenic stimulation and the capacity of follicles and sebaceous glands to respond to it. As a result of the physiological response of the sebaceous glands to androgen a complaint of increasing greasiness of the scalp is often made by women with common baldness. In all women with common baldness of rapid onset even if it be an isolated abnormality, and in women with common baldness of gradual onset, but accompanied by menstrual disturbance, hirsutism or recrudescence of acne, a full medical history and examination are essential, and in many cases endocrinological investigation is desirable.

We have observed baldness of Type IV in women without hirsutism. More extensive baldness (Types V–VIII) is always accompanied by hirsutism, and we have seen only once baldness of Type VIII, in a woman grossly masculinised by an ovarian tumour.

A special problem is presented by the patient of either sex in whom common baldness is accompanied by depression. Reluctance to establish or maintain normal social contacts may be blamed by the patient on his or her 'baldness', although repeated examination may fail to show any significant change in hair pattern. In such cases a more detailed history may bring to light other classical symptoms of depression—fatigue, lack of initiative, diminished or absent libido and a disturbed sleep cycle. In such patients reassurance alone is inadequate, for only effective management of the depression will prevent the patient from wasting his money on 'treatment' for his hair.

A different problem is the young woman in whom early baldness and the aggravation or recurrence of acne accompany or follow an episode of depression. Many such patients give a history of a marked degree of premenstrual tension since the menarche. (See Schückit et al (1975) on the relationship between premenstrual tension and depression.) Some of the patients develop amenorrhoea and hirsutism and some can later be shown to have the polycystic ovary syndrome. Others have no detectable increase of ovarian or adrenal androgen production. The relationship between the psychiatric disturbance and the androgenic cutaneous changes has not been established, but these syndromes are relatively common and in every case require careful investigation.

Diagnosis

In the male over 25 the characteristic pattern of the baldness usually makes diagnosis a simple matter, provided that the possible coexistence of hair loss of a different type is constantly borne in mind. Such a possibility is suggested by a history of recent rapid deterioration. It is frequently necessary to see the patient on several occasions over a period of some weeks before a definite conclusion can be reached, and investigations to exclude the known causes of diffuse hair loss may be required. It should also be remembered that balding men are not immune to syphilis or to alopecia areata.

In the younger male, the diagnosis may be difficult. He often complains principally not of baldness, but of increased shedding, particularly when he washes his hair. In such patients it is not always easy to determine whether shedding is really excessive or whether introspection born of depression has made him abnormally apprehensive of physiological shedding. Sometimes he may complain of baldness which is not evident to the observer. Such patients should not be dismissed with casual reassurance, but should be re-examined at intervals, after a detailed medical and social history has been taken. A strong family history may support a diagnosis of common baldness, but the absence of such a history does not exclude the diagnosis. The presence or absence of seborrhoea is not of diagnostic significance, for this is a genetic variable, and seborrhoea is evidence merely of normal sexual maturation in a susceptible subject.

In women, the diagnosis of common baldness may be difficult. In all cases it should be regarded as one of three cutaneous manifestations of androgenic stimulation and the presence of acne and/or of hirsutism should be noted. In the presence of such changes endocrinological assessment may be desirable. In their absence, particularly if there is a strong family history of baldness, the diagnosis may present no problems. However, the most frequent presentation is as a diffuse frontovertical thinning; the patient may volunteer the information that her hair has become finer and greasier. As in men the association of common baldness with other forms of hair loss is frequently encountered, and many cases require careful evaluation over a period of weeks. An accurate diagnosis is of importance in prognosis, and at times a biopsy may be useful. Common baldness should be a positive diagnosis, not a diagnosis by default.

Treatment

Effective treatment which will at least prevent the further transformation of terminal into vellus hairs can be offered to those women in whom the additional severity of their baldness beyond the physiological level is the result of a surgically reversible overproduction of androgen. In many women, however, although increased testosterone production is present, no effective surgical treatment is available because no localised lesion can be demonstrated. This is the present situation in many cases of the polycystic ovary syndrome. Their management should be discussed with endocrinologists and gynaecologists with a special interest in such problems, and falls outside the scope of this chapter.

In many young women with common baldness with or without associated hirsutism or acne, in whom the plasma testosterone level is within the upper normal range, and the menstrual cycle is regular, the possibility of prescribing an antiandrogen such as cyproterone acetate deserves consideration. Some good results have been reported (Gräf and Neumann, 1976) but it would be premature to recommend this treatment, except as part of a properly controlled trial, with the collaboration of an endocrinologist, as too little is known about possible long-term side effects.

Full discussion and explanation are essential to the humane and honest management of ordinary baldness. The accuracy of the diagnosis must of course be beyond doubt. Most men and many endocrinologically normal women will accept the situation philosophically, more particularly because in such women advance of the alopecia is usually very slow. If depression is more than mild, it should be treated, with if necessary the advice of a psychiatrist.

Surgery. There are some men, however, who because of the nature of their occupations, as entertainers or as salesmen, reasonably regard their baldness as a considerable disability. For such patients hair transplantation deserves serious consideration. One study of 50 patients who had undergone hair transplants (Clabaugh, Norwood and Pearson, 1973) showed that as compared with control subjects they were vain and assertive and mildly antisocial. Six would have been excluded from operation had they been tested earlier, but they had presented no special problems, postoperatively. Our experience suggests that nevertheless patients for operation should be very carefully selected. The operation is expensive and its results, especially in the long term, are not invariably entirely satisfactory. The patient whose real problem is his personality, rather than his baldness, should not be accepted.

Surgical treatment involves the transplantation to the bald areas of multiple small full thickness grafts from those areas of scalp still bearing predominantly terminal hairs (Orentreich, 1959; Ayers, 1964; Friedrich, 1970). The success of the procedure depends on proper selection of patients, and on the skill and experience of the operator. Postoperative complications have included bleeding, fistula formation, scarring and chronic infection (Lepaw, 1973).

Wigs. In women the baldness is usually too diffuse for transplantation surgery to be feasible. If the hair loss is extensive only a wig will conceal it.

There are various procedures by which small wigs are interwoven with persisting terminal hair; the cosmetic result is sometimes satisfactory. The patient who seeks advice from his doctor before embarking on some such procedure should be assessed in the same way as the patient considering surgery—is his baldness really his problem? If it is he should be advised to obtain from the firm he intends to employ a written statement of the probable cost of the initial procedure and of subsequent regular maintenance. Tension on the patient's surviving terminal hairs has occasionally led to patchy scarring alopecia (Perlstein, 1969).

Topical applications. There is no topical application, chemical or physical (e.g. ultraviolet or other radiation, or massage) which has been proved to alter the course of ordinary baldness.

The claim that topical testosterone induced the growth of terminal hairs in bald scalp (Papa and Kligman, 1965) has not been confirmed (Savin, 1968). Many different stimuli will induce temporary growth of certain resting follicles in some subjects, raising hopes which are false, for no cosmetically useful recovery occurs.

ALOPECIA AREATA

Aetiology

Throughout the second half of the nineteenth century the trophoneurotic theory of alopecia areata gradually supplanted the mycotic theory, which owed its long survival in part to confusion in nomenclature and in part to the inadequacies of laboratory technology. The term trophoneurotic is an invitation to loose thinking, and the theory has been adapted to successive changes in medical fashion, from focal sepsis, to psychosomatic, to 'autoimmune'. Most recent authors give qualified support to the autoimmune hypothesis, but most admit also the role of psychological factors in inducing attacks.

The findings of reputable observers in different countries in relation to so many features of alopecia areata show such marked and incompatible differences that even when allowance is made for differences in procedure and in diligence, the only reasonable assumption is that AA is a heterogeneous disorder and that its various forms occur with different relative frequency in different populations.

Heredity. Sabouraud (1929) in Paris found a positive family history of AA in 22 per cent of his cases; Brown (1929) of Glasgow, in 20 per cent. In the USA Muller and Winkelmann (1963) obtained such a history in 18 per cent of their adult cases, though in only 10 per cent of their entire series. Much lower figures are reported from south-west Europe, e.g. Portugal, 6.3 per cent (Bastos Araujo and Poiares Baptista, 1967); Italy, 4 per cent (Olivetti and Bubola, 1965); Spain, 0 per cent (Saenz, 1963). The association of AA with dark hair confidently asserted by Cockayne (1933) was not confirmed by Anderson (1950) or by Rook (1976). Many authors have suggested racial differences in the incidence of AA and such differences probably occur, but have not yet been reliably demonstrated.

Atopy. The presence of eczema or asthma or both was noted in 18 per cent of children with AA and 9 per cent of adults in a North American study (Muller and Winkelmann, 1963); 23 per cent of children with alopecia totalis were atopic. Ikeda (1965) in Japan found that 10 per cent of her patients with AA were atopic. Penders (1968) of Holland found a personal or family history of atopy in 52.4 per cent of patients with AA. In Denmark, Gip, Lodin and Molin (1969) found atopic dermatitis associated with AA in only 1 per cent of cases. These figures are very difficult to evaluate because the incidence of the atopic state in different populations is not reliably known. An estimate of 10 to 15 per cent (Rajka, 1975) should not be regarded as internationally applicable. There is however increasing evidence supporting Muller and Winkelmann (1963) and Ikeda (1965) tending to show that AA in the atopic subject is of earlier onset and greater duration and severity than in non-atopic subjects (see below, p. 237).

Autoimmunity. Many nineteenth-century clinicians recorded the association of AA with a variety of endocrine disorders and early in the present century the treatment of AA with 'thyroid extract' was advocated. When the role of organ-specific autoantibodies in certain of these endocrine disorders was demonstrated, it was suggested that an autoimmune mechanism was responsible also for the AA. The evidence, to say the least, is inconclusive. In the USA Muller and Winkelmann (1963) found thyroid disease in 8 per cent of their patients with AA. An incidence of thyroid disease of 28 per cent was found by Cunliffe et al (1969) in Newcastle, England. But Main et al (1975) could show no such association in Aberdeen, Scotland, nor could Salamon,

Musafija and Miličerić (1971) in Jugoslavia. Individual case reports associate Hashimoto's thyroiditis and AA (Klein, Weissheimer and Zaun, 1974) but prospective surveys of large numbers of patients are needed.

The association of AA with other endocrine disorders, notably diabetes mellitus and Addison's disease, has also been reported. The association of AA with vitiligo has long been recognised. Vitiligo was present in 4 per cent of cases in the USA (Muller and Winkelmann, 1963) and in Sheffield, England (Anderson, 1950). Vitiligo is itself significantly associated with thyroid disease, Addison's disease, pernicious anaemia and diabetes mellitus, although the frequency of the association varies considerably as between different series of cases.

The association of AA with lupus erythematosus (Muller and Winkelmann, 1963; Lerchin and Schwimmer, 1975) and with ulcerative colitis (Allen and Moschella, 1974) has also been noted.

The findings in autoantibody studies have not been consistent. In Newcastle, Cunliffe et al (1969) found no increase in the incidence of thyroglobulin and thyroid complement fixing antibodies as compared with control subjects. Main et al (1975) in Aberdeen similarly found no increase in thyroid auto-antibodies but a significant increase in smooth muscle antibodies. In Cambridge, Muller and Rook (1977) found no increase in any autoantibodies, including those to smooth muscle. Betterle et al (1975) had reported negative findings from Italy, but had not included smooth muscle in their investigations. However, Kern et al (1973) in North America found in 44 patients a significant association between AA and autoantibodies against thyroglobulin, cytoplasm of parietal cells and of thyroid and adrenal. It is possible that autoantibodies are present only in a highly selected group of patients with AA, and this group appears to include patients with Down's syndrome. More quantitative studies are required.

Down's syndrome. In Germany, Wunderlich and Braun-Falco (1965) found 13 cases of AA among 1000 mongols. This increased incidence of AA in Down's syndrome was confirmed when Du Vivier and Munro (1975) found 60 cases among 1000 mongols, but only one case in 1000 mentally retarded controls. The alopecia was total or universal in 25 of the 60 cases. Fourteen of the mongols with AA, 10 of them females, had fluorescent antibodies; eight had thyroid antibodies, one had parietal cell antibodies and one had antinuclear factor. In the four males with autoantibody the titre was low and probably not significant. Since 8 of the 23 female mongols with AA had antithyroid antibodies, 23 age-matched controls without AA were examined and antithyroid antibodies were found in only two. These findings cannot yet be interpreted. Thyroid antibodies are known to occur more frequently in Down's syndrome than in normal subjects, and to do so also in two other chromosomal defects, Turner's syndrome and Kleinfelter's syndrome. Mongols and their mothers are abnormally susceptible to thyroid disease (Fialkow, 1966).

Psychosomatic factors. At one extreme Panconesi and Mantellassi (1955, 1956) have claimed that 90 per cent of their patients with AA were psychologically abnormal on Rorschach testing. At the other, Ida Macalpine (1958) an experienced psychiatrist, did not consider that emotional factors played a significant role in AA. Most clinicians who have written on this subject appear to believe that stress is responsible for inducing attacks in at least some patients, or for perpetuating them. 'The perpetuating role of emotional tension states . . . is well authenticated' (Obermayer and Bowen, 1956). The question remains controversial; there are certainly many cases in which nervous stress appears on circumstantial evidence to be a provocative factor (Feldman and Rondón Lugo, 1973), but no reliable conclusions can be reached until the pathogenetic mechanism of AA is better understood. Certainly the cosmetic disability in AA may be a cause of stress (Lubowe, 1959) and the complex physical and emotional interrelations in some patients in whom AA and endogenous depression are associated have not yet been elucidated.

Age and sex incidence. Published statistics are based on hospital attendance and therefore do not necessarily reflect the true incidence. As hospital attendance is influenced by different factors in each area, apparent geographical differences cannot be accepted as true, without further evidence.

Onset between the age of 20 and 21 was recorded in 44 per cent in England (Anderson, 1950), 35 per cent in Spain (Lopez, 1951), 27 per cent in North America (Muller and Winkelmann, 1963), 32.5 per cent in Portugal (Bastos Araujo and Poiares Baptista, 1967), 35 per cent in Sweden (Gip et al, 1969). The same authors respectively recorded onset after the age of 40 in 19 per cent in England, 20 per cent in Spain, 30 per cent in North America, 20 per cent in Portugal and 25 per cent in Sweden.

The heterogeneity of AA

AA is generally regarded as a clinicopathological entity but the conflicting evidence on the frequency with which the atopic state and autoimmune disorders are associated with it, the divergent opinions on the role of stress in inducing it and the frankly contradictory claims as to its response to treatment, suggest that it may be a heterogeneous syndrome and that there may be geographical variation in the relative incidence of its different forms.

Attempts have been made in the past to differentiate various forms of AA solely on the morphology and extent of the bald areas. Ikeda (1965) of Kyoto University, Japan, studied 1989 patients with AA during the years 1946 to 1963. She classified her patients into four categories according to the presence (or absence) of certain associated disorders. A preliminary investigation established that the patients in each of these categories showed significant differences in the age of onset, clinical features and course of the AA. Ikeda's very comprehensive and detailed article should be consulted, but her principal findings may be summarised as follows:

Type I included 83 per cent of patients. This 'common' type was characterised by a lack of family or personal history of atopic disorders. The onset was usually between the ages of 20 and 40. The total course of the disease was usually under three years and individual patches tended to regrow in less than six months. Alopecia totalis developed in less than 6 per cent.

Type II included 10 per cent of patients and occurred in 'atopic' individuals. The onset was usually in childhood and the duration of the disease exceeded 10 years, alopecia totalis developing in 75 per cent. Individual patches tended to persist for over a year. Ophiasic lesions were not unusual and a reticular pattern of small bald patches also occurred. Seasonal recurrences were sometimes noted.

Type III accounted for 4 per cent of patients. Ikeda called it 'prehypertensive' because hypertension was found in one or both of the patient's parents. Most cases were in young adults, reticular alopecia was invariable and alopecia totalis developed in 39 per cent.

Type IV, with 5 per cent of patients, was called 'combined' or 'endocrine-autonomic'. We should now call it 'autoimmune'. It occurred mostly in patients over 40 and ran a prolonged course, but resulted in alopecia totalis in only 10 per cent.

The initial reaction to Ikeda's work was unfavourable, but studies along similar lines in Nijmegen (Penders, 1968; Mali, 1975) and Cambridge (Muller and Rook, 1977) suggest that many of the distinctions drawn by Ikeda are valid.

In Cambridge the records of 200 patients were analysed. These 200 were retained from a series of over 1000 cases because each patient had been followed up for at least 10 years since the first attack of AA, the patients had all been examined by the author on at least one occasion and the family history appeared to be as reliable as it can be when relatives are not available for examination. The patients were classified in five groups:

1. Personal history of atopic disorders
2. Personal history of 'autoimmune' disorders
3. Family but not personal atopic history
4. Family but not personal 'autoimmune' history
5. Neither personal nor family history of atopic or autoimmune disease.

In family histories only first and second degree relatives were included.

Our findings suggested that alopecia areata may indeed be usefully classified into at least three distinct but overlapping groups.

In Group 1 the AA tended to begin in childhood; the individual patches were persistent, reticular and ophiasic patterns were frequent, and total or universal alopecia developed in 32 per cent. The sexes were equally affected.

In Group 2 all the patients were women, and most were in middle age when the AA began. It became total in 58 per cent.

In Group 5 onset in later childhood or early adult life was usual. Single or short attacks were common and alopecia totalis developed in only 14 per cent.

Circumstantial evidence suggested that stress was often a provocative factor.

Groups 3 and 4 showed intermediate features and certainly contain cases which on longer follow-up would prove to be correctly classified in Groups 1 or 2 or 5.

The status of Ikeda's Type III (prehypertensive) is uncertain, and in our classification such cases were placed in Group 5. When the patients in this group with the clinical features of Ikeda's Type III, notably reticular alopecia, were re-examined, three of five were found in fact to be hypertensive. Penders (1968) found 4.8 per cent of his patients with AA to be prehypertensive.

Penders (1968) used slightly different diagnostic criteria; he accepted as atopic any patient who either had an atopic disease or had a family history and gave positive intradermal reactions to human dandruff and house dust. He found 52.4 per cent of his patients with AA to be atopic and only 35 per cent of Ikeda's Type I.

Pathology

The earliest histological changes are a combination of degenerative changes in connective tissue around vessels leading to the papilla, and a perivascular inflammatory infiltrate, mainly lymphocytic, around the bulb. It does not invade the papilla but may involve the internal root sheath (Van Scott, 1959). There may be spongiosis of the epidermis and lymphocytic infiltration around the openings of the follicles (Goos, 1971). The follicles are much reduced in size as the disease becomes established, and the volume of the matrix is disproportionately decreased in relation to that of the papilla (Van Scott and Ekel, 1958). These small follicles are in a phase comparable to anagen IV, beyond which they appear to be restrained from proceeding (Van Scott, 1958). Melanin granules may be seen in the papilla. In well-established lesions the inflammatory infiltration is less in evidence (Vilanova and Moragas, 1963).

Degenerative connective tissue changes in the papilla have been emphasised by some authors (Tagliavini and Dal Pozzo, 1964). An inconclusive claim has been made on the basis of studies of serial sections that the degeneration of the matrix may be attributed to a cell-mediated reaction against matrix cells (Thies, 1966). The number of mast cells in involved skin is no greater than normal (Spath and Steigleder, 1970), although the bald patches were the first to develop weals when a histamine liberator was administered (Juhlin, 1963).

The changes of AA may be more extensive than is clinically evident. Around the edge of a patch the proportion of telogen hairs and of dystrophic anagen hairs is increased, and similar but less severe changes may be found in the contralateral clinically normal scalp (Braun-Falco and Zaun, 1962; Kostanecki and Kwiatkowska, 1966). The presence of dystrophic hairs in clinically normal scalp is, however, not a constant finding (Eckert, Church and Ebling, 1968). It has been claimed that in some patients with AA of the scalp, the clinically normal skin of the upper arm shows an intense cellular infiltrate around follicles and between the lobes of sebaceous glands (Lazovic-Tepavac and Salamon, 1970).

Changes in the capillaries of affected follicles are regarded as secondary to the follicular changes and a response to the reduced circulatory requirements of the follicles (Uchiyama, 1967). Alkaline phosphate activity is diminished or absent in the papillae in early AA but as anagen becomes re-established in the miniature follicles alkaline phosphate activity becomes intense (Kopf and Orentreich, 1957). Investigations using $Na^{131}J$ suggested however that in chronic cases there may be some reduction in blood flow (Mian, 1966).

In attempts to find anatomical support for the neurotrophic theory there have been many studies of the nerve supply of affected follicles. Most authorities find no abnormality using the light microscope (Winkelmann and Jaffe, 1960; Gomez Orbaneja and Torres, 1963). However, degenerative changes are said to occur in the vegetative nervous system, but this observation requires confirmation (Gohlke and Holtschmidt, 1950). With the electron microscope degenerative changes in nerve fibres have been found in six cases of AA, but they may be a secondary phenomenon (Gay Prieto, Gonzalez and Urio-Roco, 1974).

In prolonged AA the secretory activity of sebaceous glands declines with the duration of the disease (Schweikert, 1967).

The abnormalities in the structure of the hair shaft characteristic of AA have been recognised for over a century. Pathognomonic are the exclamation-mark hairs, which are, however, not invariably present. These hairs average about 3 mm in length (Eckert et al, 1968). There are club hairs, the distal end of which is ragged and frayed but of normal calibre and pigmentation. Below their broken tips they taper towards a small but grossly normal club. Dystrophic anagen hairs are several centimetres long, but of reduced calibre and misshapen.

Electron microscopic studies of exclamation-mark hairs (Carteaud, 1969; Jackson, Church and Ebling, 1971) show that the imbricated pattern of cuticular scales is well maintained up to the point of fracture; beyond this point strands of cortical and medullary tissue are evident.

Pathodynamics. Many attempts have been made to establish the sequence of follicular events in the development of AA. Eckert et al (1968) studied hairs plucked from a series of concentric zones. Their results confirm earlier suggestions that an attack of AA begins with the premature entry of follicles into telogen at a focal point from which this process spreads outwards in a wave-like manner. However, the variations observed in the numbers of normal telogen hairs, dystrophic hairs and exclamation-mark hairs can best be interpreted if it is postulated that the follicles can respond in three different ways to the pathological trauma, depending on the latter's severity. At its greatest severity it damages and weakens the hair in the keratogenous zone, and at the same time precipitates the follicle into catagen. Such hairs break when the keratogenous zone reaches the surface of the scalp, and are later

extruded as exclamation-marks. Alternatively a follicle may simply be precipi-
tated into normal catagen and subsequently be shed as a club hair. Such
follicles may then produce dystrophic anagen hairs. Finally it is possible that
some follicles are injured just sufficiently to induce dystrophic changes,
whilst they continue to grow in the anagen phase.

If the cutaneous 'insult' ceases to act the resting follicles re-enter a normal
anagen and regrowth takes place. If the insult continues then the follicles are
restrained from passing beyond a phase of growth equivalent to anagen IV.

Clinical features

No important additions have been made to our knowledge of the clinical
features of AA except in so far as certain features can be related to prognosis.
Very marked differences in the course of AA are found in statistics from
different countries. Such differences can be explained if the relative incidence
of atopic, 'autoimmune' and simple cases varies geographically.

In Chicago (Walker and Rothman, 1950) the duration of the initial attack
was less than six months in our third, and less than one year in half, but one
third never recovered from the initial attack. The incidence of relapses in the
whole series of 230 patients was 86 per cent, but in those followed up for over
20 years it was 100 per cent. Of those developing AA before puberty 50 per
cent became totally bald and none recovered. In contrast only 25 per cent of
those developing AA after puberty became totally bald and 5.3 per cent
recovered. In the Mayo Clinic series (Muller and Winkelmann, 1963) only
1 per cent of the children and 10 per cent of adults with alopecia totalis
showed complete regrowth. The course in 140 cases in Madrid (Gomez
Orbaneja, 1963) was apparently less unfavourable, since the AA ran a short
course in 49 per cent and became total in 3.4 per cent and universal in 6.7
per cent. In Sweden (Gip et al, 1969) a 10 to 15 year follow-up showed
complete recovery in 34 per cent of males and 37 per cent of females and a
tendency for regrowth to begin earlier in females (54 per cent within six
months) than in males (34 per cent within six months). A study of 50 patients
with alopecia universalis (Schmitt, 1953) showed complete recovery in only
20 per cent with a worse prognosis in cases of prepubertal onset.

These divergent and not strictly comparable findings are difficult to
interpret intelligently. However, if the associated disorders are taken into
consideration a rational explanation of at least some of the inconsistencies
emerges. AA in the atopic subject begins early and has a poor prognosis; if
total before puberty it is unlikely to regrow completely. AA at any age may
be given a reasonably good prognosis if the patient is not atopic and has no
'autoimmune' disease, if it has remained circumscribed for over six months.
'Circumscribed' implies confined to one region of the body, usually but not
always the scalp. AA confined to the eyebrows also has a good prognosis. The
wider the involvement the more doubtful the outlook. Even in circumscribed
AA, if the patient is young and has a strong family history of atopy the

prognosis will be more guarded. If the pattern of alopecia is ophiasic the prognosis is uncertain, since most of these patients prove to be atopic subjects. The same pattern of AA occurs in sickle-cell anaemia, when it again suggests a poor prognosis (El Nasr and Roaiyah, 1954). The reticular pattern of alopecia (Fig. 7.1) also carries a poor prognosis, for it is rarely seen in simple

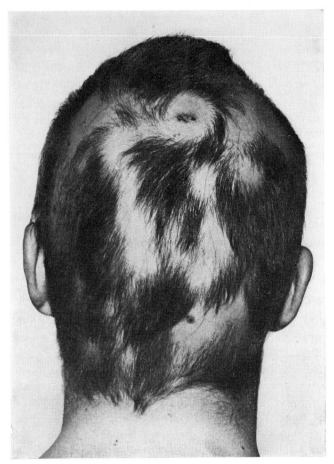

Figure 7.1   The 'reticular' form of alopecia areata. (Addenbrooke's Hospital, Cambridge)

AA. The almost unrelieved gloom of this paragraph must be brought into perspective by emphasising that in most series of cases of AA 80 per cent or more are of the simple type with a generally favourable outcome. There may be recurrences but they will usually be of relatively short duration. Nevertheless the wise dermatologist will never give a good prognosis until he has had the patient under observation for a year.

Eyes. In 58 patients with AA punctate lens opacities were no more frequent than in normal controls (Summerly, Watson and Copeman, 1966). Earlier reports on the incidence of lens opacities are mutually incompatible and must reflect the heterogeneity of AA. However, the association of cataracts with alopecia totalis is well documented (Muller and Brunsting, 1963) and in two of five adults so affected impairment of vision coincided with episodes of sudden and extensive hair loss.

Further, carefully controlled studies are needed before the association of AA with such ocular changes as Horner's syndrome, ectopia of the pupils, atrophy of the iris or tortuosity of the fundal vessels (Langhof and Lemke, 1962) can be accepted as significant. The same may be said of optic atrophy and pigmentary changes in the retina (Pisetsky and Kozinn, 1942).

Treatment

Adequately controlled therapeutic trials must match the control subjects not only for age and sex, but for duration and clinical type of AA and the presence of associated disorders. We can confirm the observations of Ikeda (1965) and Penders (1968) that in the majority of cases of AA in atopic subjects the response even to systemic steroids is disappointing and early relapse is the rule.

AA that on personal and family history and on clinical features appears to be of the simple type may safely be left untreated, or treated with a placebo if this appears to be desirable. If the patch is unsightly it is reasonable to infiltrate it with a corticosteroid suspension with the expectation that immediate relapse is unlikely. The response to intralesional triamcinolone acetonide or hexacetonide has been described as 'all or nothing'; if it occurs it is maintained for about nine months (Porter and Burton, 1971). In our experience the majority of the failures are in atopic subjects. Perhaps the most frequent indication for intralesional corticosteroid is to maintain the growth of the eyebrows, which is a cosmetic benefit even in alopecia totalis (Berger, 1961). Atrophy may be an unsightly complication of intralesional treatment: it is usually confined to the injection sites, but may follow the line of lymphatic flow over the forehead (Kikuchi and Horikawa, 1975).

In severe AA in atopic subjects systemic corticosteroids may be administered if the usual contraindications have been excluded, but only after the patient has been made aware that an effective maintenance dose may be unacceptably high and may have to be abandoned.

REFERENCES

COMMON BALDNESS

Adachi, K. (1973) The metabolism and control mechanism of human hair follicles. *Common Problems in Dermatology*, 5, 37.

Allegra, F. (1968) Histology and histochemical aspects of the hair follicles in pattern alopecia. In *Biopathology of Pattern Alopecia*, ed. Baccaredda-Boy, A., Moretti, G. & Frey, J. R., p. 155. Basel: Karger.

Allegra, F., Giacometti, L., Uno, H. & Adachi, K. (1970) Studies of common baldness in the stump-tailed macaque. III. DNA synthesis in regressing hair. *Acta dermato-venereologica*, **50**, 169.

Apostolakis, M., Ludwig, E. & Voigt, K.-D. (1965) Testosteron-, Oestrogen-, und Gonadotropenausscheidung bei diffuser weiblicher Alopecia. *Klinische Wochenschrift*, **43**, 9.

Ayers, S. (1964) Conservative surgical management of male pattern baldness. *Archives of Dermatology*, **90**, 492.

Beek, C. H. (1946) Calvities frontalis bei Frauen. *Dermatologica*, **93**, 213.

Binazzi, M. & Calandra, P. (1968) Testosterone elimination in female patients with acne, chronic alopecia and hirsutism. *Italian General Review of Dermatology*, **8**, 17.

Binazzi, M. & Wierolis, T. (1962) Les Alopécies féminines Hypooestrogéniques. *Annales de dermatologie et de syphiligraphie*, **89**, 382.

Bloom, R. E., Woods, S. & Nicolaides, N. (1955) Hair fat composition in early male pattern alopecia. *Journal of Investigative Dermatology*, **24**, 97.

Braun-Falco, O. & Christophers, E. (1968) Hair root patterns in male pattern alopecia. In *Biopathology of Pattern Alopecia*, ed. Baccaredda-Boy, A., Moretti, G. & Frey, J. R., p. 141. Basel: Karger.

Bruchner, H. A., Brown, M. & Tretsea, R. J. (1964) Baldness and emphysema. *Journal of the Louisiana State Medical Society*, **116**, 34.

Buschke, A. & Grenepert, M. (1926) Zur Kenntnis des Sexuelcharakters der Kopfhaarkleiden. *Klinische Wochenschrift*, **5**, 18.

Clabaugh, W., Norwood, O'T. & Pearson, J. (1973) Personality studies in patients receiving hair transplants for treatment of male pattern baldness. *Cutis*, **12**, 113.

Cormia, F. E. & Ernyey, A. (1961) Circulatory changes in alopecia. Preliminary report, with a summary of the cutaneous circulation of the normal scalp. *Archives of Dermatology (Chicago)*, **84**, 772.

Crovato, F., Moretti, G. & Butamino, R. (1973) 17-Betahydroxysteroid dehydrogenases in hair follicles of normal and bald scalp. A histochemical study. *Journal of Investigative Dermatology*, **60**, 126.

Damon, A., Burr, W. A. & Gerson, D. E. (1965) Baldness, fertility and number and sex ratio of children. *Human Biology*, **37**, 366.

Eliassow, A. (1926) Cholesterinstoffwerchsel und Haarwuchs. *Dermatologische Wochenschrift*, **83**, 1463.

Fazekas, A. G. & Sandor, T. (1973) The metabolism of dehydroepiandrosterone by human scalp hair follicles. *Journal of Clinical Endocrinology*, **36**, 582.

Friedrich, H. C. (1970) Indikation und Technik der operativ-plastischer Behandlung des Haarverlustes. *Hautarzt*, **21**, 197.

Garn, S. M., Selby, S. & Young, R. (1954) Scalp thickness and the fat-loss theory of balding. *American Medical Association Archives of Dermatology and Syphilology*, **70**, 601.

Giacometti, L. & Montagna, W. (1968) The nerve fibres in male pattern alopecia. In *Biopathology of Pattern Alopecia*, ed. Baccaredda-Boy, A., Moretti, G. & Frey, J. R., p. 208. Basel: Karger.

Goerttler, K. (1965) *Der menschliche Glatze im Altersformwandel der behaarten Kopfhaut.* Stuttgart: Thieme.

Gräf, K.-J. & Neumann, F. (1976) Klinische Anwendungsmöglichkeiten von Antiandrogenen in der Dermatologie. *Ärztliche Kosmatologie*, **6**, 26.

Guy, W. B. & Edmundson, W. F. (1960) Diffuse cyclic hair loss in women. *Archives of Dermatology*, **81**, 205.

Hamilton, J. B. (1942) Male hormone stimulation is prerequisite and an incitant in common baldness. *American Journal of Anatomy*, **71**, 451.

Hamilton, J. B. (1948) The role of testosterone secretions as indicated by the effect of castration in man and by studies of pathological conditions and the short life-span associated with maleness. *Recent Progress in Hormone Research*, **3**, 257.

Hamilton, J. B. (1951) Patterned long hair in man: types and incidence. *Annals of the New York Academy of Sciences*, **53**, 708.

Hamilton, J. B. (1960) Effect of castration in adolescent and young adult males upon further changes in the proportions of bare and hairy scalp. *Journal of Clinical Endocrinology*, **20**, 1309.

Harris, H. (1946) The inheritance of premature baldness in man. *Annals of Eugenics*, **13**, 172.

Jackson, D., Church, R. E. & Ebling, F. J. (1972) Hair diameter in female baldness. *British Journal of Dermatology*, **87**, 361.

Kuchinska, R. (1967) Die Beeinflüssung des Haarausfalls durch Kosmetische Präparate. *Kosmetischen Monatschrift*, **16**, 12.

Kuchinska, R. (1973) Chemische Aspekte des Haarausfalls und ihre Kosmetologischen Bedeutung. *Kosmetologie*, **5**, 177.

Kuhn, B. H. (1972) Male pattern alopecia and/or androgenic hirsutism in females. Part III. Definition and etiology. *Journal of the American Medical Women's Association*, **27**, 357.

Lattenand, A. & Johnson, W. C. (1975) Male pattern alopecia. A histopathologic and histochemical study. *Journal of Cutaneous Pathology*, **2**, 58.

Lepaw, M. I. (1973) Hair transplant complications. *Cutis*, **11**, 88.

Light, A. F. (1951) Patterned loss of hair in man: pathogenesis and prognosis. *Annals of the New York Academy of Sciences*, **53**, 729.

Ludwig, E. (1964) Die androgenetische Alopecie bei der Frau. *Archiv für klinische und experimentelle Dermatologie*, **219**, 558.

Ludwig, E. (1968) The role of sexual hormones in pattern alopecia. In *Biopathology of Pattern Alopecia*, ed. Baccaredda-Boy, A., Moretti, G. & Frey, J. R., p. 50. Basel: Karger.

Maguire, H. C. & Kligman, A. M. (1962) The histopathology of common male baldness. In *Proceedings of the XII International Congress of Dermatology*, Washington, p. 1438.

Maguire, H. C. & Kligman, A. M. (1963) Common baldness in women. *Geriatrics*, **18**, 329.

Maibach, H. I., Feldmann, R., Payne, B. & Hutshell, T. (1968) Scalp and forehead sebum production in male pattern alopecia. In *Biopathology of Pattern Alopecia*, ed. Baccaredda-Boy, A., Moretti, G. & Frey, J. R., p. 171. Basel: Karger.

Montagna, W. & Parakkal, P. F. (1974) *The Structure and Function of Skin*, 3rd edn. New York: Academic Press.

Montagna, W. & Uno, H. (1968) In *Biopathology of Pattern Alopecia*, ed. Baccaredda-Boy, A., Moretti, G. & Frey, J. R., p. 9. Basel: Karger.

Orentreich, N. (1959) Autografts in alopecias and other selected dermatological conditions. *Annals of the New York Academy of Sciences*, **83**, 463.

Osborne, D. (1916) Inheritance of baldness. *Journal of Heredity*, **7**, 347.

Papa, C. M. & Kligman, A. M. (1965) Stimulation of hair growth by topical application of androgens. *Journal of the American Medical Association*, **191**, 521.

Perlstein, H. H. (1969) Traction alopecia due to hair weaving. *Cutis*, **5**, 440.

Pierard, J., Kint, A. & Backer, J. de (1968) Sur le role probable de l'hormone male dans l'alopécie féminine. *Archives Belges de dermatologie et syphiligraphie*, **24**, 409.

Puccinelli, V. A., Caputo, R. & Casinelli, T. (1968) Electron microscopic study of the hair shaft in normal and alopecic subjects. In *Biopathology of Pattern Alopecia*, ed. Baccaredda-Boy, A., Moretti, G. & Frey, J. R., p. 129. Basel: Karger.

Rampini, E., Bertamino, R. & Moretti, G. (1968) Size and shape of sebaceous glands in male pattern alopecia. In *Biopathology of Pattern Alopecia*, ed. Baccaredda-Boy, A., Moretti, G. & Frey, J. R., p. 155. Basel: Karger.

Rassner, B., Zaun, H. T Braun-Falco, O. (1963) Zur Pathomechanismus der männliche Glatzenbildung. *Archiv. für klinische und experimentelle Dermatologie*, **216**, 307.

Salamon, T. (1968) Genetic factors in male pattern alopecia. In *Biopathology of Pattern Alopecia*, ed. Baccaredda-Boy, A., Moretti, G. & Frey, J. R., p. 39. Basel: Karger.

Salamon, T. (1971) Comparative chemical investigations on hair of various areas of the capillitium in subjects with 'normal' hair and with alopecia seborrhoeica. *Folia Medica Facultatis Medicinae Universitatis Saraeviensis*, **5**, 241.

Savin, R. C. (1968) The ineffectiveness of testosterone in male pattern baldness. *Archives of Dermatology*, **98**, 512.

Schückit, M. A., Daly, V., Herrman, G. & Hineman, S. (1975) Premenstrual symptoms and depression in a university population. *Diseases of the Nervous System*, **36**, 516.

Schwiekert, H. U. & Wilson, J. D. (1974) Regulation of human hair growth by steroid hormones. I. Testosterone metabolism in isolated hairs. *Journal of Clinical Endocrinology*, **38**, 811.

Setty, L. R. (1970) Hair patterns of the scalp of white and Negro males. *American Journal of Physical Anthropology*, **33**, 49.

Silvestri, U. (1967) Studio físico del Capello in Casuistica de Alopecia su base seborroica. *Archivio Italiano di Dermatologia, Venereologia, e Sessuologia*, **34**, 405.

Singh, M. & McKenzie, J. (1961) The histology and histochemistry of the diseases of hairy and non-hairy parts of the human skin with special reference to baldness. *Journal of Anatomy*, **95**, 569.

Smith, M. A. & Wells, R. S. (1964) Male type alopecia, alopecia areata and normal hair in women. *Archives of Dermatology*, **89**, 95.

Snyder, L. H. & Yingling, H. C. (1935) The application of the gene frequency method of analysis to sex-influenced factors with especial reference to baldness. *Human Biology*, **7**, 608.

Stüttgen, G. & Goerz, G. (1968) Non-sexual hormones and male pattern alopecia. In *Biopathology of Pattern Alopecia*, ed. Baccaredda-Boy, A., Moretti, G. & Frey, J. R., p. 61. Basel: Karger.

Thiele, F. A. J. (1975) Chemical aspects of hair loss and its cosmetological significance. *British Journal of Dermatology*, **92**, 355.

Vadasz, E. & Debreczeni, M. (1967) Untersuchungen zur Ätiologie der androgenetischen Alopecia der Frau. *Hautarzt*, **18**, 454.

ALOPECIA AREATA

Allen, H. B. & Moschella, S. L. (1974) Ulcerative colitis associated with skin and hair changes. *Cutis*, **14**, 85.

Anderson, I. (1950) Alopecia areata: a clinical study. *British Medical Journal*, **2**, 1250.

Bastos Araujo, A. & Poiares Baptista, A. (1967) Algunas Consideraciones sobre 300 Casos de Pelada. *Trabakos da Sociedade Portugesa de Dermatologia e Venereologia*, **25**, 135.

Berger, R. A. (1961) Alopecia areata of eyebrows—corticosteroids. *American Medical Association Archives of Dermatology*, **83**, 151.

Betterle, C., Pesserico, A., Dal Prete, G. & Trisotto, A. (1975) Autoantibodies in alopecia areata. *Archives of Dermatology*, **111**, 927.

Braun-Falco, O. & Zaun, H. (1962) Uber die Beteiligung des gesamten Capilitiums bei Alopecia areata. *Hautarzt*, **13**, 342.

Brown, W. H. (1929) The aetiology of alopecia areata and its relationship to vitiligo and possibly sclerodermia. *British Journal of Dermatology*, **41**, 299.

Carteaud, J.-P. (1969) Cheveux de plaques peladiques examinés en microscope électronique par balayage; *Bulletin de la Société française de dermatologie et de syphilographie*, **76**, 660.

Cockayne, E. A. (1933) *Inherited Abnormalities of the Skin and Appendages*, p. 354. Oxford: University Press.

Cunliffe, W. C., Hall, R., Stevenson, C. J. & Weightman, D. (1969) Alopecia areata, thyroid disease and autoimmunity. *British Journal of Dermatology*, **81**, 879.

Du Vivier, A. & Munro, D. D. (1975) Alopecia areata, autoimmunity and Down's syndrome. *British Medical Journal*, **1**, 191.

Eckert, J., Church, R. E. & Ebling, F. J. (1968) The pathogenesis of alopecia areata. *British Journal of Dermatology*, **80**, 203.

El Nasr, H. S. & Roaiyah, M. F. A. (1954) Prognosis of alopecia areata. *Journal of the Egyptian Medical Association*, **37**, 476.

Feldman, M. & Rondón Lugo, A. J. (1973) Considerations psicosomaticas en la alopecia areata. *Medicina Cutanea*, **7**, 95.

Fialkow, P. J. (1966) Autoimmunity and chromosomal aberrations. *American Journal of Human Genetics*, **18**, 93.

Gay Prieto, J., Gonzalez, G. & Urio-Roco, A. (1974) Inervación del folículo piloso de las alopecias universales. *Actas Dermo-Sifiliográficas*, **65**, 477.

Gohlke, & Holtschmidt (1950) Neurohistologische Studien bei Alopecia areata. *Archiv. für Dermatologie und Syphilologie*, **191**, 527.

Gomez, Orbaneja, J. (1963) Modalidades clínico evolutivas de la Alopecia areata. *Actas Dermo-Sifiliograficas*, **54**, 353.

Gomez Orbaneja, J. & Torres, A. de C. (1963) Inervación del folículo pilosebacea en la Alopecia areata. *Actas Dermo-Sifiliograficas*, **54**, 387.

Goos, M. (1971) Zur Histopathologie der Alopecia areata. *Archiv. für Dermatologische Forschung*, **240**, 160.

Gip, L., Lodin, A. & Molin, L. (1969) Alopecia areata. *Acta dermato-venereologica*, **49**, 180.

Ikeda, T. (1965) A new classification of alopecia areata. *Dermatologica*, **131**, 421.

Jackson, D., Church, R. E. & Ebling, F. J. (1971) Alopecia areata hairs. A scanning electron microscopic study. *British Journal of Dermatology*, **85**, 242.

Juhlin, L. (1963) Reactions to infusion of a histamine liberator. *Archives of Dermatology*, **88**, 771.

Kern, F., Hoffmann, W. H., Hambrick, G. W. & Bizzard, R. M. (1973) Alopecia areata: immunologic studies and treatment with prednisone. *Archives of Dermatology*, **107**, 407.

Kikuchi, I. & Horikawa, S. (1975) Perilymphatic atrophy of the skin. *Archives of Dermatology*, **111**, 795.

Klein, V., Weissheimer, B. & Zaun, H. (1974) Simultaneous occurrence of alopecia areata and immunothyroiditis. *International Journal of Dermatology*, **13**, 116.

Kopf, A. W. & Orentreich, N. (1957) Alkaline phosphates in alopecia areata. *American Medical Association Archives of Dermatology*, **76**, 288.

Kostanecki, W. & Kwiatkowska, E. (1966) Uber Wachstums und Melanogenese-Störungen der Haare bei Alopecia areata. *Archiv. für klinische und experimentelle Dermatologie*, **226**, 21.

Langhof, H. & Lemke, L. (1962) Ophthalmologische Befunde bei Alopecia areata. *Dermatologische Wochenschrift*, **146**, 585.

Lazovic-Tepavac, O. & Salamon, T. (1970) Uber die Histopathologie der Alopecia areata. *Dermatologische Monatschrift*, **156**, 665.

Lerchin, E. & Schwimmer, B. (1975) Alopecia areata associated with discoid lupus erythematosus. *Cutis*, **15**, 87.

Lopez, B. (1951) Contribucion al conocimiento de la etiopatogenia y tratamiento de la Pelada. *Actas Dermo-Sifiliográficas*, **42**, 589.

Lubowe, I. I. (1959) The treatment of alopecia universalis with methyl prednisolone (Medrol) associated with vitiligo involving arms, forearms, neck and thigh. *American Medical Association Archives of Dermatology*, **79**, 665.

Macalpine, I. (1958) Is alopecia areata psychosomatic? *British Journal of Dermatology*, **70**, 117.

Main, R. A., Robbie, R. B., Gray, E. S., Donald, D. & Horne, C. H. W. (1975) Smooth muscle antibodies and alopecia areata. *British Journal of Dermatology*, **92**, 389.

Mali, J. W. H. (1975) Alopecia areata. *British Journal of Dermatology*, **93**, 605.

Mian, E. U. (1966) Sull'irrorazione del cuoio capelluto nell'alopecia areata. *Giornale Italiano di Dermatologia*, **107**, 919.

Muller, K. & Rook, A. J. (1977) To be published.

Muller, S. A. & Brunsting, L. A. (1963) Cataracts in alopecia areata. *American Medical Association Archives of Dermatology*, **88**, 202.

Muller, S. A. & Winkelmann, R. K. (1963) Alopecia areata. *Archives of Dermatology*, **88**, 290.

Obermayer, M. E. & Bowen, E. T. (1956) Trichotillomania and alopecia areata. *Pediatric Clinics of North America*, **3**, 639.

Olivetti, L. & Bubola, D. (1965) Osservazioni cliniche su 160 Casi de Area Celsi. *Giornale Italiano di Dermatologia*, **106**, 376.

Panconesi, E. & Mantellassi, G. (1955) Fattori psichici nella etiopatogenesi dell'area Celsi. *Rassegna di Dermatologia e Sifilografia*, **8**, 121.

Panconesi, E. & Mantellassi, G. (1956) Ulteriori risultati di indageni psicodiagnostiche nella alopecia areata. *Rassegna di Dermatologia e Sifilografia*, **8**, 205.

Penders, A. J. M. (1968) Alopecia areata and atopy. *Dermatologica*, **136**, 395.

Pisetsky, J. E. & Kozinn, P. J. (1942) Total alopecia associated with ocular disorders. *American Journal of Diseases of Children*, **64**, 80.

Porter, D. & Burton, J. L. (1971) A comparison of intralesional triamcinolone hexacetonide and triamcinolone acetonide in alopecia areata. *British Journal of Dermatology*, **85**, 272.

Rajka, G. (1975) *Atopic Dermatitis*. Vol. 3 in the Series *Major Problems in Dermatology*. London: Saunders.

Sabouraud, R. (1929) Lecons et démonstrations des jeudis. *Archives Dermato-Syphiligraphiques de la Clinique de l'Hôpital Saint-Louis*, **1**, 31.

Saenz, H. (1963) Neuvo contribucion ad Estudio de la Alopecia areata en España. *Actas Dermo-Sifiliograficas*, **54**, 357.

Salamon, T., Musafija, A. & Miličerić, M. (1971) Alopecia Areata und Erkrankungen der Thyreoidea. *Dermatologica*, **142**, 62.

Schmitt, C. L. (1953) Trauma as a factor in the production of alopecia universalis. (Preliminary report.) *Pennsylvania Medical Journal*, **56**, 975.

Schweikert, H. U. (1967) Quantitatin Untersuchungen über die Telgdrüsenfunktion bei Alopecia areata. *Archiv für klinische und experimentelle Dermatologie*, **230**, 96.

Späth, U. & Steigleder, G. K. (1970) Zahl der Mastzellen bei Alopecia areata. *Zeitschrift für Haut und Geschlechtskrankheiten*, **45**, 435.

Summerly, R., Watson, D. M. & Copeman, P. W. M. (1966) Alopecia areata and cataracts. *American Medical Association Archives of Dermatology*, **93**, 411.

Tagliavini, R. & Dal Pozzo, V. (1964) Osservazioni istochemische in Alcuni Casi di Area Celsi. *Giornale Italiano di Dermatologia*, **105**, 195.

Thies, W. (1966) Vergleichende histologische Untersuchungen bei Alopecia areata und narbig-atrophierenden Alopecia. *Archiv für klinische und experimentelle Dermatologie*, **227**, 541.

Uchiyama, M. (1967) Histological and histochemical studies of alopecia areata. *Japanese Journal of Dermatology*, **72**, 281.

Van Scott, E. J. (1958) Morphologic changes in pilosebaceous units and anagen hairs in alopecia areata. *Journal of Investigative Dermatology*, **31**, 35.

Van Scott, E. J. (1959) Evaluation of disturbed hair growth in alopecia areata and other alopecias. *Annals of the New York Academy of Sciences*, **83**, 480.

Van Scott, E. J. & Ekel, T. M. (1958) Geometric relationships between the matrix of the hair bulb and its dermal papilla in normal and alopecic scalp. *Journal of Investigative Dermatology*, **31**, 281.

Vilanova, X. & Moragas, J. M. de (1963) Alopecia areata (injertos e histologia). *Actas Dermo-Sifiliograficas*, **54**, 337.

Walker, S. A. & Rothman, S. (1950) Alopecia areata. A statistical study and consideration of endocrine influences. *Journal of Investigative Dermatology*, **14**, 403.

Winkelmann, R. K. & Jaffe, M. O. (1960) Nerve network of the hair follicles in alopecia areata. *Archives of Dermatology*, **82**, 750.

Wunderlich, C. & Braun-Falco, O. (1965) Mongolismus und Alopecia areata. *Medizinische Welt*, **i**, 477.

8
TUMOURS OF THE SKIN

John H. Epstein   Richard W. Sagebiel   Richard C. Connors
Bernard Ackerman

The subject of recent advances in the field of cutaneous tumour formation is far too extensive to be summarised adequately within the confines of one chapter. The present discussion will therefore present specific aspects of cutaneous tumour formation and behaviour on which relatively new information is available. Since the subjects are not closely related they are presented in three distinct sections with individual bibliographies. These include an examination of the current concepts concerning malignant melanomas, a discussion of recently recognised pseudomalignancies of the skin, and a review of experimental epidermal carcinogenesis.

MALIGNANT MELANOMA

Richard W. Sagebiel

May you live in interesting times.
Old adage

Investigators involved in the recent changes regarding malignant melanoma can certainly claim to live in interesting times. During the past five years significant progress has been made in the understanding of the different biological forms of malignant melanoma and some progress has been made towards relating their clinical and histological features to therapy and prognosis.

A major portion of this advance has been the relation of the levels of invasion of the tumour within the skin to prognosis, and, more recently, a similar correlation with the maximum thickness of the primary neoplasm measured on the microscope slide. This concept, in turn, helps to dictate not only primary surgical therapy but also defines the so-called 'high risk primary' patient in whom various adjunct therapeutic procedures are now attempting to affect the progression of the disease.

Although malignant melanoma represents only 1 to 2 per cent of all cancer, it appears to be increasing in certain populations of the world (Beardmore and Davis, 1975). Moreover, it affects a relatively younger age group than many cancers and is present on the surface of the skin, and thus attracts the attention of both physician and patient. The incidence of 1 to 5 per 100 000 individuals appears to be affected strongly by geographical and racial considerations. The increased susceptibility of individuals of Celtic origin, particularly when they have been transplanted to areas of high sunlight exposure, accounts for the highest incidence in the world reported from the Queensland Melanoma Project in Australia (Beardmore and Davis, 1975). Darkly pigmented individuals have a low rate of cutaneous melanoma, although there are certain local peculiarities of malignant melanoma involving the sole of the foot and relatively non-pigmented mucosal surfaces (Fleming et al, 1975).

Overall, more than 90 per cent of malignant melanomas are cutaneous in origin. An additional 9 per cent arise in the eye and the balance are accounted for by unusual sites where pigment cells are known to occur, such as the mucosal surfaces of the upper respiratory, genitourinary or gastrointestinal tracts. In all instances the model of neoplastic transformation appears to be the same; that is, a malignancy of the melanocyte or pigment-producing cell.

This review describes first, the classification of biological forms of malignant melanoma and the definition of their levels of invasion; secondly it

Table 8.1 Distribution of malignant melanoma (University of California Melanoma Clinic, 1972–75)

Superficial spreading	253 (65%)
Nodular	91 (23%)
Lentigo maligna	25 (6%)
Not otherwise classified	25(6%)
Total	394

considers the histological features related to prognosis and, finally it discusses a brief clinical staging scheme.

Classification

The current classification (Clark et al, 1969) of the three biological forms of malignant melanoma is:

1. Superficial spreading malignant melanoma
2. Nodular malignant melanoma
3. Lentigo maligna melanoma

All three types of malignant melanoma may be seen at any level of invasion, so that the terms in themselves are not a guide to prognosis.

1. *Superficial spreading malignant melanoma* (SSM). This form of melanoma accounts for approximately 70 per cent of the total numbers seen in a large series of malignant melanomas (Table 8.1). It is characterised by a biphasic growth pattern. The first phase, which may exist for many years in some cases and for at least several years in most, consists of a radial growth of malignant cells within the epidermis and superficial dermis. At some point in time the

cells in one or more areas penetrate deeper into the dermis in what is referred to as a vertical growth phase. This deeper invasion is associated with a marked worsening of the five year prognosis, and may be thought of as a form of 'tumour progression'.

2. *Nodular malignant melanoma* (NM). Nodular malignant melanomas are thought of as arising in the vertical growth phase without a pre-existing radial growth phase. Nodular melanomas make up approximately 20 per cent of the total numbers of melanomas. Many of them assume protuberant or polypoid forms, which must, in order to account for their relatively bad prognosis, be evaluated according to cross-sectional tumour load or maximum tumour thickness rather than depth of invasion. Nodular melanoma occurs at any age and in any location, in general increasing in incidence with age.

3. *Lentigo maligna melanoma*. The third type of malignant melanoma, arising in association with a lentigo maligna or so-called Hutchinson's melanotic freckle, accounts for something less than 10 per cent of the total numbers of malignant melanomas. It is almost certainly related to sunlight exposure and is found primarily on the head and neck of elderly individuals. It is characterised by the longest period of radial growth, up to 20 years or more in most instances, before the onset of the vertical growth phase. In general it seems to have a somewhat better prognosis at all levels of invasion, although metastasis and death from this form of melanoma have been reported.

Levels of invasion (McGovern et al, 1973)

Level I. Malignant melanocytes confined to the epidermis. The concept of 'malignant melanoma in situ' is currently being used as a research diagnosis only. In practice the histological diagnosis applied to this process has been 'atypical melanocytic hyperplasia' with a comment as to the extent of the lesion, the degree of cytological atypicality, and the host response. It is assumed that complete exicsion of an intraepidermal atypical lesion should result in 100 per cent cure, although these relatively infrequent lesions have not yet been completely evaluated.

Level II. Invasion by malignant melanocytes into the papillary dermis. In general this may take two forms. The first consists of tumour cells closely associated with a dense cellular host response consisting primarily of lympho-cytes and occasional histiocytes. This may increase the thickness of the papillary dermis between two and ten times. A second form is associated with individual tumour cells without significant cellular or other host response. Occasionally the papillary dermis becomes fibrotic and contains pigmented macrophages or prominent small vessels. In these forms the papillary dermis is usually not greatly thickened. Level II invasion with a maximum tumour thickness less than 0.75 mm is associated with an excellent (95 per cent) five year survival following local re-excision alone (Breslow, 1970; Wanebo, Woodruff and Fortner, 1975).

Level III. Tumour cells at the junction of papillary and reticular dermis.

This level is the most difficult to evaluate and the most important from the point of view of prognosis. Level III invasion does not occur when the first cell touches the junction, but rather when the tumour cells fill entirely the papillary dermis and abut against the reticular dermal collagen. In many instances this results in some compression of the underlying thick bundles of reticular dermal collagen. Frequently the cellular host response is absent at Level III. Breslow (1972) has calculated that when Level III invasive tumours become thicker than 0.76 mm the prognosis worsens. Wanebo et al (1975) have confirmed this, again measuring maximum tumour thickness. In some areas of the body such as the neck and scalp, the site of the papillary–reticular dermal interface is difficult to determine in normal skin, whereas on the trunk and extremities, this junction is much more easily identified and the level of the tumour is therefore much easier to assess. The estimation of anatomic levels combined with measurement by ocular micrometer probably offer the best criteria for estimating the prognosis of the tumour.

Level IV. Malignant melanocytes within the reticular dermis. When tumour cells are in association with reticular dermal collagen, with or without a cellular host response, the tumour is classified as Level IV. In earlier years it seemed useful to differentiate between invasion of the upper and the lower halves of the reticular dermis, but this has not proven to be of practical importance, and the entire reticular dermis appears to act as one unit from the point of view of prognosis at this level of invasion.

Level V. Invasion into the subcutaneous fat. Invasion at this level from either SSM or NM results in a less than 30 per cent five year survival regardless of the form of therapy. It is not yet entirely known whether Level V LMM is associated with a similar poor prognosis.

Clinical features related to prognosis (Mihm et al, 1973)

1. *Superficial spreading malignant melanoma*. In general when first seen these tumours are small with varied outlines, pigmentation, and colour. The two most important colours are red, resulting from the erythema and cellular host response and blue reflecting pigmentation deep in the dermis. The radial growth phase may show central or eccentric areas of regression with normal or hypopigmented areas. They may become crusted and patients may report either pruritus or a tingling sensation. During the period of vertical growth phase one or more nodules may result in an elevated dome-shaped papule or nodule frequently reddish-brown in colour or relatively less pigmented than the surrounding and occasionally ulcerated. The vertical growth phase is associated with deep invasion and a worsened prognosis.

2. *Nodular malignant melanoma*. These tumours are probably the most frequently misdiagnosed. Even with a high index of suspicion, the astute physician may fail to diagnose this neoplasm correctly (Kopf, Minitzis and Bart, 1975). Its period of growth is generally somewhat shorter than that of SSM. The lesion may be noted for the first time by the examining physician.

It may vary in pigmentation from flesh or dull red to black and may be uniform in colour and outlines. It may be dome-shaped, protuberant, or even polypoid in configuration. By the time a nodular melanoma has become polypoid it frequently is ulcerated and occasionally has an inflamed base. These lesions are unfortunately often neglected. The smaller ones may be confused with pigmented basal carcinomas, Spitz naevi (benign juvenile melanomas), benign naevi, dermatofibromas, or seborrhoeic keratoses. Nodular malignant melanoma tends to invade deeply from the onset. Larger protuberant or pedunculated lesions have a five year prognosis of levels IV to V tumours (i.e. 30–40 per cent five year survival) by virtue of their large cross-sectional area or tumour thickness (see below).

3. *Lentigo maligna melanoma*. This form is probably the easiest to diagnose in its very early stages. Histological distinction from the so-called adult or 'senile' lentigo is sometimes difficult and subjective. It revolves almost entirely around the cytological atypicality of individual melanocytes, and the presence of areas of regression within the papillary dermis. Clinically the tumour is irregular in outline and faintly pigmented in its early stages. It evolves by centrifugal spread with increasingly irregular pigmentation and outlines. Areas of regression are commonly seen in later stages. Ultimately after a varying but usually long period of evolution the nodule of vertical growth can be seen (Clark and Mihm, 1969). The macular lesion characteristically extends down pilosebaceous units and sweat glands, a feature which is dramatically emphasised when superficial forms of therapy for the early lentigo maligna are attempted and recurrence results from the deeper layers around appendages (Litwin et al, 1975).

MISCELLANEOUS FEATURES OF ALL THE ABOVE TYPES

Size and duration. In general the size of the lesion is roughly correlated with prognosis in the three forms of malignant melanoma, i.e. the larger the lesion the worse the prognosis. This may in fact be merely restating the relationship to depth of invasion and/or tumour cross-sectional area. In general larger lesions have been either neglected or allowed to grow through their normal evolution for a longer period of time so that duration and size may be considered as two features of the same phenomenon, both related to depth of invasion.

Site. There is some correlation between the site and the ultimate prognosis. In general it helps to explain some of the earlier literature in which head and neck malignant melanoma was thought to have a better prognosis. These reports included large numbers of lentigo maligna melanomas which indeed have a better prognosis or at least a slower natural history. In general, site per se is probably not related to prognosis as closely as are other features. The predilection of SSM for the upper back in men and the calf in women could affect prognosis. Clinical awareness of this distribution of higher risk areas in individuals of light complexion and poor tanning ability, may result in earlier diagnosis before the onset of the vertical growth phase. Similarly in darkly pigmented individuals sites of major importance for examination and early diagnosis are the relatively non-pigmented areas, especially the sole of the foot, the subungual areas and the oral mucosae.

Elevation. A protuberant or polypoid malignant melanoma has a worse prognosis than its apparent level of invasion would suggest (Little, 1972). This is probably related to two factors. The first is that the overall cross-sectional area or tumour load is generally large; greater than 1 cm in both dimensions. Moreover, the collagen at the base of the protuberant lesion is usually a desmoplastic tumour stroma rather than normal reticular dermal collagen. This would appear to offer a simple explanation for the fact that the elevated or protuberant lesion behaves in the manner of a deeply invasive Level IV or V tumour.

Colour. In general the colour is helpful in diagnosis but not prognosis. Deeply pigmented primary neoplasms can have either amelanotic or melanotic metastases. Histologically malignant melanoma may have little apparent pigment, but the descriptive term 'amelanotic melanoma' has no prognostic significance and is really a misnomer. Even these tumours show some pigment formation when viewed by the electron microscope.

Age of patient. The incidence of malignant melanoma increases with advancing age. This is true for both men and women except for a peculiar increase in incidence of malignant melanoma of the calf in women between 35 and 45 years of age. This striking pehnomenon is not merely a question of overdiagnosis, as the mortality figures of such lesions also indicate increased incidence. Relationships to sunlight and/or trauma have been suggested. However, the reasons for this distribution remain speculative.

Halo formation. The presence of halos around primary malignant melanomas is well known. Moreover, zones of depigmentation around other naevi in patients with primary malignant melanoma have been documented (Epstein et al, 1973). Both phenomena appear to be of great theoretical interest but currently have not been proven to be of prognostic value. In general the halos associated with malignant melanoma are less distinct and somewhat more irregular in outline than the normally rather dramatically circular outline of the benign halo naevus.

Preceding lesion. In approximately 20 to 40 per cent of primary malignant melanomas examined histologically for this feature an association with pre-existing benign naevi is found (Little, 1972). On the other hand, a history of pre-existing pigmented spots sometimes of many years' duration, before the onset of change, is given by as many as 50 to 80 per cent of patients. The presence of a pre-existing naevus is not directly related to prognosis.

Family history. Familial malignant melanoma appears to have a special evolution and prognosis (Anderson, 1971). The patients usually develop the lesions early, frequently before the age of 30, and melanomas are often multiple. The genetic penetrance of this trait within a family may be strong but the mortality appears to be somewhat less than that of malignant melanoma in general. It is known that perhaps only 5 per cent of patients with malignant melanoma will develop a second primary whereas these are commonly found in the familial form (Beardmore and Davis, 1975).

Histological cell type. The variance within primary neoplasm of cells with spindle-shaped outlines, epithelioid cell patterns, mixed patterns or small naevoid cell variance are not yet known to have significant prognostic value (Little, 1972).

Mitoses. Numbers of mitotic figures have been correlated with five year prognosis by the Queensland Melanoma Project. Large numbers of mitotic figures within the primary neoplasm tend to be associated with a worse prognosis (Little, 1972).

Host reaction. Preliminary studies of the cellular host reaction to the primary neoplastic cells have suggested some relationship to prognosis (Wanebo et al, 1975), but the data have not yet been completely evaluated. There is some suggestion that a uniform band-like infiltrate beneath tumour cells is a good prognostic feature, however a lymphocytic–histiocytic host response has not yet been proven to be associated with a favourable progress. The presence of plasma cells has been associated with a significantly bad prognosis (Little, 1972). Tissue reactions include mesenchymal host response with fibrosis, angioneogenesis, stromal pigmentation and macrophages present in varying amounts. These factors remain to be evaluated.

Clinical staging

Although a generally accepted definitive staging system has not been instituted for malignant melanoma, the following represents a preliminary staging system evolved through the Malignant Melanoma Clinical Cooperative Group. This includes the following categories:

Stage   I   Local disease
Stage II   Regional draining nodes
Stage III   Disseminated disease.

Included in the local disease category are primary lesions with satellites within 5 cm or local recurrence within 5 cm of the primary site. Regional spread on the same extremity can also be classified as local disease; palpable regional nodes not histologically examined do not exclude the patient from the local disease category. Regional disease includes patients with histologically positive regional lymph nodes. Disseminated malignant melanoma involves remote cutaneous and/or lymph node sites and visceral spread.

This clinical staging system hopefully will allow the uniform recording of the biology and prognosis of the malignant melanoma so that various therapeutic procedures can be adequately evaluated.

RECENT RECOGNISED PSEUDOMALIGNANCIES OF THE SKIN

Richard C. Connors   A. Bernard Ackerman

There are a variety of cutaneous lesions whose microscopic features strongly suggest malignancy, but whose biological behaviour is benign. The best known of these is the keratoacanthoma. Other well-established cutaneous pseudomalignancies are the spindle and epithelioid cell naevus (Spitz, 1948), trichoepithelioma, seborrhoeic keratosis with intraepidermal nests (Mehregan and Pinkus, 1964), nodular fasciitis (Konwaler, Keasbey and Kaplan, 1955; Hutter, Stewart and Foote, 1962), and pseudocarcinomatous epidermal hyperplasia overlying dermatofibromas and granular cell tumours.

During the past 15 years, additional pseudocancers of the skin have been described. Though these cannot be confidently classified histogenetically in all instances, they may be tentatively grouped as in Table 8.2.

Table 8.2   Recently recognised pseudomalignancies of the skin

A.	*Pilar:*	Proliferating trichilemmal cyst
B.	*Melanocytic:*	Recurrent melanocytic naevus
C.	*Fibroblastic:*	Atypical fibroxanthoma
D.	*Inflammatory:*	
		1. Actinic reticuloid
		2. Lymphomatoid papulosis
E.	*Vascular:*	Angiolymphoid hyperplasia with eosinophils

The essential clinical and histological attributes of these pseudocancers are the subject of this review.

Pilar

Proliferating trichilemmal cyst

The proliferating trichilemmal cyst typically presents as a slowly enlarging growth on the scalp of an elderly woman. It may occur in younger women, and, infrequently, in men or in areas other than the scalp. Its largest diameter is usually between 1 and 5 cm, but may be greater than 25 cm. The smaller lesions are often indistinguishable clinically from routine pilar cysts, while the larger lesions are frequently fungating and ulcerated and suggest carcinoma (Lund, 1957; Wilson-Jones, 1966; Reed and Lamar, 1966; Dabska, 1971; Christophers and Spelberg, 1973).

Microscopically, there is a well-demarcated intradermal tumour composed of sharply defined, interweaving strands and nests of squamous epithelium (Fig. 8.1). A band of homogeneous eosinophilic material surrounds some of these epithelial aggregates, and many of them show central accumulations of keratin. The dominant method of keratinisation is identical to that seen in trichilemmal cysts, i.e. the peripheral cells progressively enlarge, develop pale-staining cytoplasm, lack clear intercellular bridges, do not develop a granular layer, and abruptly lose their nuclei to form compact cornified cells (Pinkus, 1969).

The following histological changes also may occur, either focally or diffusely: squamous eddies, individual keratotic cells, basaloid cells, abortive hair papillae and bulbs, calcium deposition, granulomatous inflammation, foci of necrosis, and atypical epithelial cells (Fig. 8.2). Horn-filled channels from the tumour to the skin surface may be demonstrable with serial sectioning.

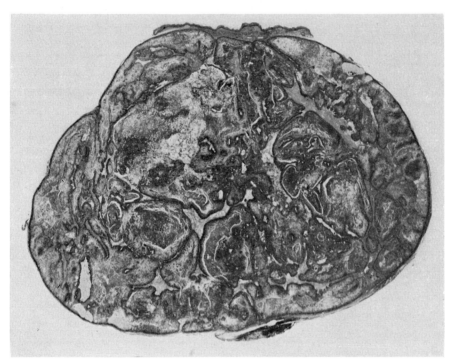

Figure 8.1 The proliferating trichilemmal cyst shows sharp demarcation both of the entire tumour and of the component epithelial aggregates. × 594

This pilar growth clearly derives from the trichilemmal portion of the outer root sheath. Whether it develops via epithelial proliferation within an antecedent trichilemmal cyst, or whether it represents a trichilemmal neoplasm, *sui generis*, is undetermined. The designation 'proliferating trichilemmal cyst' is tentative, but it is probably more accurate than many of the other appellations applied to this lesion.

Quite certain, on the other hand, is the biological benignancy of this growth. Simple excision is curative, local recurrence is rare, and metastasis never occurs.

The histological differentiation of proliferating trichilemmal cyst from squamous cell carcinoma rests primarily on the architectural pattern of the lesion, i.e. the sharp circumscription both of the entire tumour and of its component epithelial aggregates. Additionally helpful are the trichilemmal keratinisation, the horn-filled channels to the surface, the peripheral eosinophilic bands, and the predominant cytological typicality. The benignancy that these microscopic features suggest is corroborated if the lesion has originated from the scalp of an older woman.

Inadequate biopsy of a proliferating trichilemmal cyst may not allow accurate microscopic identification, and this lesion may then be erroneously

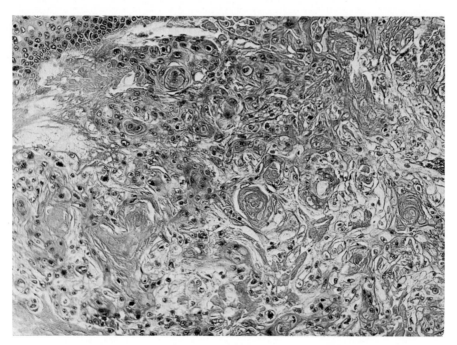

Figure 8.2   A higher power view of the proliferating trichilemmal cyst in Figure 8.1 reveals cytological atypia and structural disarray, mimicking squamous cell carcinoma. × 138

interpreted, as probably occurred often in the past (Bishop, 1931; Peden, 1948; Welch, 1958), as a squamous cell carcinoma arising in a cyst.

Melanocytic

Recurrent melanocytic naevus

When a melanocytic naevus is incompletely removed and subsequently recurs, the resultant lesion often exhibits considerably more melanocytes within and above the epidermal basal cell layer than were present in the original naevus (Schoenfeld and Pinkus, 1958; Cox and Walton, 1965; Lewis, 1971; Kornberg and Ackerman, 1975). Some of these intraepidermal melanoyctes may be cytologically atypical, and there may be marked variation in the size and shape of the melanocytic nests, as well as confluence of these nests. The ensemble of these changes may simulate the intraepidermal component of a superficial spreading malignant melanoma (Fig. 8.3).

There is, nevertheless, both direct and circumstantial histologic evidence against malignancy. The direct evidence is the sharp lateral demarcation of the intraepidermal melanocytic hyperplasia (Fig. 8.4). The circumstantial evidence is the fibrosis within the papillary and/or reticular dermis, testimony to earlier surgical manipulation, and the commonly concurrent intradermal melanocytic naevus, residue of the original lesion.

History of prior surgery should be pursued when one is confronted by these histological changes. If this history is obtained, the previous biopsy material must be reviewed in order to confirm its benignancy. Should histological material from the initial surgical specimen not be available, it may not be possible to designate the intraepidermal melanocytic hyperplasia within the recurrent lesion as unequivocally benign.

Fibroblastic

Atypical fibroxanthoma

Atypical fibroxanthoma generally occurs as a nodule on the head or neck of an elderly individual with sun-damaged skin. The ears, cheeks or nose are most frequently involved. The lesion is usually less than 3 cm in diameter. Its surface may be intact, or there may be ulceration and episodic minor bleeding. Occasionally the nodule is friable and highly vascular and suggests a pyogenic granuloma. The age of the growth varies from weeks to years. It develops somewhat more commonly in men and almost exclusively in caucasoids. It may present in younger patients, often on the trunk or extremities. Symptoms of pain or tenderness are unusual, and a history of antecedent trauma to the affected site is obtained in only a small percentage of cases. Simple excision is curative, but local recurrence after inadequate removal may occur (Halpert and Hackney, 1949; Bourne, 1963; Helwig, 1963; Kempson and McGavran, 1964; Reed, 1967; Kroe and Pitcock, 1969; Hudson and Winkelmann, 1972; Fretzin and Helwig, 1973).

Histologically, atypical fibroxanthoma demonstrates a non-encapsulated cellular mass within the dermis, frequently either contiguous with the overlying epidermis or separated from it by only a narrow band of collagen (Fig. 8.5). The epidermis may be hyperplastic, thin, or ulcerated. In lesions from exposed sites, copious solar elastotic material in the surrounding dermis and cytological atypicality in the overlying epidermis are common. The tumour sometimes expands into the subcutis, but never into the deeper tissues. Its cellular constituents are varied in structure and haphazard in array. Plump spindle cells with large nuclei, some vesicular, others hyperchromatic, are dispersed irregularly or arranged in ill-defined fascicles. Cells polyhedral in configuration are also numerous and are often markedly atypical. Their

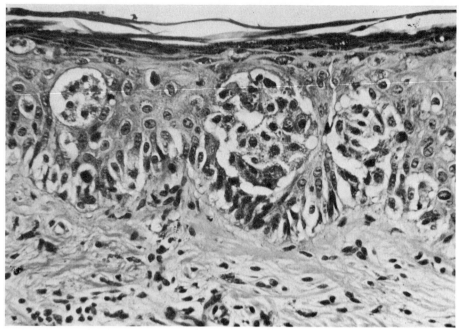

Figure 8.3 Atypical melanocytes at all levels of the epidermis, both singly and in nests of varying sizes and shapes, are present in this recurrent melanocytic naevus, thus suggesting a superficial spreading malignant melanoma. × 342

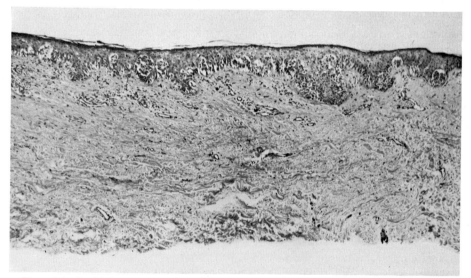

Figure 8.4 In this lower power view of the recurrent melanocytic naevus in Figure 8.3, sharp circumscription of the intraepidermal melanocytic proliferation and fibrosis within the upper dermis are evident. Intradermal malanocytic nests, a common but not invariable feature of recurrent melanocytic naevi, are absent. × 58

nuclei are voluminous and vesicular; nucleoli prominent; and cytoplasm abundant and either granular or vacuolated in appearance. Scattered strikingly amongst this cytological collage are bizarre giant cells with single or multiple nuclei and foamy cytoplasm (Fig. 8.6). Fat-laden histiocytes are also common, as are mitotic figures, many aberrant in form. The percentages of these different cells vary considerably from lesion to lesion and even among sections from the same specimen.

Collagen formation is usually minimal, and significant mucin deposition or necrotic foci are rare. Vascular proliferation, however, is often marked,

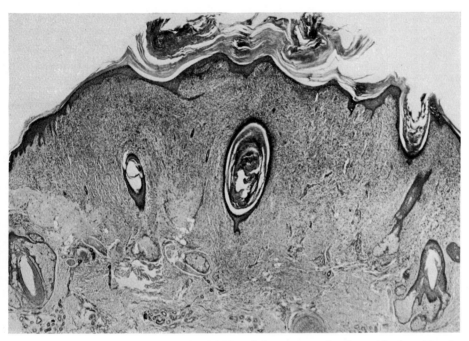

Figure 8.5 Atypical fibroxanthoma is a highly cellular tumour, often located in the mid and upper dermis and commonly in contact with the overlying epidermis. × 26

generally in the form of numerous small endothelial-lined spaces. Telangiectatic vessels are occasionally evident, as are extravasated red blood cells. Extension of the cellular proliferation into vascular lumina does not occur. Fat stains reveal intracytoplasmic lipid in histiocytes, polyhedral cells, and giant cells.

Atypical fibroxanthoma must be differentiated microscopically from a diverse group of biologically malignant lesions. Dermatofibrosarcoma protuberans is a monomorphous spindle cell neoplasm without numerous markedly atypical cells, giant cells, or foam cells, but with prominent collagen formation and fascicles of cells arranged in a distinctively whirling pattern.

Malignant melanoma exhibits intraepidermal proliferation of atypical melanocytes, melanin production and absence of foam cells. Spindle cell squamous carcinoma commonly demonstrates focal squamous differentiation, such as individually cornified cells or squamous pearl formation. Some of these spindle cell carcinomas, nevertheless, especially among those which develop secondary to roentgen ray exposure (Sims and Kirsch, 1948; Underwood, Montgomery and Broders, 1951; Rachmaninoff, McDonald and Cook,

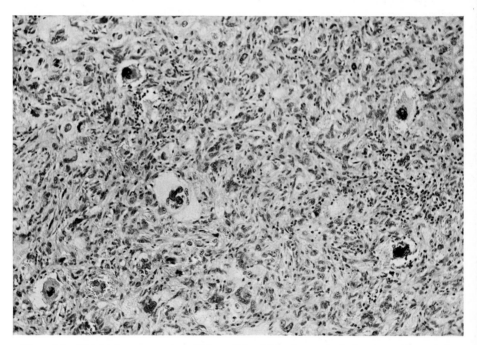

Figure 8.6 This higher power view of Figure 8.5 exhibits the cytological potpourri frequently found in atypical fibroxanthoma: spindle cells, foam cells, polyhedral cells, giant cells, and prominent nuclear atypia. × 135

1961), cannot be reliably distinguished histologically from those atypical fibroxanthomas in which spindle cells predominate.

The histogenesis of atypical fibroxanthoma is entirely unknown. Whether it is epithelial or mesenchymal in origin, whether it is truly neoplastic or simply reactive: both basic issues are moot. Although solar induction of these lesions is often suggested both clinically and microscopically, the mechanism of such induction is undetermined. The relationship of atypical fibroxanthoma to fibrous histiocytoma or to the histologically similar pseudosarcoma of the upper respiratory and digestive tracts (Lane, 1957; Grigg, Rachmaninoff and Robb, 1961) is unclear. The latter lesion develops in association with and, presumably, in response to an overlying in situ or invasive squamous cell carcinoma. Similarly, as noted above, atypical fibroxanthoma commonly has overlying intraepidermal cellular atypia.

This absence of understanding of the pathogenesis of atypical fibroxanthoma and its relative infrequency make it difficult to lay down criteria for its microscopic diagnosis. Accordingly, only lesions that are both histologically and clinically characteristic should be unequivocally diagnosed as atypical fibroxanthoma. Thorough study of multiple sections and correlation with the clinical data are essential. A history of prior roentgen therapy to the involved site, for example, precludes a definitive designation of atypical fibroxanthoma, for postradiation spindle cell malignancies, as noted above, may be indistinguishable microscopically from the spindle cell variant of atypical fibroxanthoma.

The two cases reported of alleged atypical fibroxanthoma which metastasised should not have been so categorised. One of these cases demonstrated at its primary site cellular invasion of the walls of medium-sized veins (Fretzin and Helwig, 1973). The other case occurred in an area of chronic radiodermatitis and microscopically exhibited extension into cartilage (Jacobs, Edwards and Ye, 1975). Such features exclude the diagnosis of atypical fibroxanthoma and demand total excision of the lesion.

Inflammatory

Actinic reticuloid

Actinic reticuloid refers to a severe, persistent photodermatitis occurring nearly exclusively in older men; commonly extending to non-exposed areas; significantly responsive only to total avoidance of natural light; associated with photosensitivity extending through the longwave ultraviolet, often into the visible light range; and simulating a lymphoma both clinically and histologically (Ive et al, 1969).

The clinical resemblance to lymphoma derives from the grotesque pachydermatous plaques which may develop in light-exposed sites. Biopsies from such lesions frequently reveal a dense, predominantly perivascular infiltrate of lymphocytes and histiocytes, as well as variable numbers of eosinophils, plasma cells, and mast cells (Fig. 8.7). Scattered histiocytic giant cells may occur. A minority of the mononuclear cells are large and have hyperchromatic nuclei. Some of the inflammatory cells may be present focally within the epidermis. Spongiosis is slight or absent. The papillary dermis is markedly thickened by hypertrophied collagen bundles associated with prominent oval and stellate fibroblasts (Fig. 8.8). This fibrosis may also involve much of the reticular dermis. Vascular channels are increased in number and lined by plump endothelial cells.

The polymorphous inflammatory infiltrate and proliferative vascular changes are indicative of a benign lymphoid hyperplasia or pseudolymphoma (Bluefarb, 1960; Caro and Helwig, 1969). The fibrosis is secondary to the chronic intense rubbing which this severely pruritic eruption elicits. The occasional spongiosis and the inflammatory cells focally within the epidermis suggest that the process is basically a spongiotic dermatitis.

This suggestion is supported by biopsies of non-plaque lesions from either light-exposed or non-exposed skin and of experimentally induced lesions. Spongiosis is common in such biopsy material. Mononuclear cells are present within the epidermis. There is a dense superficial perivascular, often band-like infiltrate of lymphocytes and histiocytes. A concomitant deep, though less

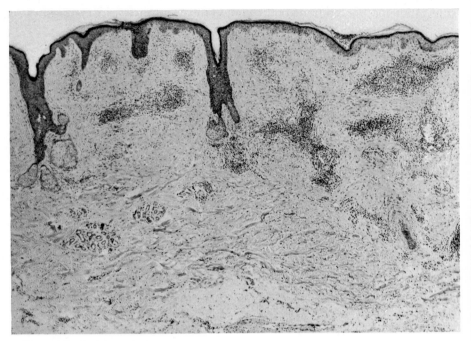

Figure 8.7   Actinic reticuloid typically displays, as in this lesion, a dense, predominantly perivascular inflammatory cell infiltrate and marked thickening of the papillary dermis by hypertrophied collagen bundles. × 37

dense perivascular infiltrate often occurs. Some of the mononuclear cells have hyperchromatic nuclei. Papillary dermal fibrosis is mild or absent.

The dense superficial infiltrate with cells within the epidermis may mimic early mycosis fungoides, but the spongiosis and scant cytological atypicality argue for benignancy. Clinical correlation confirms this interpretation.

Actinic reticuloid, then, is initially a spongiotic process with a superficial and deep perivascular infiltrate of lymphocytes and histiocytes. With chronic photoexacerbation and rubbing, the spongiosis wanes, but a dense polymorphous infiltrate and pronounced dermal fibrosis develop. Though a single immunological investigation reaches a contrary conclusion (Menter,

McKerran and Amos, 1974), these histological alterations in actinic reticuloid are most consistent with a photoallergic dermatitis in its progression from acute to chronic stages.

The differentiation of either the early or the late microscopic changes of actinic reticuloid from lymphoma can usually be made with assurance. Uncertainty is generally eliminated both by the clinical picture and by additional biopsies.

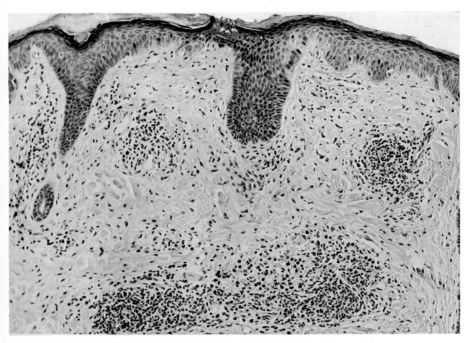

Figure 8.8 Higher power examination of Figure 8.7 highlights the papillary dermal fibrosis and the numerous associated large, often stellate fibroblasts. Atypical mononuclear cells are present within the inflammatory cell infiltrate. × 138

The one report of lymphoma occurring in a patient with actinic reticuloid provides, unfortunately, a paucity of histological and clinical information (Jensen and Sneddon, 1970). The diagnosis of reticulum cell sarcoma was based solely on a skin biopsy. The single photomicrograph presented of the allegedly lymphomatous skin lesion is not adequate for substantive diagnostic interpretation. No note is made of systemic disease either at the time of diagnosis or during the 18 months of follow-up, though the only therapy was local irradiation. In sum, the evidence provided that this patient with actinic reticuloid actually developed lymphoma is unconvincing.

Lymphomatoid papulosis

Lymphomatoid papulosis denotes an eruption of papules and small nodules, primarily on the trunk and extremities, which reveal histologically highly atypical mononuclear cells. The lesions begin as erythematous macules. Many progress to papules with central purpura. Some develop a fine scale, others a small crust. Still others become necrotic, ulcerate, and heal with scars. The lesions may be few or numerous. They typically recur in crops, heal spontaneously, and are not significantly symptomatic. The eruption is

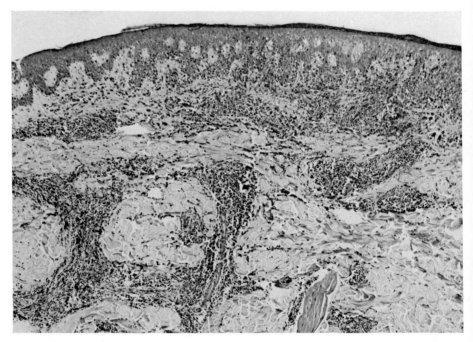

Figure 8.9 This section from a lesion of lymphomatoid papulosis shows a dense superficial and deep perivascular infiltrate of mononuclear cells, many of which, even at this relatively low power, are clearly atypical. The mononuclear cells obscure the dermoepidermal interface and are present within the epidermis. × 63

frequently protracted, lasting many years, but there is no detectable systemic involvement. Young adults seem somewhat preferentially afflicted, but patients 8 and 68 years of age have been reported (Dupont, 1965; Verallo and Haserick, 1966; Macaulay, 1968; Black and Wilson-Jones, 1972; Valentino and Helwig, 1973).

Lymphomatoid papulosis cannot be differentiated clinically from Mucha–Habermann's disease. Its distinctive feature is cytological atypicality.

The microscopic changes in lymphomatoid papulosis are usually well demarcated, reflecting the circumscription of the clinical lesions. Typically, a mononuclear cell infiltrate surrounds blood vessels at all levels of the dermis, fills the papillary dermis, obscures the dermoepidermal junction and extends into the epidermis (Figs. 8.9, 8.10). Extravasated red blood cells, intra- and subepidermal oedema, and epidermal necrosis are common. Macular and early papular lesions may show only a superficial band-like infiltrate of mononuclear cells with little or no epidermal involvement, whereas necrotic and ulcerated lesions often display a dense infiltrate that extends to the depths of the dermis.

The percentage of cells within this infiltrate which have atypical morphological features often varies from lesion to lesion. They are usually prominent

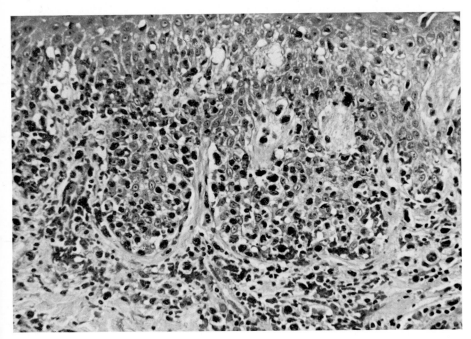

Figure 8.10 Markedly atypical mononuclear cells are scattered throughout the epidermis in this more detailed view of Figure 8.9. × 276

in the oedematous, crusted, or ulcerated papules, but less numerous in slightly scaly papules and resolving lesions. The atypical cells are considerably larger than their normal cohorts. Their nuclei are voluminous, distinctly hyperchromatic and bizarrely shaped. Mitotic figures, some abnormal in configuration, and giant cells with multiple nuclei may occur.

Though inflammatory cells are often seen traversing vessel walls, necrotic vascular changes are restricted almost exclusively to immediately beneath ulcerations and are presumably a secondary phenomenon. Primary necrotising vasculitis is rare.

To summarise, the histological attributes of lymphomatoid papulosis, except for the cytological abnormalities, are, like the clinical features, basically identical to those of Mucha–Habermann's disease. The available clinical and microscopic evidence favours the essential unity of these two processes. Unfortunately, this does not elucidate the histogenesis of lymphomatoid papulosis, for the origins of Mucha–Habermann's disease are wholly unclear. Equally obscure is the meaning of the atypical cells in lymphomatoid papulosis.

The differentiation of lymphomatoid papulosis from a malignant haematological process involves both microscopic and clinical considerations. Leukaemias and systemic lymphomas do not produce lichenoid dermal infiltrates, as found in lymphomatoid papulosis, and the patients generally have detectable internal disease at the time of cutaneous involvement. Mycosis fungoides often exhibits microscopically a polymorphous cellular infiltrate and, more significantly, it dies not present the clinical picture of lymphomatoid papulosis.

Confidence in these guidelines, nevertheless, must necessarily be tempered by the reports of two patients with seeming lymphomatoid papulosis who proceeded to develop systemic lymphoma. At the time the lymphoma become evident, each patient had had a chronic eruption, one for seven years (Kawada et al, 1969), the other for 16 years (Borrie, 1969; Black and Wilson-Jones, 1972), which clinically and histologically was wholly consonant with lymphomatoid papulosis. The development of strikingly large, nodular and ulcerated skin lesions, as well as lymphadenopathy, heralded the lymphomatous disease. Both patients rapidly succumbed. One was autopsied, and there was widespread lymphoma.

These two reports certainly cloud an already murky matter. Lymphomatoid papulosis has only recently been described. Its cause is not even remotely comprehended. Empirically, it has been found that, in spite of the disturbing histologic picture, the vast percentage of lymphomatoid papulosis patients do not develop lymphoma. Still, in light of the above two cases, these patients must be regularly re-evaluated, and significant change in the character of their skin lesions or in their general well-being or the development of lymphadenopathy requires immediate investigation.

Vascular

Angiolymphoid hyperplasia with eosinophils

Angiolymphoid hyperplasia with eosinophils presents clinically as papules or nodules which range in diameter from 0.2 to 10.0 cm; these occur predominantly about the head and neck, especially on or around the ears; and number from one to thirty lesions. They are somewhat more common in females and develop most often during the third to the fifth decades of life, though they have been reported in individuals as young as 14 and as old as 84. Primarily dermal lesions are often overtly vascular, bleed with mild trauma, and may be pruritic. Subcutaneous nodules are simply firm, asymptomatic swellings. Both types of lesions may be present in the same patient (Summerly, 1963; Peterson, Fusaro and Goltz, 1964; Fattah and Fahmy, 1968; Wells and

Whimster, 1969; Wilson-Jones and Bleehen, 1969; Wilson-Jones and Marks, 1970; Mehregan and Shapiro, 1971; Reed and Terazakis, 1972).

Angiolymphoid hyperplasia with eosinophils may resolve spontaneously after many months, but more often persists for years. Excision is curative, but recurrence following partial removal or destruction is common. A peripheral blood eosinophilia occasionally occurs, but there are no other known systemic manifestations, and prolonged follow-up has proven these curious growths to be benign.

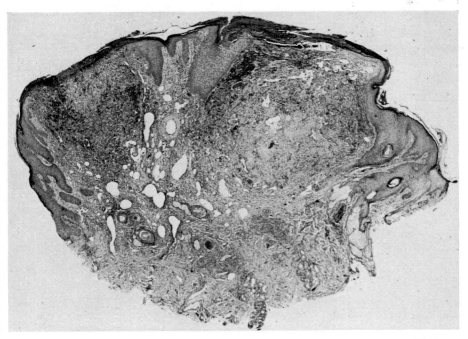

Figure 8.11 This traumatised nodule of angiolymphoid hyperplasia with eosinophils has within the dermis numerous irregularly shaped vascular channels and a variably dense inflammatory cell infiltrate. There is overlying crust and ulceration. × 20

The dominant histological alteration in angiolymphoid hyperplasia with eosinophils is a fairly circumscribed mixture of vascular channels and inflammatory cells (Fig. 8.11). These may localise exclusively within the dermis or within the subcutis or may involve both. Rarely, there is extension into underlying fascia and muscle. Serial sections through the same lesion frequently reveal remarkable variation in the relative amounts of vascular vis-à-vis inflammatory-cell components.

The vascular element comprises both thick-walled vessels and lumina lined only by endothelial cells. These endothelial cells often are strikingly large, project prominently into the vascular channels, and demonstrate distinctive cytoplasmic vacuoles (Fig. 8.12). Collections of endothelial cells without vessel formation are also common. The lumina of many of the variously sized and shaped vascular channels are clear. Some contain lightly eosinophilic, homogeneous material, resembling lymph. Others contain erythrocytes.

Interspersed among these vascular proliferations are variably dense infiltrations of lymphocytes, histiocytes, eosinophils and mast cells. Lymphoid

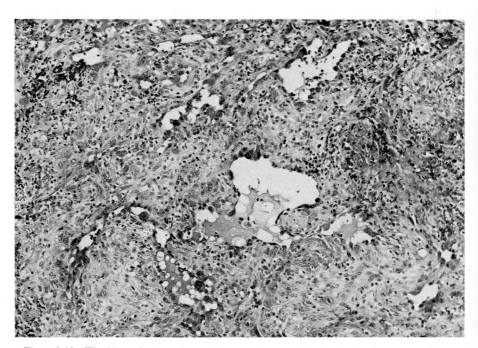

Figure 8.12 The bizarrely shaped vessels in angiolymphoid hyperplasia with eosinophils are often lined, as shown here, by large plemorphic cells which project into the lumina and many of which display prominent intracytoplasmic vacuoles. The stroma contains plump fibroblasts and a polymorphous inflammatory cell infiltrate in which eosinophils are plentiful. ×138

follicles may occur, especially within the subcutis. Eosinophils are usually numerous.

The stromal setting for these changes often contains mucin deposits and prominent fibroblasts. Extravasated erythrocytes and haemosiderin are evident.

The pronounced hyperplasia of endothelial cells and vascular spaces may simulate angiosarcoma. Cutaneous angiosarcoma usually occurs in the scalp of an elderly individual and displays histologically anastomosing vascular channels lined by markedly atypical endothelial cells, some in mitosis (Wilson-Jones, 1964; Reed et al, 1966). These cells are often heaped in several layers, narrowing or obliterating the lumina. They may also form confluent cellular masses. Angiolymphoid hyperplasia with eosinophils is less diffuse in its architectural pattern than angiosarcoma, does not exhibit comparable cytological atypicality, and possesses a prominent inflammatory cell component, absent from angiosarcoma. Nevertheless, a small or fragmented biopsy specimen may not allow conclusive differentiation.

The histogenesis of angiolymphoid hyperplasis with eosinophils is uncertain. It is not clear whether it is reactive or neoplastic. This uncertainty, as well as the varying clinical presentations depending on the intracutaneous locus predominantly involved, have resulted in a plethora of designations. The basic histological similarity, however, whether the process be primarily dermal or subcutaneous in localisation, argues convincingly for nosological unity.

Finally, the relationship between angiolymphoid hyperplasia with eosinophils and 'Kimura's disease' is unsettled. The latter condition is reported from Japan and China as cutaneous nodules or patches developing predominately in young men; demonstrating lymphocytic and eosinophilic infiltrations, but with limited vascular proliferation; and consistently associated with significant peripheral blood eosinophilia (Chang and Chen, 1962; Fujita, 1963; Kawada, Takahashi and Anzai, 1965). Radiotherapy or systemic corticosteroids are required to resolve the lesions. Whether 'Kimura's disease' is a variant of angiolymphoid hyperplasia with esoinophils or a different disease has not been determined.

Conclusion

These closing comments concern the clinical approach to all the cutaneous pseudomalignancies, both those just discussed and those long recognised.

High-quality biopsy material is essential. The differentiation of the pseudomalignant from the truly malignant is too challenging and too critical to be made on the basis of poor biopsy material. The clinician must remove adequate and representative tissue without traumatising it. The pathologist must insist that excellent sections are prepared.

The clinician must know the microscopical features, and the microscopist must know the clinical manifestations. Most cutaneous pseudocancers have rather typical clinical presentations. Thus, the dermatologist often should consider the relevant pseudomalignancy in his clinical differential diagnosis and so alert the pathologist. In addition, whenever the dermatologist receives a seemingly inappropriate diagnosis of malignancy from the pathologist, the possibility of a pseudomalignancy should be considered, and the case thoroughly reviewed with the pathologist. The pathologist, at the same time, must be knowledgeable in cutaneous gross pathology, i.e. clinical dermatology. Competence in dermatopathology cannot be achieved without such knowledge. Accordingly, the pathologist should require the submitting dermatologist to describe on the biopsy form the in vivo lesion, recording both its history and its physical attributes. Prepared in this fashion, the histologist should be able to recognise the cutaneous pseudomalignancies and so avoid incorrect diagnoses of malignancy.

Clinical follow-up is imperative. The dermatologist, on receipt of a pseudo-malignant diagnosis, should appropriately re-examine and follow the patient. Only in this way can the veracity of the pseudomalignant designation be determined.

Finally, if there is doubt about the diagnosis and more tissue remains, a further biopsy should be made. No organ is as easily sampled as the skin. The cutaneous clinician and pathologist should always obtain more tissue, if possible, when confronted with difficult and significant diagnostic problems. Diagnosis of a cutaneous pseudomalignancy is often difficult and always significant, so there should be no hesitation to do additional biopsies.

EXPERIMENTAL STUDIES RELATED TO EPIDERMAL TUMOUR FORMATION: ULTRAVIOLET TUMOUR FORMATION

John H. Epstein

The skin, expecially that of rodents, has been used as one of the primary sites for evaluation of carcinogenic stimuli. As a result there is a vast catalogue of agents ranging from aromatic hydrocarbons to viruses and rare earths which have proven to be tumourogenic in this organ. However, as yet only a very few of these have been found related to human skin neoplasms. Of such stimuli, light energy is by far the most important and most extensively studied (Blum, 1959; Epstein, 1970).

The role of sunlight in the development of the common human skin cancers, that is the basal cell epithelioma and squamous cell carcinoma, and even the much less common malignant melanoma, have been supported by astute observations and epidemiological studies. However, investigations confirming this association, as well as the determination of the action spectrum and the required energy levels, have been confined to animal experimentation for both practical and ethical reasons. Practically, it would take too long to make cancers in humans and ethically it would be improper.

Action spectrum studies. Determination of the offending wavelengths or action spectrum for the formation of cutaneous cancers has presented a most difficult task primarily due to problems in methodology. A number of studies using various light sources and filters determined that ultraviolet (u.v.) rays shorter than 320 nm will produce cancers in a variety of experimental animals. Rays between 280 and 320 nm (u.v. B) were more efficient than shorter ultraviolet (u.v.) wavelengths (u.v. C) (reviewed in Blum, 1959; Epstein, 1970). Freeman, Hudson and Carnes (1970) confirmed these findings with a monochromatic source. Thus the spectrum responsible for the usual photo-toxic erythema reaction also appears to contain the primary carcinogenic spectrum. It should be noted that the longer u.v. rays between 320 and 400 nm (u.v. A) will produce phototoxic reactions and cutaneous cancers in the presence of appropriate exogenous photosensitisers (Griffin, Nakim and Knox, 1958; Urbach, 1959).

Recently Forbes (1973) reported that a light source containing large amounts of u.v. A as well as u.v. B produced more cancers than that containing u.v. B with less u.v. A. Though the amount and duration of delivery of this energy were extremely large the study does suggest that these long rays may participate in sunlight induced cutaneous carcinogenesis. This concept gains more importance in view of recent studies demonstrating that u.v. A markedly augments the acute phototoxicity induced by u.v. B (Willis, Kligman and Epstein, 1972). Thus both u.v. B and u.v. A may be important to the development of human skin cancers.

Development of u.v.-induced Cancers

Quantitative investigations. Obtaining quantitative data relating to cutaneous cancer formation was almost as difficult as determining the carcinogenic action spectrum because of the remarkable number of variables involved. Nevertheless the monumental work of Blum and his co-workers has supplied extensive experimental information concerning time and u.v. dose relationships. These investigators demonstrated that u.v. carcinogenesis followed the law of reciprocity (reviewed in Blum, 1959). Increasing the dose or shortening the intervals between exposures accelerated tumour formation but did not alter the shape of the incidence curve. Further Blum (1950) and Rusch, Kline and Baumann (1941) demonstrated that skin cancers will develop if enough energy is delivered for a sufficient period of time. However, tumours would not appear no matter what energy was used if it was not applied over an adequate number of days. From the accumulated data, Blum (1959) surmised that u.v.-induced cancer formation is a continuous process beginning with the initial exposure, and that appearance of tumours within the lifetime of the experimental animal depended upon sufficient acceleration of the growth process. In support of this concept, Epstein and Roth (1968), and subsequently Pound (1970), reported the production of squamous cell carcinomas in mouse skin with 1 u.v. exposure when croten oil promotion was utilised. Recently Harber et al (quoted in Urbach, Epstein and Forbes, 1974, p. 262) produced cutaneous tumours with 1 u.v. exposure alone. However, the growths were primarily papillomas which appeared on the edge of u.v.-induced ulcers and may have represented non-specific epidermal hyperplasia secondary to severe skin damage and may have no bearing on human skin carcinogenesis.

Qualitative investigations. Many of the studies relating to findings associated with the presence of skin cancers were accomplished with human tissue. Unfortunately these studies could supply only a static view of the problem.

Evaluation of changes occurring during u.v.-induced tumour development required an experimental model for the production of epidermal cancers which are the primary growths produced in human skin by the sun's energy.

For many years the ears of albino mice and rats were the primary sites for study of experimental u.v.-induced tumours because these areas lacked the inhibitory effects of hair, pigment and a thick stratum corneum. The basic tumour produced was a sarcoma which was quite adequate for quantitative studies. Recently the hairless mouse was found to provide an excellent model for evaluation of qualitative as well as quantitative development patterns of epidermal cancer formation, since squamous cell carcinomas can be produced in these animals almost to the exclusion of sarcomas. In addition these animals proved useful in studying the effect of u.v. on melanoma formation.

UV-induced squamous cell carcinomas

Evaluation of the progressive development of frank invasive squamous cell carcinomas from u.v.-induced benign hyperplasia and actinic keratosis stages was accomplished in the hairless mouse model (Epstein, Fukuyama and Dobson, 1969). Histochemical techniques demonstrated a number of striking anatomical changes in both the dermis and epidermis. These included an accumulation of acid mucopolysaccharides and a loss of insoluble collagen in the upper dermis and proliferation of fibrocytes and mast cells associated with progressive epidermal hyperplasia and eventual dysplasia. One of the most notable changes occurred in the epidermal–dermal basement membrane (BM). A periodic acid Schiff (PAS) stain revealed a progressive thickening of the structure with the development of epidermal hyperplasia. As anaplasia and abnormal epidermal cell proliferation occurred the BM became thicker, irregular, clumped and frayed in appearance and with frank invasive malignancy it disappeared altogether. Interestingly immunochemical studies done with pemphigoid serum BM antibodies (Jecot, Cram and Epstein, 1973) demonstrated a relatively normal regular BM structure throughout the hyperplasia and premalignancy phases, despite anaplasia, indicating that the PAS staining BM differed antigenetically from the immunochemically demonstrated material. Both BM structures disappeared at the point of invasion. Similar breaks in the BM have been noted with the invasion of human skin cancers (Cawley, Hsu and Weary, 1966) and chemically induced experimental tumours (Dobson, 1963). Electron microscopic studies have suggested that microprojection of cells through the basal lamina may represent the earliest stage of tumour invasion (Ashworth, Stembridge and Luibel, 1961).

Epidermal cell kinetics associated with the development of malignancy were accomplished with radioactive tracer techniques (Epstein et al, 1969). These studies revealed a progressive increase in the number of germinative basal cells synthesising DNA and dividing with a reduction of the G2 and DNA synthesis periods associated with the epidermal changes. In addition a progressive reduction of the cell transit time through the epidermis despite its increasing thickness was noted. With frank cancer formation the germinative cell layer disappeared and many abnormal as well as normal appearing mitoses were present throughout the tumour mass. Thus the process of carcinogenesis was characterised by acceleration, cell formation, maturation and turnover. Further, the epidermal germinative basal cell appeared to be the primary or initial site of abnormal proliferation.

Malignant melanoma

The role of sunlight in melanoma formation has not been conclusively demonstrated. Epidemiological studies have suggested that these tumours in certain anatomical locations may be induced or aggravated by this radiation. However, a number of factors continue to cloud the picture. Recent data indicate that u.v. energy is capable of producing malignant melanocytic growths in experimental animals.

The induction of benign non-invasive melanocytic tumours has been accomplished primarily in hamsters and pigmented mice with topical polycyclic hydrocarbon carcinogens. Ghadially, Illman and Barker (1960) were unable to produce malignant transformation of these lesions with a variety of traumatic procedures. More recently this transformation was induced in hairless mice with u.v. energy shorter than 320 nm (Epstein et al, 1967). Repeated irradiation of the benign tumours over a period of several months resulted in the production of invasive melanocytic tumours with light and electron microscopic characteristics of malignancy, many of which metastasised to the regional lymphnodes. These results indicate that malignant melanoma formation can be induced by u.v. energy. Whether a similar process occurs in human skin remains to be determined.

Immune Responses

Within the past two to three decades the importance of immunological control of cancerous growth has received a great deal of attention. As with other neoplasms tumour-specific antigens have been demonstrated in chemically induced cutaneous epitheliomas (Tuffrey and Batchelor, 1964). Also a loss of tissue-specificity has been demonstrated in experimentally induced animal skin cancers (Carruthers and Baumler, 1965) as well as in human cutaneous neoplasms (Nairn et al, 1960). More recently De Moragas, Winkelmann and Jordan (1970) using pemphigus sera containing intercellular antibodies and BM antibodies present in pemphigoid sera noted that both intercellular and BM antigenic material varied inversely with the degree of epidermal cell anaplasia in human squamous cell carcinomas. In experimental animals it has been possible to examine these antigenic materials as they relate to the transformation from a benign to a malignant state. In u.v. and chemically induced cutaneous carcinogenic responses the intercellular antigenic material disappeared when the epidermal cells reached the premalignant phase (Muller and Sutherland, 1971). The BM antigenic response was diminished or lost when invasion occurred (Muller and Sutherland, 1971; Jecot et al, 1973). These results support the concept that antigenic deletion may play an important role in the transformation and invasion of malignant cells.

Studies on the importance of immunologic surveillance in the control of cutaneous epidermal cancers have been sparse to date. However, Nathanson, Forbes and Urbach (1973) demonstrated that injections of mouse anti-lymphocyte serum accelerated the appearance and incidence of u.v.-induced tumours in hairless mice. Thus cell mediated immune control may well be important to the inhibition of cutaneous cancer formation.

Xeroderma Pigmentosum (XP) and u.v. Carcinogenesis

Perhaps one of the most intriguing aspects of u.v. carcinogenesis concerns the relationship between acute phototoxic effects and eventual cancer formation. As noted, light-induced carcinogenesis occurs only in systems in which acute phototoxic effects can be demonstrated. In addition, cancer formation begins with the initial radiation exposure. The immediate or early changes which lead to cancerisation remain undetermined. However, the most intriguing findings to date relating acute photoinjury to cutaneous carcinogenesis have developed from the study of DNA repair systems and the genetic disease xeroderma pigmentosum (XP). XP is a rare genodermatosis in which the basic problem appears to be an extreme sensitivity to the carcinogenic effects of the sun's rays. In 1968 Cleaver described an apparent defect in the enzymatic excision of u.v.-induced thymine dimers in the DNA of cultured fibroblasts from patients with XP. Subsequent studies confirmed these tissue culture findings (Setlow et al, 1969; Cleaver, 1971). Further the defect was demonstrated to be present in the epidermal cells (Epstein et al, 1970; Jung, 1970) and circulating lymphocytes of patients with this disease (Burk, Lutzner and Robbins, 1969).

More recently complementation studies have demonstrated five genetic types of XP with distinct excision repair defects (Robbins et al, 1974; Cleaver and Bootsma, 1975). In addition Lehman et al (1975) described a defect in postreplication DNA repair in three cell lines from patients with clinical evidence of XP but no deficiency in the excision repair system. Since an inability to repair u.v.-damaged DNA would be expected to result in an increased somatic mutation rate, a relationship between these defects and cutaneous carcinogenesis presents an attractive hypothesis. However, a definitive correlation of these acute responses with eventual cancer formation has not been established. Further even if these defects are responsible for the skin cancer susceptibility of XP patients, they would not relate to skin cancers in the general public unless they could be acquired, perhaps through repeated photoinjury.

REFERENCES

MALIGNANT MELANOMA

Anderson, D. E. (1971) Clinical characteristics of the genetic variety of cutaneous melanoma in man *Cancer*, **28**, 721–725.

Beardmore, G. L. & Davis, N. C. (1975) Multiple primary cutaneous melanomas. *Archives of Dermatology*, **111**, 603–609.

Breslow, A. (1970) Thickness, cross-sectional areas and depth of invasion in the prognosis of cutaneous melanoma. *Annals of Surgery*, **172**, 902–908.

Breslow, A. (1972) Tumor thickness, level of invasion and node dissection in stage I cutaneous melanoma. *Annals of Surgery*, **182**, 572–575.

Clark, W. H. Jr, From, L., Bernadino, E. A. & Mihm, M. C. (1969) The histogenesis and biologic behaviour of primary human malignant melanomas of the skin. *Cancer Research*, **29**, 705–727.

Clark, W. H., Jr & Mihm, M. C. (1969) Lentigo maligna and lentigo-maligna melanoma. *American Journal of Pathology*, **55**, 39.

Esptein, W. L., Sagebiel, R. W., Spitler, L., Wybran, J., Reed, W. B. & Blois, M. S. (1973) Halo nevi and melanoma. *Journal of the American Medical Association*, **225**, 373–377.

Fleming, I. D., Barnawell, J. R., Burlison, P. E. & Rankin, J. S. (1975) Skin cancer in black patients. *Cancer*, **35**, 600–605.

Kopf, A. W., Minitzis, M. & Bart, R. (1975) Diagnostic accuracy—malignant melanoma. *Archives of Dermatology*, **111**, 1291–1292.

Little, J. H. (1972) Histology and prognosis in cutaneous malignant melanoma. In *Melanoma and Skin Cancer*, ed. McCarthy, W. H., pp. 107–119. Sydney, Australia: VCN Blight, Government Printer.

Litwin, M. S., Krementz, E. T., Mansell, P. W. & Reed, R. J. (1975) Topical chemotherapy of lentigo maligna with 5-fluorouracil. *Cancer*, **35**, 721–733.

McGovern, V. J., Mihm, M. C., Jr., Bailly, C., Booth, J. C., Clark, W. H., Cochran, A. J., Hardy, E. G., Hicks, J. D., Levene, A., Lewis, M. G., Little, J. H. & Milton, G. W. (1973) The classification of malignant melanoma and its histologic reporting. *Cancer*, **32**, 1446–1457.

Mihm, M. C., Jr, Fitzpatrick, T. B., Lane Brown, M. M., Raker, J. W., Malt, R. A. & Kaiser, J. S. (1973) Early detection of primary cutaneous malignant melanoma. *New England Journal of Medicine*, **289**, 989–996.

Wanebo, H. J., Woodruff, J. & Fortner, J. G. (1975) Malignant melanoma of the extremities: a clinicopathologic study using levels of invasion (microstage). *Cancer*, **35**, 666–676.

PSEUDOMALIGNANCIES

Bishop, E. L. (1931) Epidermoid carcinoma in sebaceous systs. *Annals of Surgery*, **93**, 109–112.

Black, M. M. & Wilson-Jones, E. (1972) 'Lymphomatoid' pityriasis lichenoides: a variant with histologic features simulating a lymphoma. *British Journal of Dermatology*, **86**, 329–347.

Borrie, P. F. (1969) Lymphomatoid papulosis. *Proceedings of the Royal Society of Medicine*, **62**, 159–161.

Bourne, R. G. (1963) Paradoxical fibrosarcoma of skin (pseudosarcoma). A review of 13 cases. *The Medical Journal of Australia*, **1**, 504–510.

Chang, T. & Chen, C. (1962) Eosinophilic granuloma of lymph nodes and soft tissue. *Chinese Medical Journal*, **81**, 384–387.

Christophers, E. & Spelberg, H. (1973) Proliferating trichilemmal cysts. *Hautarzt*, **24**, 377–380.

Cox, A. J. & Walton, R. G. (1965) The induction of junctional changes in pigmented nevi. *Archives of Pathology*, **79**, 428–434.

Dabska, M. (1971) Giant hair matrix tumour. *Cancer*, **28**, 701–706.

Dupont, A. (1965) Slowly progressive and clinically benign reticulopathy with histologic structure of highest grade malignancy. *Hautarzt*, **16**, 284–286.

Fattah, A. A. & Fahmy, A. (1968) Subcutaneous lymphoid hyperplasia wth eosinophils. *Dermatologica*, **137**, 220–224.

Fretzin, D. F. & Helwig, E. B. (1973) Atypical fibroxanthoma of the skin. A clinicopathologic study of 140 cases. *Cancer*, **31**, 1541–1552.

Fujita, K. (1963) A syndrome composed of soft tissue tumours, lymphadenopathy, and eosinophilia. *Japanese Journal of Dermatology*, **73**, 367.

Grigg, J. W., Rachmaninoff, N. & Robb, J. M. (1961) Pseudosarcoma associated with squamous cell carinoma of the larynx: report of a case. *Laryngoscope*, **71**, 555–561.

Halpert, B. & Hackney, V. C. (1949) Fibrosarcoma of the helix of the ear. *Archives of Pathology*, **48**, 218–220.

Helwig, E. B. (1963) Atypical fibroxanthoma. *Texas State Journal of Medicine*, **59**, 664–667.

Hudson, A. W. & Winkelmann, R. K. (1972) Atypical fibroxanthoma of the skin: a reappraisal of 19 cases in which the original diagnosis was spindle-cell squamous carcinoma. *Cancer*, **29**, 413–422.

Hutter, R. V. P., Stewart, F. W. & Foote, F. W. (1962) Fasciitis: a report of 70 cases with follow-up proving the benignity of the lesion. *Cancer*, **15**, 992–995.

Ive, F. A., Magnus, I. A., Warin, R. P. & Wilson-Jones, E. (1969) 'Actinic reticuloid': a chronic dermatosis associated with severe photosensitivity and the histological resemblance to lymphoma. *British Journal of Dermatology*, **81**, 469–485.

Jacobs, D. S., Edwards, W. D. & Ye, R. C. (1975) Metastatic atypical fibroxanthoma of skin. *Cancer*, **35**, 457–463.

Jensen, N. E. & Sneddon, I. B. (1970) Actinic reticuloid with lymphoma. *British Journal of Dermatology*, **82**, 287–291.

Kawada, A. K., Takahashi, H. & Anzai, T. (1965) Eosinophilic folliculosis of the skin (Kimura's disease). *Japanese Journal of Dermatology*, **76**, 61–72.

Kawada, A. K., Anekoji, K., Miyamoto, M. & Nakai, T. (1969) Unusual manifestations of malignant reticulosis of the skin: cutaneous lesions simulating parapsoriasis guttata. *Dermatologica*, **138**, 369–378.

Kempson, R. L. & McGavran, M. H. (1964) Atypical fibroxanthomas of the skin. *Cancer*, **17**, 1463–1471.

Konwaler, B. E., Keasbey, L. & Kaplan, L. (1955) Subcutaneous pseudosarcomatous fibromatosis (fasciitis). *American Journal of Clinical Pathology*, **25**, 241–252.

Kornberg, R. & Ackerman, A. B. (1975) Pseudomelanoma: recurrent melanocytic nevus following partial surgical removal. *Archives of Dermatology*, **111**, 1588–1590.

Kroe, D. J. & Pitcock, J. A. (1969) Atypical fibroxanthoma of the skin: report of ten cases. *American Journal of Clinical Pathology*, **51**, 487–492.

Lane, N. (1957) Pseudosarcoma (polypoid sarcoma-like masses) associated with squamous-cell carcinoma of the mouth, fauces, and larynx. Report of ten cases. *Cancer*, **10**, 19–41.

Lewis, B. L. (1971) Junctional activity recurring over an incompletely removed balloon cell naevus. *Archives of Dermatology*, **104**, 513–514.

Lund, H. Z. (1957) In *Tumors of the Skin, Armed Forces Institute of Pathology Atlas of Tumor Pathology*, Section 1, Fascicle 2, p. 246. Washington, DC.

Macaulay, W. L. (1968) Lymphomatoid papulosis. *Archives of Dermatology*, **97**, 23–30.

Mehregan, A. H. & Pinkus, H. (1964) Intraepidermal epithelioma: a critical study. *Cancer*, **17**, 609–636.

Mehregan, A. H. & Shapiro, L. (1971) Angiolymphoid hyperplasia with eosinophils. *Archives of Dermatology*, **103**, 50–57.

Menter, M. A., McKerron, R. A. & Amos, H. E. (1974) Actinic reticuloid: an immunological investigation providing evidence of basement membrane damage. *British Journal of Dermatology*, **90**, 507–515.

Peden, J. C. (1948) Carcinoma developing in sebaceous cysts. *Annals of Surgery*, **128**, 1136–1147.

Peterson, W. C., Fusaro, R. M. & Goltz, R. W. (1964) Atypical pyogenic granuloma. *Archives of Dermatology*, **90**, 197–201.

Pinkus, H. (1969) 'Sebaceous cysts' are trichilemmal cysts. *Archives of Dermatology*, **99**, 544–555.

Rachmaninoff, N., McDonald, J. R. & Cook, J. C. (1961) Sarcoma-like tumors of the skin following irradiation. *American Journal of Clinical Pathology*, **36**, 427–437.

Reed, R. J. & Lamar, L. M. (1966) Invasive hair matrix tumors of the scalp. *Archives of Dermatology*, **94**, 310–316.

Reed, R. J., Palomeque, F. E., Hairston, M. A. & Krementz, E. T. (1966) Lymphangio-sarcomas of the scalp. *Archives of Dermatology*, **94**, 396–402.

Reed, R. J. (1967) Atypical fibroxanthomas and spindle cell carcinomas of the skin. *Bulletin of the Tulane Medical Faculty*, **26**, 75–89.

Reed, R. J. & Terazakis, N. (1972) Subcutaneous angioblastic lymphoid hyperplasia with eosinophilia (Kimura's disease). *Cancer*, **29**, 489–497.

Schoenfeld, R. J. & Pinkus, H. (1958) The recurrence of nevi after incomplete removal. *Archives of Dermatology*, **78**, 30–35.

Sims, C. F. & Kirsch, N. (1948) Spindle cell epidermoid epithelioma simulating sarcoma in chronic radiodermatitis. *Archives of Dermatology and Syphilology*, **57**, 63–68.

Spitz, S. (1948) Melanomas of childhood. *American Journal of Pathology*, **24**, 591–609.

Summerly, R. (1963) Subcutaneous lymphoid hyperplasia with eosinophils. *Proceedings of the Royal Society of Medicine*, **56**, 728–729.

Underwood, L. J., Montgomery, H. & Broders, A. C. (1951) Squamous-cell epithelioma that simulates sarcoma. *Archives of Dermatology and Syphilology*, **64**, 149–158.

Valentino, L. A. & Helwig, E. B. (1973) Lymphomatoid papulosis. *Archives of Pathology*, **96**, 409–416.

Verallo, V. M. & Haserick, J. R. (1966) Mucha–Habermann's disease simulating lymphoma cutis. *Archives of Dermatology*, **94**, 295–299.

Welch, J. W. (1958) Carcinoma arising in sebaceous cysts. *Archives of Surgery*, **76**, 128–132.

Wells, G. C. & Whimster, I. W. (1969) Subcutaneous angiolymphoid hyperplasia with eosinophils. *British Journal of Dermatology*, **81**, 1–15.

Wilson-Jones, E. (1964) Maglignant angio-endothelioma in the skin. *British Journal of Dermatology*, **76**, 21–39.

Wilson-Jones, E. (1966) Proliferating epidermoid cysts. *Archives of Dermatology*, **94**, 11–19.

Wilson-Jones, E. & Bleehen, S. S. (1969) Inflammatory angiomatous nodules with abnormal blood bessels occurring about the ears and scalp (pseudo or atypical pyogenic granuloma). *British Journal of Dermatology*, **81**, 804–816.

Wilson-Jones, E. & Marks, R. (1970) Papular angioplasia: vascular papules of the face and scalp simulating malignant vascular tumors. *Archives of Dermatology*, **102**, 422–427.

EXPERIMENTAL STUDIES

Ashworth, C. T., Stembridge, V. A. & Luibel, F. J. (1961) A study of basement membranes of normal epithelium, carcinoma in situ and invasive carcinoma of uterine cervix using miroscopic and histochemical methods. *Acta cytologica*, **5**, 369–378.

Blum, H. F. (1950) On the mechanism of cancer induction by ultraviolet radiation. *Journal of the National Cancer Institute*, **11**, 463–495.

Blum, H. F. (1959) *Carcinogenesis by Ultraviolet Light*. New Jersey: Princeton University Press.

Burk, P. G., Lutzner, M. A. & Robbins, J. H. (1971) Ultraviolet-stimulated thymidine incorporation in xeroderma pigmentosum lymphocytes. *Journal of Laboratory and Clinical Medicine*, **77**, 759–767.

Carruthers, C. & Baumler, A. (1965) Immunochemical staining with fluorescein labelled antibodies as an aid to study skin cancer formation. *Journal of the National Cancer Institute*, **34**, 191–200.

Cawley, E. P., Hsu, Y. T. & Weary, P. E. (1966) The basement membrane in relation to carcinoma of the skin. *Archives of Dermatology*, **94**, 712–715.

Cleaver, J. E. (1968) Defective repair replication of DNA in xeroderma pigmentosum. *Nature*, **218**, 652–656.

Cleaver, J. E. (1971) Repair of damaged DNA in human and other eukaryotic cells. In *Nucleic Acid–Protein Interactions—Nucleic Acid Synthesis in Viral Infection*, ed. Ribbons, D. W., Woesner, J. F. & Schultz, J., pp. 87–112. Amsterdam: North-Holland.

Cleaver, J. E. & Bootsma, D. (1975) Xeroderma pigmentosum, biochemical and genetic characteristics. *Annual Review of Genetics*, **9** (in press).

De Moragas, J. M., Winkelmann, R. K. & Jordan, R. E. (1970) Immunofluorescence of epithelial skin tumours. Parts I and II. *Cancer*, **25**, 1399–1407.

Dobson, R. L. (1963) Anthramine carcinogenesis in the skin of rats. *Journal of the National Cancer Institute*, **31**, 841–859.

Epstein, J. H. (1970) Ultraviolet carcinogenesis. In *Photophysiology*, ed. Giese, A. C., Vol. V, pp. 235–273. New York: Academic Press.

Epstein, J. H. & Roth, H. L. (1968) Experimental ultraviolet light carcinogenesis. *Journal of Investigative Dermatology*, **50**, 387.

Epstein, J. H., Epstein, W. L. & Nakai, T. (1967) Production of melanomas from DMBA induced blue naevi in hairless mice with ultraviolet light. *Journal of the National Cancer Institute*, **38**, 19.

Epstein, J. H., Fukuyama, K. & Dobson, R. L. (1969) Ultraviolet light carcinogenesis. In *The Biologic Effects of Ultraviolet Radiation*, pp. 551–568. New York: Pergamon Press.

Epstein, J. H., Fukuyama, K., Reed, W. B. & Epstein, W. L. (1970) Defect in DNA synthesis in skin of patients with xeroderma pigmentosum demonstrated in vivo. *Science*, **168**, 1477–1478.

Forbes, P. D. (1973) Influence of long wave u.v. on photocarcinogenesis. In *Book of Abstracts* for the American Society for Photobiology. First Annual Meeting, 10–14 June, Sarasota, FL, p. 136.

Freeman, R. G., Hudson, H. T. & Carnes, R. (1970) Ultraviolet wavelength factors in solar radiation and skin cancer. *International Journal of Dermatology*, **9**, 232–235.

Ghadially, R. N., Illman, O. & Barker, J. F. (1960) The effect of trauma on the melanocytic tumours of the hamster. *British Journal of Cancer*, **14**, 647–650.

Griffin, A. C., Hakim, R. E. & Knox, J. (1958) The wavelength effect upon erythemal and carcinogenic response in psoralen treated mice. *Journal of Investigative Dermatology*, **31**, 289–295.

Jecot, K., Cram, D. L. & Epstein, J. H. (1973) Immunologic basement membrane changes and ultraviolet induced skin cancer. *Clinical Research*, **21**, 246.

Jung, E. G. (1970) Investigations on dark repair in various light-sensitive inherited disorders. *Humangenetik*, **9**, 191–192.

Lehman, A. R., Kirk-Bell, S., Arlett, C. F., Paterson, M. C., Lohman, P. H. M., de Weerd-Kastelein, E. A. & Bootsma, D. (1975) Xeroderma pigmentosum cells with normal levels of excision repair have a defect in DNA synthesis after ultraviolet irradiation. *Proceedings of the National Academy of Science, U.S.A.*, **72**, 219–223.

Muller, H. K. & Sutherland, R. C. (1971) Epidermal antigens in cutaneous dysplasia and neoplasia. *Nature*, **230**, 384.

Nairn, R. C., Richmond, H. G., McEntegart, M. G. & Fothergill, J. E. (1960). Immunologic differences between normal and malignant cells. *British Medical Journal*, **2**, 1335–1340.

Nathanson, R. B., Forbes, P. D. & Urbach, F. (1973) Ultraviolet photocarcinogenesis: modification by antilymphocytic serum or 6-mercaptopurine. *Proceedings of the American Association for Cancer Research*, **14**, 46.

Pound, A. W. (1970) Induced cell proliferation and the initiation of skin tumour formation in mice by ultraviolet light. *Pathology*, **2**, 269–275.

Robbins, J. H., Kraemer, K. H., Lutzner, M. A., Festoff, B. W. & Coun, H. G. (1974) Xeroderma pigmentosum, an inherited disease with sun sensitivity, multiple cutaneous neoplasms and abnormal DNA repair. *Annals of Internal Medicine*, **80**, 221–248.

Rusch, H. P., Kline, B. E. & Baumann, C. A. (1941) Carcinogenesis by ultraviolet rays with reference to wavelength and energy. *Archives of Pathology*, **31**, 135–146.

Setlow, R. B., Regan, J. D., German, J. & Carrier, W. L. (1969) Evidence that xeroderma pigmentosum cells do not perform the first step in the repair of ultraviolet damage to their DNA. *Proceedings of the National Academy of Science, U.S.A.*, **64**, 1035–1041.

Tuffrey, M. A. & Batchelor, J. R. (1964) Tumour-specific immunity against murine epitheliomas induced with 9,10-dimethyl-1,2-benzanthracene. *Nature*, **204**, 349–351.

Urbach, F. (1959) Modification of ultraviolet carcinogenesis by photoactive agents. *Journal of Investigative Dermatology*, **32**, 373–378.

Urbach, F., Epstein, J. H. & Forbes, P. D. (1974) Ultraviolet carcinogenesis: experimental, global and genetic aspects. In *Sunlight and Man*, ed. Pathak, M. A., Harber, L. C., Seiji, M. & Kukita, J. S., pp. 259–283. Tokyo: University of Tokyo Press.

Willis, I, Kligman, A. & Epstein, J. H. (1972) Effects of long ultraviolet rays on human skin: photoprotective or photoaugmentative. *Journal of Investigative Dermatology*, **59**, 416–420.

9
TOPICAL THERAPY

A. W. McKenzie   D. S. Wilkinson

Only three years have passed since Polano (1973) reviewed the advances in topical therapy that had taken place over the preceding 10 years. Though new ideas have not been lacking in the short time that has passed subsequently, these have not always been satisfactorily translated into practice. Some therapeutic agents that were of promising value in 1973 have failed to be accepted widely; others have produced an unwelcome rate of sensitisation. Perhaps the greatest general 'advance' has been a better realisation of the value of older remedies or improvements in their application and a return to the old principle that it is better to know and to use proplerly a few well-tried remedies and to retain a certain scepticism about the claims of new products. There has also been a welcome retreat from the overuse of those very valuable agents the fluorinated steroids and a greater emphasis on the formulation of substitutes which rely on modification of the base or in a weaker concentration of the active agents.

We shall not, therefore, attempt to cover the whole field of topical therapy but shall concentrate on certain aspects in which there has been a shift of emphasis or experimental work which appears to justify inclusion. No doubt, in the next edition, many of these will have been re-evaluated and will suffer the same fate as their predecessors.

Bases and Emollients

Despite continuing interest in the composition and effect of bases for topical agents, the choice remains very much an empirical one. Absorption studies cannot always be equated with clinical efficiency and unexpected idiosyncratic reactions by the patient may influence the acceptability of a preparation that should in theory be entirely applicable to a given dermatological situation. Such reactions are non-immunological and can be regarded as 'intolerance' rather than 'irritancy' to avoid confusion with reactions to known irritants. They are not uncommonly seen even with cosmetics, where great care is obviously taken to avoid the use of known irritants. Such states of intolerance have been little studied but are subject to great variation in any one individual. We have seen the phenomenon in a marked degree in 'unstable' psoriatics who, at time of active spread, become unable to tolerate many simple bases that they have until then been using without ill-effect. The facial skin is especially liable to show this effect to bases that are well tolerated elsewhere.

An explanation may be found in the studies of Sarkany and Gaylarde (1973) and Gaylarde and Sarkany (1973). They found that propylene glycol, Carbowax 1500, FAPG base and emulsifying ointment BP caused acanthosis and even erythema in the guinea-pig skin. Christophers (1970) had found similar effects with white soft paraffin and Delactétaz, Etter and Emah (1971) noted erythema (and parakeratosis) with a stearate ester of polyethylene gycol 300. These effects match the comedogenic activity of common cosmetic bases obtained by Kligman and Mills (1972). But we do not yet know what governs the erratic and individual nature of the response and its variation in a given subject.

Nevertheless, closer attention to the formulation of bases, particularly those designed for corticosteroids, has enhanced the effect or allowed a more effective absorption of a weaker concentration (Beare, 1971). These are discussed elsewhere in this chapter. The incorporation of urea has a logical basis, especially in patients with dry or ichthyotic skin, as it is a polar binder of water and non-allergenic. Once its instability in water and its unattractive odour was overcome, it became available for incorporation in bases and, though long-term studies may not show any significant advantages in general use, we have found it more valuable than conventional hydrocortisone preparations in selected cases, e.g. mild atopics with dry skins, patients with dry forms of hand eczema and in the xerosis of the aged.

An emollient is, by definition, a substance designed to 'soften' the skin. But this carries two meanings in dermatology, which are not always well defined— the physical softening of hardened and dry keratin, as in cracks and fissured skin and the 'feel' (in cosmetic terms) of an agent that provides an oily or greasy texture to its surface. Trials of these agents have mostly been carried out on ichthyotics (Pope, et al, 1972), and a urea formulation (Calmurid) has been found to be more effective than other preparations tested. Almeya and Burt (1974) also reported favourably on a similar preparation containing hydrocortisone 1 per cent (Alphaderm). In a personal comparison of different emollients given in the winter to patients with various problems of 'dry skin', we have found considerable differences in acceptability between patients in different groups and, to some extent, between the sexes. No doubt cultural factors influenced this necessarily subjective assessment but we feel that more detailed and careful studies are needed in a field that has been less studied by dermatologists than by cosmeticians.

Keratolytics

The relative ineffectiveness of standard keratolytics in extreme situations (tylosis, hyperkeratotic eczema, etc.) has prompted further studies. Those concerned with a range of α-hydroxy acids are discussed elsewhere in this chapter. Baden and Goldsmith (1972) found that a strong (40 to 60 per cent) aqueous solution of propylene glycol was effective under occlusion for ichthyosis. An ethanol-cellulose gel was more acceptable cosmetically (Baden and Alper, 1973). With the addition of 6 per cent salicylic acid this was also useful in softening hyperkeratotic psoriatic plaques prior to subsequent treatment and in preparing warts for paring and liquid nitrogen (Baden, 1974).

Meanwhile, an explanation for the keratolytic effect of salicylic acid was given by Marks, Davies and Catell (1975). They found the changes to be most marked in the stratum corneum with a possible direct solubilising effect on intercellular cement. Changes in the Malpighian layer occurred only with increasing concentrations.

Retinoic Acid

This interesting agent ('Vitamin A acid', 'Retin-A', 'Tretinoin') has attracted a good deal of attention in recent years. Polano (1973) reviewed the earlier work in acne and psoriasis and further references occur in the appropriate sections of this volume. But the biphasic action of retinoic acid, the increased germinative layer activity and the dehiscence of Malpighian cell attachments has led to its use in a wide variety of skin lesions, from callosities to lichen planus. Its action is unfortunately limited by its irritant effect, though this may be suppressed by the concomitant or subsequent application of corticosteroids. There have been a large number of reports on its effect on these diverse conditions (Symposium, 1975) but we believe that it will be some time before the results of properly controlled trials are sufficiently persuasive to be able to state what value to attribute to retinoic acid in therapy of conditions other than acne.

Vitamin A acid has not been considered to be a sensitiser despite widespread use. However, Jordan, Higgins and Dvorak (1975) have made out a case for true sensitivity in two prison volunteers who were undergoing usage trials. As the reactions occurred on initial testing, the authors suggest a prior sensitisation may have occurred by unknown cross-sensitisation unique to the environment.

Antibacterials and Germicides

Though antibiotics are widely used, alone and in combination with steroids, for superficial infections of the skin and mucosae, there are often situations in which a non-antibiotic antibacterial agent is preferred, e.g. in intertriginous areas, where the bacterial growth is likely to be mixed or associated with yeasts. Moreover, the sensitising capacity of neomycin and related antibiotics has created some distrust among dermatologists. Among alternatives, the hydroxyquinolines are probably the most widely used, especially chloriodo-hydroxyquinoline (Vioform, Chinoform, clioquinol). We use this antibacterial, with hydrocortisone, for most cases of balanitis and vulvitis and have seldom encountered sensitivities. As an impregnated bandage it is widely used in many clinics as a dressing for leg ulcers. Despite pressure and occlusion by an over-bandage, clinical sensitivity is uncommon, though we have noticed an increase in this in recent years in patch-testing these patients. Controlled trials on this group of agents are few but Konopka et al (1975) found a combination of Locorten and Vioform more effective in suppressing penicillin-resistant staphylococci than Vioform alone.

The presence of *Staphylococcus aureus* in atopic skin was felt to be a neglected aetiological component by Leyden, Marples and Kligman (1974), who investigated the bacteriology of chronic plaques and exudative lesions in this disease by quantitative aerobic cultures. Although clinical signs of infection were usually lacking, they found that *Staph. aureus* was present in 90 per cent of plaque lesions (45 per cent having a density exceeding $1 \times 10^6/cm^2$), whilst in the exudative disease the same organisms, with a mean density of $14 \times 10^6/cm^2$, were present in every case. They contrasted this finding with the uncommon occurrence of *Staph. aureus* in normal skin, except in the perineum (Noble, Valkenburg and Wolters, 1967) and compared oral and topical antibiotic treatment in relation to the diminution of the *Staphylococcus*. Thirteen patients with lichenified lesions were treated with 1 per cent neomycin cream b.d. for seven days and 11 similar patients were given 1 g of erythromycin per day. In the neomycin group *Staph. aureus* was eradicated in six patients, with a much lower bacterial density in the others, and in the erythromycin group three showed complete eradication of *Staph. aureus*, with reduced bacterial density in the others. Retrospective clinical analysis showed that those patients who showed improvement, judged by lessening of pruritus, erythema and excoriations, had initially more than 1 million organisms/cm², with a drastic fall in the number after treatment. These findings, the authors suggest, provide a plausible rationale for the use of antibiotics in the initial treatment of atopic dermatitis and may indicate that *Staph. aureus* in high numbers can aggravate existing disease. The high density of *Staph. aureus* in atopic skin must certainly be considered of importance in relation to public health and familial spread of infection.

Zaynoun, Matta and Uwayda (1974) report an interesting study on the use of topical antibiotics in pyodermas. In 46 patients suffering from a variety of superficial pyogenic infections, mainly primary staphylococcal impetigo but including infection secondary to other lesions, they conducted a double blind trial of 0.1 per cent gentamicin cream b.d. against a placebo cream, with each group instructed to wash the lesions with 2 per cent hexachlorophane soap twice daily to remove crusts. All organisms isolated from the lesions were sensitive to gentamicin, but at the end of one week there was no statistical difference between the gentamicin and placebo groups when the clinical results were graded from excellent to poor. On the basis of these results the authors cast doubt on the necessity or wisdom of using topical antibiotics in superficial infections and attribute their results to washing and the removal of crusts. They do not comment on the bacteriostatic effect of the hexachlorophane soap.

Since the last edition of this work, hexachlorophane has fallen into disfavour. The daily washing of newborn infant rhesus monkeys, using only 5 ml of a 3 per cent suspension, was shown to cause vacuolar cerebellar changes after 90 days. After one week's exposure, the blood levels were found to be $1.5\,\mu g/ml$ (Lockhart, 1972). But the warning note was sounded some years earlier when elevated serum levels and convulsions occurred in burn patients (Larson, 1968). Two children with burns and two others with ichthyosis, who were bathed routinely with hexachlorophane, died in hospital with extensive vacuolar degeneration of the white matter, similar to those seen in rats fed hexachlorophane orally. It will be noted that all cases had some degree of skin damage favouring absorption. But this was not all. Examination of the brains of 7 out of 69 infants who died in the perinatal period were shown to have similar findings: 2 ml of the 3 per cent emulsion had been used in and around the umbilicus for up to 19 applications (Powell et al, 1973). Further studies in premature and full-term infants (Curley et al, 1971; Kopelman, 1973; Abbot et al, 1972) suggest that in infants even modest exposure can cause appreciable blood levels. Rather surprisingly, absorption and a high death rate also occurred in a group of French infants accidentally exposed to 6 per cent hexachlorophane in the form of a powder.

There is little evidence that the moderate and sensible use of hexachlorophane by adults carries any risk, though even surgical personnel, using it with frequent scrubbing, showed appreciable blood levels (Butcher et al, 1973) and prolonged or extensive use by dermatological patients should be discouraged. Even though absorption is likely to be minimal, there seems little justification for its widespread use as a facial cleanser in patients with acne, especially those who are obsessional by nature. The incorporation of hexachlorophane in steroid ointments may also lead to absorption and blood levels that may be unacceptable (Bye, Morison and Rhodes, 1975) and this combination should be reviewed.

Chlorhexidine, previously used less widely, became the natural successor to hexachlorophane in the medical field, as trichlorcarbanilide did to tetrachlorsalicylanilide in the toiletry field. It has been partiuclarly studied by Lowbury and Lilly (Lilly and Lowbury, 1971; Lowbury and Lilly, 1973; Lowbury, Lilly and Ayliffe, 1974), who found a 0.5 per cent alcoholic solution of chlorhexidine to be more effective in reducing the skin flora than hexachlorophane, without the addition of chlorocresol (which alone was also effective). A detergent solution was even more active, giving an immediate reduction of 86.7 per cent of the skin flora. Finally (Lowbury et al, 1974), a single application of 10 ml of 0.5 per cent chlorhexidine in 95 per cent alcohol gave a 97.9 per cent reduction, greater than that given by the 4 per cent detergent solution. Equally good results were achieved by a 0.1 per cent tetrabrom-*o*-methyl phenol solution in alcohol, widely used for disinfection of surgeon's hands in Germany. Other preparations were somewhat less effective but would, nevertheless, be perfectly adequate for routine skin use.

The early work of Shelanski and Shelanski (1956) had shown that, in combination with povidone (polyvinylpyrrolidone), iodine forms a complex in which it is still active and yet free from the toxic and irritating effects of the free tincture. Frank (1959) and Greenberg (1961) found it effective in seborr- hoeic dermatitis, and a wide range of uses were presented at a symposium held at the University of Miami in 1972. Recently, Hudson (1973) has shown that it compares favourably with hexachlorophane as a skin cleanser for patients with acne in not affecting the skin's ability to recover its 'acid mantle' for 3 h after washing. It has been advocated for use under plaster of Paris to reduce bacterial and fungal contamination (Boroda and Monzas, 1974). Personal use as an ointment or liquid application for leg ulcers has shown that it is well tolerated and has, so far, a low rate of sensitisation. But Erikson (quoted by Hjorth, 1974) showed that four out of seven patients sensitive to potassium iodide reacted to 2.5 per cent povidone-iodine (aqueous). In the treatment of burns, povidone-iodine ointment (10 per cent) compared well with mafenide acetate (Sulfamylon) and silver sulphadiazine (Georgiade and Harris, 1972). Gilmore and his colleagues (Gilmore and Martin, 1974; Gilmore and Sanderson, 1975) found that an aerosol spray, containing 5 per cent available iodine, reduced infection in postappendicectomy wounds by half and was better than a standard antibiotic spray used hitherto. If these experiences are substantiated, a wide use may lead to a reduction in the high present rate of neomycin sensitivity. But a warning note has been sounded by Pietsch and Meakins (1976), whose two patients with extensive burns treated with povidine- iodine developed a severe metabolic acidosis and a very high serum-iodine concentration, requiring haemodialysis. As in all topically applied medica- ments, the effects of absorption through damaged (or absent) epidermis, create a totally different metabolic situation from that encountered in normal use.

Topical Antivirals and Photo-inactivation

Many viral infections still successfully resist pharmacological and immuno- therapeutic attack. Their intracellular localisation gives them an entrenched position, isolating them from circulating antiviral agents. Advances in therapy are slow and made difficult to assess because of the variability of the course of the disease and the influence of ill-understood psychological or immuno- logical factors. Nevertheless, there have been some small advances in recent years.

Idoxuridine (5-iodo-2-dioxyuridine, IDU) is a halogenated synthetic thymidine analogue and, acting as a thymidine competitor, inhibits viral DNA synthesis and viral replication. Herrmann (1961) reported the inhibition of plaque formation of vaccinia and herpes simplex virus by IDU in vitro.

Kaufman (1962) reported its successful use clinically in herpetic keratitis. When it was evaluated in cutaneous herpes simplex the initial conflicting reports were probably due to its low solubility in water and the relative difficulty in penetrating skin. Hall-Smith, Corrigan and Gilkes (1962) treated recurrent cold sores and reported excellent results using a 0.1 per cent lotion or a 0.5 per cent cream applied frequently, but Juel-Jensen and MacCallum (1964) and Kibrick and Katz (1970) failed to show any therapeutic effect from idoxuridine in a cream base. With the better appreciation of the pharmacology of dimethylsulphoxide (DMSO) (Kligman, 1965), idoxuridine was found to be soluble and stable in this, and MacCallum and Juel-Jensen (1966) in a double-blind trial found the drug to shorten healing time in a 5 per cent concentration in 10 per cent DMSO in cases of recurrent cutaneous herpes simplex. In herpetic whitlows Juel-Jensen (1970) reported some response to a 5 per cent solution of idoxuridine, but a better response to a 40 per cent solution in DMSO. We have used such preparations of IDU in our own hospital practice, particularly for genital herpes and can confirm its value, if used early and frequently in the attack, as well as its freedom from side effects (though soreness and irritation may occur if used for more than three days). Juel-Jensen and MacCallum (1972) and Juel-Jensen (1974) point out that since IDU simulates thymidine, a DNA precursor, it is therefore only effective on the replicating virus. They emphasise the need to start treatment as early as possible in an attack. The only commercially available preparation of idoxuridine in DMSO is Herpid (IDU 5 per cent, DMSO to 100 per cent), the manufacturer's main therapeutic indication being herpes zoster (see below). Though by no means ideal, it is probably the best available topical agent for general use.

The recurrent nature of most herpes simplex skin infections is a tiresome nuisance to the patient, and while IDU in DMSO produces benefit in reducing the discomfort and duration of the lesions, it does nothing against potential reactivation of the virus which, in the case of recurrent eruptions in the second and third divisions of the trigeminal nerve, probably results from latency of the virus in the trigeminal ganglion (Baringer and Swoveland, 1973). The suppressive nature of IDU in DMSO, is, however, of greater potential importance in circumstances where trivial reactivations can lead to marked extension of the eruption, e.g. the abnormal immune system of lymphomata and the immunosuppression after renal transplantation (Lynfield, Farhangi and Runnels, 1969; Montgomerie et al, 1969).

A further recent and interesting approach to the treatment of herpes simplex infections is through the process of photo-inactivation. This is based on the work of Wallis and Melnick (1964, 1965) who demonstrated that the irreversible binding of certain heterotricyclic dyes to herpes virus in vitro is followed by complete inactivation of the virus if there is brief subsequent exposure to fluorescent light. The most active dyes are neutral red, proflavine and toluidine blue. Using this in vitro finding Felber et al (1973) in a double-blind study ruptured early herpes simplex vesicles, painted them with an aqueous solution of 0.1 per cent neutral red and subsequently exposed the lesions to fluorescent light for 15 min. In the actively treated patients most expressed symptomatic improvement superior to any other medication, and in almost all a 50 per cent improvement in healing time was noted. A decreased recurrence rate was also claimed. Cheng, Fiumara and Weinstein (1975) reported photo-inactivation of herpes virus induced by methylene blue and, using it in genital herpes, reported that 70 per cent of 36 patients improved with a shortening in duration of the attack. Cheng and Weinstein (1975) used the same preparation in a unilateral trial in one case of eczema herpeticum. One half of the child's face was exposed to a daylight fluorescent lamp with two 15 W tubes at a distance of 15 cm for 15 min and the treatment repeated in 4 h. Virus culture was negative 24 h after the first application on the treated side only and healing was obtained in four days. The dyes appear to have an affinity for the guanine base portions of DNA, causing disruption of the molecule on exposure to light. The clinical effect is due to photo-sensitisation of intracellular replicating herpes virus and the fluorescence of the alcohol-based solution compared to the non-fluorescence of the aqueous solution is not material to the end result (Jarratt and Felber, 1975).

It is too early to evaluate this seemingly simple form of treatment. In enthusiastic hands it appears to be as valuable as IDU—and certainly much cheaper. But there have not yet been enough controlled trials in a notoriously variable disease to decide on its general effectiveness.

The use of IDU has been shown to reduce the very appreciable morbidity resulting from herpes zoster. Juel-Jensen et al (1970) reported both a shortening of the healing time of the vesicles and the duration of herpetic pain. A beneficial effect was achieved by the intermittent application of 5 per cent IDU in 100 per cent DMSO and this effect was enhanced when 40 per cent IDU in 100 per cent DMSO was applied continuously for four days; the IDU was applied on lint which was rewetted with this solution daily for four days and the dressing kept in place by a bandage. The benefits of the treatment must be weighed against the cost, which may be up to £60 per patient (Juel-Jensen, 1973).

Dawber (1974) treated 118 patients with zoster of less than six days duration, and reported that 5 per cent idoxuridine in 100 per cent DMSO in the form of Herpid produced shortening of the vesicular phase, the healing time and the duration of pain. Herpid was brushed on to the visible lesions 4-hourly for four days, and no added benefit was achieved when the concentration of IDU was increased to 25 per cent with the preparation applied 2-hourly. In reply to this paper, Juel-Jensen and MacCallum (1974) wrote that they advocated application of IDU to the whole of the affected dermatome and that further work had shown that concentrations of 20 per cent and 5 per cent IDU applied continuously were inferior to a 40 per cent strength.

Benefit appears to result from IDU in herpes zoster when treatment is started within six days of onset. The optimum method and timing of application may well be influenced by convenience and economics. IDU is teratogenic and should not be used in children under 12 years or when pregnancy is present or potential. IDU in DMSO may produce a stinging sensation and a transient wealing due to histamine release by DMSO. Clinical trials have not yet clarified the possible reduction in incidence or severity of post-herpetic neuralgia in the elderly.

Antifungal Preparations

Imidazole derivatives

Though there has been no dramatic advance in topical antifungal therapy, the place of *miconazole* (1-[2,4-dichloro-β-(2,4-dichlorobenzyloxy)phenethyl]-imidazole nitrate) and of *clotrimazole* (bis-phenyl(2-chlorophenyl)-1-imidazolyl methane) are assured. These compounds have a broad spectrum of activity against both yeasts and dermatophytes, including *Aspergilli, Cryptococcus neoformans, Histoplasma capsulatum* and *C. immitis*. They can also be given by mouth (Marger and Adam, 1971) and (miconazole) by intravenous drip infusion. Topically, they have been shown to be clinically as effective as pre-existing agents with, as yet, no reports of resistance. Clotrimazole was effective vaginally against both *Candida* and *Trichomonas*, 'curing' 82 per cent of 663 women within six days. Cultures were said to have remained negative after six weeks in over 90 per cent of patients (Kunicki, 1974). In a much more limited experience we have also found it useful and well tolerated, though relapses have occurred when appropriate oral therapy was not given at the same time. A careful assessment of clotrimazole was carried out by Clayton and Connor (1973). They compared a 1 per cent clotrimazole cream with nystatin and Whitfield's ointment (3 per cent salicylic and 6 per cent benzoic acid). All 17 patients with candidiasis cleared and remained clear four weeks later; eight patients with erythrasma were cleared with clotrimazole. In 31 patients with pityriasis versicolor, clotrimazole and Whitfield's ointment were equally effective but the former was more acceptable. Of 32 patients with ringworm infections who completed the trial, the clinical results were equal but fungus regrew with both forms of treatment in a significant proportion of patients after both preparations. Further studies on miconazole by Botter (1972) appeared to substantiate his earlier work on its value, under occlusion, in fungal infections of the nails. A varnish has become available (though not marketed in the UK). Though research studies have continued to be encouraging, we must await further well-conducted, long-term studies before this attractive possibility can be regarded as an advance in therapy. The precise identification of the causative organism is the desirable prerequisite in treating ringworm and yeast infection, but where the infections are suspected and where mycological or bacteriological facilities are limited, the broad spectrum of activity possessed by clotrimazole makes it a very useful drug.

The only cutaneous side effects appear to be transient burning or irritation immediately after application of the product.

Another imidazole derivative (2-thiazol-4-ylbenzimidazole) has been known as an antifungal agent for 15 years (Robinson, Silber, Graessia, 1969) but has always been overshadowed by other antimycotics. It has aroused renewed interest lately. Knight (1973) found it effective in a human model and Battistini et al (1974) tested it on a number of clinical varieties of ringworm infection. At 10 per cent concentration in a vanishing cream base, it effectively cleared tinea corporis and cured 17/18 patients with tinea capitis—though not those affected by *Microsporum audonini*—in 80 days. It was ineffective in onychomycosis and tinea pedis. However, Carr and Lewis (1975) found it effective within two weeks against tinea nigra palmaris caused by *Cladosporium werneckii*. Though undoubtedly effective in some clinical situations, it may owe some of its popularity in certain countries to its reputation in other fields and is likely to remain of limited value as an antifungal agent.

Griseofulvin

The outstanding effect of oral griseofulvin on ringworm infections and the relative lack of effect topically has again been investigated by Epstein et al (1975) without any definite answer to the paradox. They found that the topical application of 0.45 per cent grisefulvin in alcohol resulted in very high concentrations of griseofulvin in the stratum corneum with persistence for four or more days after application. The griseofulvin prevented experimentally induced *Trichophyton mentagrophytes* infection but had no effect therapeutically on an established infection. To test the possibility that the griseofulvin was in an inactive form in the stratum corneum, cellophane tape strippings of the treated stratum corneum were analysed and the dilemma was compounded by the finding of drug with in vitro antifungal activity in every specimen.

Tolnaftate

Clinical experience has substantiated the effectiveness of this drug in the treatment of infection by *Epidermophyton*, *Microsporum* and *Trichophyton* species. The product does not inhibit to any clinically significant degree the growth of *Candida albicans* (*British Medical Journal*, 1967). Good clinical results are obtained in infection of the toe-webs and groins, but the results in the scaling foot and hand infections by *T. rubrum* are disappointing. Tolnftate in powder form was used by Gentles, Evans and Jones (1974) to control the incidence of tinea pedis in a swimming bath. When supplied in individual sachets and applied between and under the toes after bathing, the overall incidence of tinea pedis decreased from 8.5 to 2.1 per cent over a $3\frac{1}{2}$ year period. Contact dermatitis due to tolnaftate is uncommon but does occur Gellin, Maibach and Wachs, 1972; Emmett and Marrs, 1973).

Sodium omadine (a 1-hydroxypyrydine-2-thione derivative)

This broad spectrum antimycotic agent (Risold and Peguegnot, 1969) has been chiefly of interest in antidandruff formulations (see below). But Knight (1973) found it as effective as thiabendazole in experimental infection in human models. This author rightly points out the difficulty in relating in vitro with in vivo findings in this field. Fungi are highly discerning of their environment and, like lichens, mosses and mushrooms, depend on a delicate balance of adjuvant factors for their survival and propagation. The presence of an apparently potent adversary does less to discourage them than do adverse environmental conditions. Kligman and Marples (1974) have demonstrated this well in their study of 'athlete's foot' and suggest that simple agents that reduce or control moisture and maceration will by themselves prevent the emergence of fungal infections.

Corticosteroids

During the three years that have elapsed since Polano (1973) wrote his excellent and informative review, there has been no basic changes in the principles governing the indication for the use of these preparations. The advantage of corticosteroids in steroid responsive dermatoses is accepted and inevitably the number of available compounds has increased, each being heralded by papers indicating their usefulness and superiority over other products. Many dermatologists, however, will differ when a relative pecking order of efficacy is attempted, but most are unanimous in pointing out certain disadvantages which have gradually appeared. The efforts of the drug industry are now directed, not only to producing very potent corticosteroids such as clobetasol propionate (Sparkes and Wilson, 1974), but to the introduction of other products which are effective without incurring those cutaneous disabilities and biochemical abnormalities which have been so much publicised in the medical and lay press. These products will be indicated after a brief discussion of the systemic and local side-effects of topical corticosteroids.

Systemic side-effects. Polano (1973) mentioned the earlier evidence which indicated systemic absorption of corticosteroids when applied with or without polythene occlusion to human skin. These experiments showed not only that topically applied ^{14}C-labelled steroids could be recovered in the urine, but that adrenal suppression, implied by diminished urinary 17-ketosteroids, occurred when steroids were applied to skin under occlusive dressings (Scoggins, 1962). Subsequently this potentially serious side-effect was investigated in terms of plasma cortisol and the integrity of the hypothalamo-pituitary–adrenal axis under a variety of conditions and with differing steroid preparations. Reassuringly, it was found that only a small number of patients had lower than normal plasma corticosteroid levels during and after treatment with topical steroids (Fry and Wight, 1965; Wilson, Williams and Marsh, 1973; Munro and Clift, 1973). James, Munro and Feiwel (1967) showed in six patients that when a potent steroid such as betamethasone-17-valerate was used on widespread skin disease under polythene occlusion for 14 days, there was presumptive evidence in all of adrenal suppression in a diminution of urinary and plasma steroids, but that there was a quick return to normal values a few days after cessation of treatment. The response to metyrapone after treatment did not differ significantly from controls, but hypothalamo-pituitary–adrenal function was 'slightly inhibited' when tested by the stress of hypoglycaemia. The fact that topical corticosteroids can produce a fall in plasma cortisol has led to the screening of new preparations as these are introduced. Thus, in a study of 34 patients treated by Walker et al (1974) over a period of two to four weeks, clobetasol propionate induced a fall in plasma cortisol in only five patients at some stage of the investigation. When large amounts of clobetasol ointment were used (more than 100 g/week) on six patients with a significant proportion of the body surface involved by disease (20–80 per cent), only two had lowered plasma corticosteroid levels, and in four there was no evidence of adrenal suppression.

While there can be no doubt, therefore, about the possible suppression of hypothalmic–pituitary–adrenal function by powerful topical steroids, this ability has probably been overstated in the literature and, with the possible exception of infants and young children (Feiwel, Munro and James, 1967), small quantities of steroid ointments, used on unoccluded skin, carry a negligible risk from systemic absorption. The fact that biochemical abnormalities can be induced has led to modified treatment schedules when widespread and persistent skin disease is being treated (see below).

Local side-effects. Polano (1973) commented on the atrophy which local corticosteroid preparations can cause. This has been observed to be an effect proportional to the potency of the steroid used. With the widespread use of steroids, probably the commonest side-effect is the diagnostic difficulty they produce when they change the morphology of eruptions before a definitive diagnosis is made. Ive and Marks (1968) reported suppression of the signs of fungus infection, while Macmillan (1972) commented upon the morphological changes induced in scabies by fluorinated steroids.

The adverse effect of fluorinated steroids is seen at its worst when they are used on facial skin in women. The loss of dermal collagen with increasing erythema, telangectasia, papule and pustule formation when they are used on rosacea (Sneddon, 1969) has been accompanied by the appearance of perioral dermatitis (Sneddon, 1972; Weber, 1972) and steroid rosacea (Leydon and Kligman, 1974) when they are used over long periods for banal dermatoses on facial skin.

The appearance of pustular psoriasis is a recognised complication of the withdrawal of systemic steroid therapy in psoriasis. Boxley, Dawber and

Summerly (1975) have described the occurrence of two instances of generalised pustular psoriasis after the withdrawal of a potent topical fluorinated steroid, clobetasol propionate.

Adverse effects. Atrophy, erythema and striae are now well documented. But other reactions continue to be described. The gluteal granuloma of Tappeiner and Pfleger has been related to the use of fluorinated corticosteroids under conditions of maceration and occlusion (Bazex et al, 1972; Maleville et al, 1973). Leucoderma following intralesional injections is well recognised (Dupré and Fournié, 1973) but it was also seen following the use of Cordran (Haelan) tape (Kestel, 1971). Kligman has made use of the less pronounced tendency of topical corticosteroids without occlusion to produce a lightening of skin colour in his formulation of depigmenting agents (see Depigmenting Agents).

Recent topical corticosteroids

The ideal topical corticosteroid is one which combines potency with an absence of adverse local reactions and negligible systemic absorption. Much recent work has been directed to this goal, with the introduction of new compounds, the manipulation of the hydrocortisone molecule, and the formulation of new bases designed to enhance percutaneous absorption. An international controlled trial of clobetasol propionate (Dermovate) (Sparkes and Wilson, 1974), demonstrated its undoubted pre-eminence over other potent topical steroids in eczema, and especially psoriasis. Routine clinical use has confirmed the effectiveness of the preparation, but appreciation of its usefulness has been paralleled by its production of profound skin atrophy and by reports of appreciable signs and symptoms from systemic absorption. Staughten and August (1975) found sustained reduction of plasma cortisol levels in four patients treated with the preparation, and three patients showed not only signs and symptoms of adrenal insufficiency on withdrawal of the drug but rebound activation of psoriasis with pustulation. Pustular psoriasis on withdrawal of clobetasol propionate was also reported by Tan and Samman (1974) and Boxley et al (1975).

Feldman and Maibach (1974), using the urinary recovery of ^{14}C, demonstrated a two-fold increase in the skin penetration of hydrocortisone when combined with 10 per cent urea in a cream base. Hydrocortisone has been combined with urea at a compatible near neutral pH by absorbing the urea on to a polysaccharide powder matrix dispersed in an anhydrous medium. The product (Alphaderm) has been compared clinically against betamethasone 17-valerate (Betnovate) (Jacoby and Gilkes, 1974). In trials which were not double blind, the preparation was shown to be 'at least as effective' as the betamethasone, although there was no statistical difference between the two treatments. Almeyda and Burt (1974) compared the same two preparations in a double-blind controlled study of the treatment of atopic eczema and clinical evaluation indicated equal potency. Statistical evaluation showed 'a trend in favour of the U-Hc. powder-cream'. The same authors compared the new neutral pH product with an acidic 10 per cent urea/1 per cent hydrocortisone cream (Calmurid-H.C.) and demonstrated a statistically significant superiority in the former. The superiority was claimed to be due to the urea remaining in a hypermolar concentration (12 M) on the inert powder matrix, thus maintaining an enhanced keratolytic activity.

Hydrocortisone with a butyryl radical at the 17-position (Locoid) has been shown to be effective clinically. Ashurst (1972) reported results comparable to those obtained with fluocinolone acetonide in eczema and psoriasis, while Alexander and Lyne (1973) found it as effective as betamethasone 17-valerate in the same conditions. Polano and Kanaar (1973) reported that 0.1 per cent hydrocortisone butyrate gave significantly better therapeutic responses in eczema than 0.1 per cent triamcinolone acetonide and 1 per cent hydrocortisone acetate. Sneddon (1973) alluded to these indices of potency in reporting that its use did not prevent the beneficial effect of tetracycline in rosacea and perioral dermatitis induced by fluorinated steroids.

Hydrocortisone in a base formulation founded on propylene glycol and a critical proportion of an aqueous solution of sodium lauryl sulphate (Dioderm) has been subjected to clinical trials in a wide variety of eczematous skin disease. At a 0.1 per cent concentration, it was found to be more effective than 0.1 per cent hydrocortisone cream BPC (Whitfield and McKenzie, 1975).

Flurandrenole (Haelan, Cordran) tape, an adhesive tape of a copolymer of acrylate ester and acrylic acid containing flurandrenole 4 μg/cm^2 has provided an elegant and effective method of applying a medium-strength steroid under occlusion to a small lesion. The adhesive properties are good and it has been particularly effective in our hands in facial lesions of lupus erythematosus and lymphocytic infiltration, and in localised lesions of discoid eczema and lichen planus elsewhere. Atrophy can occur as with other steroids applied under occlusion, though we have not seen this occur in less than three weeks' continuous use.

Munro and Wilson (1975) discussed hypothalamic–pituitary–adrenal (HPA) suppression by topical corticosteroids and comment this may be seen when any potent steroid, whether or not containing halogen atoms, is applied at length and in large quantities to the 'broken' cutaneous barrier of skin disease. They report a new corticosteroid, clobetasone butyrate (Molivate) with a low systemic activity (thymus involution) and a topical (vasoconstriction) activity below that of betamethasone 17-valerate, and very much less than clobetasol proprionate. In clinical double-blind trials, 0.05 per cent clobetasone butyrate had greater topical anti-inflammatory activity than 1 per cent hydrocortisone. HPA function was minimally affected when the ointment was used in large quantities and under total body polythene occlusion. In an animal model, the product caused less epidermal thinning than other steroids tested with the exception of hydrocortisone.

The exact position of these new preparations awaits further study and experience. It is all too easy to compare new topical agents that suppress inflammatory reactions on patients whose dermatoses would respond equally well to rest, soothing non-steroid cream and reassurance. In such trials the weakest steroid appears as effective as the strongest; in both cases an 'over-kill' situation may exist. It behoves all dermatologists presented with glowing accounts of 'equal efficiency' of one product versus another to look carefully at the condition treated. Contact eczema should never appear in such comparisons—by definition the contact allergen has been removed. Atopic dermatitis responds to the simplest measures in hospital. Nature and its healing propensities (when left alone) are often overlooked in the vanity of man's aspiration to perform miracles.

Modified treatment regimes with topical corticosteroids

From the above it will be seen that there is a deceleration in the quest for more powerful local steroids. In clinical practice there is a tendency, always implicit but now necessary, to modify treatment regimes in order to lessen cutaneous and systemic side-effects. Care is necessary in the prescription of the more potent products, e.g. betamethasone 17-valerate and clobetasol propionate, and if their active anti-inflammatory properties are to be used, it would appear wise to limit the total quantity applied on diseased skin to 50 to 60 g per week. Walker et al (1974) recommend that short courses of highly active steroids should be given and, with suppression, the steroid should be withdrawn until a relapse occurs. Alternatively, the manufacturers of a new double halogenated steroid (Halcinonide) recommend restriction of treatment to b.d. application for three weeks, with a non-steroidal preparation used during the quiescent phase. In practice, many dermatologists find it helpful to use the more potent preparations for short periods of relapse and to rely on products of lesser potency for maintenance therapy. All would agree on the need to restrict the use of active fluorinated steroids on the facial skin of women. The clinical picture will obviously dictate practice, but any of the simple modifications of regime imply a degree more of patient–doctor co-operation and a change in one of the habits of the past which have lead to complications, i.e. repeat prescriptions. Modification in the frequency of application of steroids to the skin might lead to a diminution in dosage without the sacrifice of efficacy. Eaglstein, Farzad and Caplan (1974) set out to determine if more frequent application of corticosteroids would lead to an enhanced therapeutic effect. In 12 patients with bilaterally symmetrical psoriasis or eczema, they found no difference in response on the side treated six times a day compared with the side treated three times a day. In the context of frequency of application of local steroids required to produce a therapeutic response, the paper on acute tolerance to their vasoconstrictive action (tachyphylasis) is of interest (du Viver and Staughton, 1975). The authors speculate on the relationship of this finding in normal skin to the clinically observed resistance to a topical steroid after constant use on diseased skin. The observation does have clinical significance but to a degree which will depend upon further investigation. Many preparations available in the United Kingdom are recommended by the manufacturers to be used for two to four applications per day. It seems to us that twice daily application is usually sufficient and that more frequent applications are useful only for the emollient effect of the corticosteroid base.

Corticosteroid dilutions and bases

The vogue for the dilution of commercially available corticosteroids, although still with us, is less popular than formerly. Mooney (1974) has indicated the compatibility problems involved in the practice and has stressed the care required for sterility to be maintained and for topical effectiveness to to be preserved. If an alkaline vehicle such as Boots E.45 cream is used as a diluent of fluocinolone acetonide, oxidative degradation occurs at the 11 and 21 positions and a 20 per cent dilution of the steroid loses 50 per cent of its steroid concentration after one month at 23°C. The choice of preservative is also important since they may be rendered inactive if bound or absorbed by the non-ionic emulsifiers usually used in corticosteroid creams. Similarly, the degree of preservation usually depends on the availability of the preservative in the aqueous phase and this may be upset if oils are added leading to shift into this phase. If dilutions are required, the rules suggested by Mooney are (1) use simple, adequately preserved diluents (see British Pharmaceutical Codex); (2) make small batches; (3) do not keep longer than is necessary for patient treatment; (4) use aseptic mixing techniques. The same author casts doubt on the therapeutic desirability or pharmaceutical stability of mixtures containing corticosteroids, coal tar, cade oil, etc.

The incidence of cutaneous sensitivity reactions to lanolin bases and paraben preservatives has led to the introduction of new steroids in synthetic bases which, while designed primarily to enhance steroid absorption, have the dual advantages of being lanolin-free and containing their own inherent preservative in the form of propylene glycol. Thus, fluocinonide (Metosyn) is dissolved in propylene glycol with fatty acids added to give the product the spreading properties of a cream and the emollient effects of an ointment. Fluclorolone acetonide (Topilar) is dissolved in a combination of propylene glycol and fatty alcohols (FAPG cream base), while clobetasol propionate (Dermovate) has propylene glycol as a solvent in both cream and ointment bases.

Any drug formation must ensure that there is maximum release when in contact with the skin, and at a given concentration release of a drug is always faster from a vehicle in which the drug is entirely solubilised. Malone et al (1974), using the standard alcoholic constrictor test and the in vitro release of ^{14}C-labelled steroid, fluclorolone acetonide, demonstrated optimum availability of the drug when it was completely solubilised, poorest availability when it was poorly dissolved (suspension) and intermediate availability when the solubiliser was in excess of that required to dissolve the steroid. In correlating solubility, release and in vivo response, the authors point to the prophetic value of these in vitro studies in the investigation of vehicle efficacy. Similar studies using the vasoconstrictor assay were reported for clobetasol proprionate by Sparkes and Wilson (1974). Maximum vasoconstriction was found from ointments with formulations containing only sufficient propylene glycol to dissolve the steroid. With creams of nearly saturated solution of the steroid in the aqueous phase (propylene glycol in water) gave optimum release.

Jet injection of corticosteroids

The introduction of a convenient apparatus for multiple jet injection (the Port-o-Jet) has enlarged the scope of topical corticosteroid therapy, not so much in the range of diseases treated but in the ease with which multiple injection can be performed. Verbov and Abell (1970) found it effective in alopecia areata and discoid lupus erythematosus and Abell (1972) extended its use to the nail-folds in the treatment of psoriatic nail involvement. Cheloids in particularly may be helped because of the difficulty of infiltration by the conventional needle (though this can be overcome by the use of a dental syringe and vial in which the lignocaine is replaced by triamcinolone). Complete clearance of granuloma annulare was achieved in 68 per cent of cases (Sparrow and Abell, 1975) and five cases of necrobiosis lipoidica also responded well. But most dermatologists would agree with Bleeker (1974) that the advantages of this technique lie in its speed and relative painlessness, especially when large numbers of patients are being treated and in unduly sensitive areas such as the nail-folds.

Dithranol

The mechanism of the action of dithranol (anthralin) is still the subject of active research. It is believed that enzyme inactivation and mitotic inhibition are involved, the former perhaps due to increased lipoid peroxidisation leading to cross-linking of enzyme protein (Diezel, Meffert and Sönnichsen, 1975). Using the mouse tail test, Wrench and Britten (1975) could not induce granular layer formation using 10 per cent dithranol in an ointment base or in Lassar's paste. They suggested that the primary action of dithranol might lie elsewhere but the strength used was high and other reactions may have been masked. An immediate and paradoxical 'acanthogenic' effect preceding a decrease in the mitotic count has been reported by Braun-Falco, Bury and Schoefinius (1971) and Cox and Watson (1972). Fisher and Maibach (1975) studied the effect of dithranol (anthralin) and its separated components and found that anthralin alone was able to reduce mitotic activity. A diminution of DNA uptake had also been confirmed by Liden and Michalesson (1974) following the earlier work of other authors.

There have been continuing studies in the prevention of oxidisation of dithranol (especially in zinc oxide paste) to pink inactive anthrone and the prevention of this by salicylic acid (Luckacs and Braun-Falco, 1973; Panec-Waelsch and Hulsebosch, 1974; Raab and Gmeiner, 1974). The protective effect of salicylic acid appears to consist in the neutralisation of hydroxyl ions in an alkaline medium and perhaps by its reaction with the free zinc ions to prevent the formation of inactive zinc-dithranol complex. Raab and Gmeiner (1974) found that not only dithranol but zinc ions and salicylic acid also inhibited glucose-6-phosphate dehydrogenase and in combination with zinc and dithranol, had an increased, though not additive effect. So there is every justification for the time-honoured combination even though the total inhibiting effect may eventually be reduced by the formation of complexes mentioned. This work emphasises the need for the paste to be reasonably fresh and stored in a dry cool atmosphere.

Meanwhile, attempts have continued to try to improve the practical aspects of dithranol therapy. Seville (1975) omitted ultraviolet light and tar baths and formulated a 'stiffened' dithranol ointment, which was easier for the patients to use and which, over a number of years, had proved as effective as the standard paste hitherto employed. The formula must be followed exactly:

Dithranol	0.5 per cent (or as required)
Salicyclic acid	0.5 per cent
Chloroform	2.5 per cent
Hard paraffin BP	
White soft paraffin BP	} aa ad 100 per cent

The hard paraffin should have a melting point of 53/55°C, the soft paraffin one of about 49°C (for UK). The paraffins are heated until just melted, then triturated until smooth and brilliant white (38°C). The chloroform mixture is added and the wax triturated until cool. The ointment is labelled 'Rub on slab until smooth. Store in dark'. The preparation appears to have a shelf life of more than a year—comparing favourably with the short shelf-life reported for dithranol-zinc oxide pastes (Panec-Waelsch and Hulsebosch, 1974).

A 'dithranol stick', formulated in beeswax base, was assessed by us on 14 patients. The strength of dithranol (0.5 per cent) was not sufficiently liberated or absorbed and the overall effect was that of a 0.1 to 0.25 per cent paste. But it was accepted favourably by patients with psoriasis of the face. An improved formulation, incorporating a higher strength dithranol, may well be of value for localised lesions.

Cytostatic Agents

Polano (1973) gave a complete account of 5-fluorouracil as an inhibitor of thymidylate synthetase, together with indications for its clinical use. In the form of a 5 per cent w/w cream (Efudix) it now has an established place in the treatment of diffusely distributed solar keratoses of the face and neck, but lesions on the arms and the thick skin of the hands often require the use of the drug under polythene occlusion to give comparable effects. Acceptable results are obtained in Bowen's disease, but in basal cell and squamous carcinomata the results are much inferior to conventional surgery or radiotherapy. The mechanism of action of the drug in actinic keratoses was investigated and reported by Eaglstein, Weinstein and Frost (1970). While, clinically, the preparation appears to have a selective action on tumour tissue, a 1 per cent concentration induces electron microscopic changes in the keratinocytes of normal skin (Zelickson, Mottaz and Weiss, 1975). The drug's use requires close clinical supervision and patients should be warned about its potential phototoxicity and an ultraviolet filter prescribed under appropriate circumstances. Burnett (1975) described two instances of herpes simplex of the lips which were superimposed on the inflammation induced by fluorouracil on facial skin.

Goette (1974) reported the successful treatment of erythroplasia of Querat with topical fluorouracil. Almeida Concalves (1975), using it for digital warts, found that a varnish containing fluorouracil 5 per cent and salicylic acid 10 per cent gave a cure rate of 50 per cent over nine weeks compared with a cure rate of 4 per cent when the varnish contained only 10 per cent salicylic acid. Shelley (1972) reported reversible onycholysis when periungual warts were treated with topical fluorouracil.

There has been some advance in the use of topical nitrogen mustard, which remains a useful and convenient treatment for mycosis fungoides, despite the frequency of sensitisation (see Mycosis Fungoides, below). A new therapeutic group, the nitrosourea compounds, have been reported on favourably by Zackheim (1972) and Zackheim and Epstein (1975). Of the preparations tried, carmustine (1,3-bis-(2-chloroethyl)-nitrosourea) was preferred to lomustine (1,(2-chloroethyl)-3-cyclohexyl-1-nitrosourea), which was more apt to give bone marrow depression. The technique of application is very important, as carmustine has a half-life of only 15 min. Cross-reaction with mechlorethamine does not occur.

Cytotoxics

The unacceptable rate of sensitisation to topical mechlorethamine hydrochloride has led to attempts at desensitisation (Van Scott and Kalmanson, 1973). A simplified approach has recently been proposed by Constantine, Fuks and Farber (1975). They applied each day increasing strengths of nitrogen mustard, starting at 0.01 mg/100 ml and achieved tolerance to 20 mg/100 ml in three of their five patients. Though much slower than intravenous methods, this procedure can be more easily carried out on an ambulant basis by any intelligent patient.

Coal Tar

The long history of the therapeutic effect of coal tar has not been matched by an equivalent interest in the mechanism of its action (Muller and Kierland, 1964). Several attempts have been made recently to isolate the fractions of this complex natural substance which are responsible for its effect. The higher phenolic fraction of high temperature tar (a wide range of substituted poly-hydroxyphenols and their isomers) produced orthokeratosis in mouse tail skin (Wrench and Britten, 1975a, b). This appears to be due to a direct effect on the granular layer, perhaps by release of lysosomes at that level. This is followed by mitotic stimulation. A suitable vehicle that restrained the action of the phenolics to this level might bring about the former without stimulating the latter. A similar study of a synthetic proprietary tar preparation containing significant amounts of naphthalene, phenanthrene, phenol, carbazole and anthracene was found to cause epidermal thickening without granular layer induction (Wrench and Britten, 1975c). This may be because of the low content of phenolics. Young (1970) also found the synthetic tar to be without value.

The action spectrum of coal tar was studied by Tanenbaum et al (1975) who commented on the paucity of the important u.v.a. band in most conventional 'sunlamps'. Tar is a relatively weak photosensitiser in comparison with topical methoxalen (minimum phototoxic doses $7.7–17.4 \text{ J/cm}^2$ and 0.25 J/cm^2 respectively).

The effect of adding u.v.l. to a coal tar regime, therefore, remains uncertain and requires further study. Tring (1973) thought that a systemic factor might be released.

Dinitrochlorbenzene

The therapeutic use of DNCB in patients deliberately sensitised to it has continued to attract some support. Sensitisation is easily achieved and the effect of inducing a lymphocytic response and stimulation of cellular immunity at the site of skin lesions has led to a number of experimental studies (Remy and Stuttgen, 1972; Malek-Mansour, Castermans-Elias and Lapière, 1973; Helm, 1974). Two cases of Dubreuilh's precancerous melanosis and one of parapsoriasis lichenoides were treated with excellent temporary effect by the application of a 1 to 10 per cent solution (Heid, Grosshans and Basset, 1975). It may be of value in Bowen's disease of the vulva (Sanderson, 1975). In disseminated malignant malanoma, individual lesions regressed without affecting the natural course of the disease. Its use in the treatment of common warts poses more serious ethical considerations, even though it may continue to be shown to be effective (see Warts, below).

Depigmenting Agents

The topical use of chemical substances to achieve depigmentation of the human skin is relatively recent and the results have, on the whole, been unsatisfactory. Cultural as well as medical demand has stimulated research into new agents of potential value (Bleehen et al, 1968) but these have usually been found to be melanocidal or too sensitising to allow a safe and controlled effect. Hydroquinone, which probably acts by interupting the tyrosine–tyrosinase pathway of melanin synthesis, has been widely used in a 2 to 5 per cent concentration with varying success. At best, the results are slow to appear and inconstant. It does not, however, damage the melanocytes and sensitisation is uncommon (Spencer, 1965). Arndt and Fitzpatrick (1965) regarded it as an effective depigmenting agent. Its mechanism of action was investigated by Jimbow et al (1974) who reported that it affected the formation, melanisation and degradation of melanosomes and, eventually, the destruction of the membranous organelles in melanocytes. In contrast, the monobenzyl (and monomethyl) ethers of hydroquinone were shown by Riley (1969, 1970) to damage melanocytes irreversibly, probably by free radical production causing lipid peroxidation of the cell membrane. Becker and Spencer (1962) could not achieve a uniform or predictable depigmentation of black skin at a strength of 1 to 20 per cent of the monobenzyl ether. About half their patients developed a long-lasting ectopic depigmentation and a confetti-like leukoderma of the treated site was persistent in a third of the subjects. It is also a potent contact sensitiser; a bizarre appearance occurs when postsensitisation inflammatory hyperpigmentation surrounds the often patchy but persistent hypopigmentation resulting from treatment. There was, therefore, every reason to seek for more effective agents. But the most promising of 33 substances studied by Bleehan et al (1968), 4-isopropyl-catechol, was also a sensitiser. The phenolic compounds responsible for industrial leukoderma, notably p-tertiary butyl phenol, have the same destructive action on the melanocyte, ectopic spread and capacity for allergic sensitisation (Malten et al, 1971).

In a recent carefully conducted study Kligman and Willis (1975) have devised a new approach, based on two observations in the course of treatment of other conditions. They noted some degree of lightening of the skin of patient with acne treated with vitamin-A acid and confirmed the findings of Cahn (1972) of loss of pigment at the site of intralesional injections of corticosteroids. Using, eventually, a formula consisting of vitamin A acid 0.1 per cent, hydroquinone 5 per cent and dexamethasone 0.1 per cent (or other corticosteroid) in either a hydrophilic ointment or an ethanol-propylene glycol base, they achieved excellent depigmentation of freckles and melasma in 23/27 patients. Postinflammatory pigmentation in the dark skin was sometimes less responsive, due to the presence of dermal melanin-laden histiocytes but 12 out of 18 patients gave a satisfactory report. Unlike Spencer (1965), using hydroquinone alone, they were unable to depigment senile lentigines of the hands of white subjects.

All three ingredients must be present—an interesting example of therapeutic synergism—and the solution must be reasonably fresh. With twice daily applications, a uniform depigmentation was achieved in black skin in three to seven weeks and rather longer in white subjects. There was no spread of effect outside the treated areas and no reduction in the melanocyte count. Some irritation and initial erythema is common but tolerable. Normal pigmentation returns rapidly after treatment ceases and may be excessive. Sunscreen agents might reduce the accelerating effect of u.v. light in this process.

The authors rightly state that the strength of the ingredients are somewhat arbitrary and that further experience and study will be necessary before a satisfactory regime is worked out. Though the action of hydroquinone can be accepted, that of the other two constituents is conjectural. Nevertheless, this combination promises to provide a new stimulus for dermatologists to offer effective help to patients concerned with problems of local hyperpigmentation —notably melasma associated with pregnancy or the contraceptive pill.

Light Barriers and Screens

Protection of the photosensitive skin was, until recently, on a very empirical basis. Certain chemicals were known to be effective against shortwave u.v. penetration, for instance, cinnamates, para-aminobenzoic acid and quinine salts. But three developments stimulated a more critical appraisal of the chemistry and formulation of such screening agents: the increasing accuracy of exact diagnosis made possible by the use of monochromators, the greater incidence (or recognition) of exogenous photosensitisers and changes in cultural habits of dress and holiday patterns. Photosensitive patients are no longer content to sit in the shade with gloves and parasols. This need has not been lost on the cosmetic industry, whose research workers have also contributed, to the search for safe and effective screening agents.

MacLeod and Frain-Bell (1971) have noted the importance of relating the action spectrum involved in the absorption spectrum of the agent to be used as a screen, and to the need to compare the in vivo effect with that obtained in vitro. It has long been recognised that chemical screens are effective against short u.v. light (< 320 nm) and that protection fails when the photosensitive action spectrum includes longer wavelengths, even if not confined to these.

Short u.v. protection

Mexenone had superseded PABA in general use until Pothak, Fitzpatrick and Frenk (1969) showed that PABA and, in particular, its esters, were the most effective agents available. Further studies by Katz (1970) and Langner and Kligman (1972) suggested that a 5 per cent hydro-alcoholic solution of PABA was best; but opinion was divided on the role of exercise and bathing in diminishing the protection afforded. MacLeod and Frain-Bell (1975) made a detailed study of a number of different preparations of PABA, dimethyl-aminobenzoate and mexenone in alcohlic solutions with and without glycerol. They concluded that the best protection against the sunburn u.v. range was given by a mixture of PABA and the ester and that this was not enhanced by mexonone; that a 70 per cent ethanol 30 per cent water vehicle was the most effective and that glycerol did not improve the effect (though propylene glycol might do so); and that showering (or swimming) but not exercise reduced the effectiveness, even if this was delayed 2 h after application. This was contrary to the findings of Willis and Kligman (1970). A suitable formula consisted of

PABA	5 per cent
Ester	2.5 per cent
(Mexenone	0.5 per cent)
Ethanol	70 per cent
Water to	100 per cent

They pointed out that the strengths of the active agents might well be reduced and still give adequate protection to normal fair-skinned subjects.

Dihydroxyacetone and lawsone (2-hydroxy-1,4-naphthaquinone) was used by Johnson and Fusaro (1972), with apparent success in a wide variety of photosensitivity eruptions, including erythropoietic protoporphyria, in which they obtained 12-fold increase in light tolerance (Fusaro and Dunge, 1970). They claim that the compound is easy to apply, binds well to the stratum corneum and resists washing. They also claim that the addition of lawsone (0.25 per cent) to 3 per cent DHA in 50 per cent aqueous isopropanol gives immediate protection against u.v.l. (Fusaro and Johnson, 1975).

MacLeod and Frain-Bell (1971) give the following formula for a combined long and shortwave protective cream:

Titanium dioxide	20 per cent
Zinc oxide	6 per cent
Kaolin	2 per cent
Red ferric oxide	1.0 per cent
Mexenone	4 per cent
Cream to	100 per cent

The effect may be modified with brown ferric oxide or more mexenone cream.

Joó and Simon (1974) used 2-hydroxyphenyl-benztriazol derivatives, which are highly intensive absorbers of u.v.l., especially from 300 to 370 nm. They found that a combination of two derivatives, to a total of 20 per cent in a sorbitan–wool fat–wax base was best. There were two cases of sensitisation in 145. But this figure might rise to unacceptable levels with increased use.

Insect Repellants

Despite the stimulus afforded by events in the Far East, a wholly satisfactory repellant against disease-bearing mosquitoes and ticks has not been evolved. This is not so much the fault of the chemical nature of the repellant as of the physical and physiological limitations in actual use. Maibach, Khan and Akers (1974), in their excellent review stress the disparity of in vitro and in vivo testing. Not only must an effective be irritating to the mosquito's taste and smell perceptions but it must volatilise enough to create a barrier zone sufficiently wide to deflect the insect in its zig-zag approach to the skin. If the repellant is not used over the whole body surface, the zone will be penetrated. But volatility (associated with a low b.p.) must be equated with persistence and Feldman and Maibach (1970) found that the percutaneous absorption of a widely used repellant was significant—and greater than had been expected. The higher the ambient temperature, the shorter the protection given (Khan, Maibach and Skidmore, 1973). Hexamethylene-imine butane sulphonamide was best in this respect. Wind velocity, washing, sweating (Khan, Maibach and Skidmore, 1969) and friction and abrasion from clothing and exercise were also found to be limiting factors. But there is great individual variability in 'attractiveness' to mosquitoes and this remains the most important limiting feature in the effectiveness of insect repellants.

The older and still widely used dimethylphthalate has given way to 'Deet'— N,N-diethyl-m-toluamide—which, theoretically at least, offers protection for about 4 h (Maibach et al, 1974). Other repellants that have been tested include ethyl hexane diol and triethylene glycol monohexyl ether. No single one combines the qualities needed for perfect protection—persistence on the skin, sustained volatility and lack of toxicity.

Antiperspirants

Many attempts at providing an effective and safe antiperspirant mentioned by Polano (1973) have proved uncertain in effect or sensitising in action and the search for an absolute remedy for this distressing complaint continues. Agents active theoretically or *in vitro* cannot always be formulated successfully for general use. An increasing demand for aerosols rather than 'roll-on' types of application have added further problems of stability and effectiveness and the need for perfumes has at times confused the issue of acceptability. Accurate methods of testing antiperspirants are difficult to devise. Aluminium chlorhydrate has remained the mainstay of formulations, though certain zirconium salts, such as the chlorhydroxide, free from the danger of granuloma formation, have made a significant 'come-back' in recent years. Cullen (1975) claimed to have reduced sweating significantly in 14 of 26 patients with 5 per cent methenamine in a solid gel base, using a double-blind method of assessment. But this was used on the palms and soles and methenamine, a condensation of ammonia and formaldehyde, has a bad reputation of sensitisation in the rubber industry (Cronin, 1924). Its action is due to the formation of a keratotic plug, unlike that of the aluminium salts, and its suppressive action is lost after skin stripping. Abell and Morgan (1974) reviewed the unsatisfactory previous methods of sweat control and investigated glycopyrronium bromide and tap water iontophoresis. Glycopyrronium bromide is a quaternary ammonium compound with marked anticholinergic properties and these authors reported promising results in palmar and plantar skin with periods of dryness varying from 14 days to 3 months. They suggest that iontophoresis introduces the drug into both the epidermis and sweat duct, but were unable to explain the prolonged effect. All patients experienced some symptoms from systemic absorption of the drug, some mild and others unacceptable. The method gave disappointing results in axillary hyperhidrosis. Cunliffe, Johnson and Williamson (1972) used poldine methanosulphate (Nacton) successfully in three cases of unilateral hyperhidrosis. But none of these agents has achieved general acceptance for this common condition.

Shelley and Hurley (1975), in their excellent review, state that 'there is not a single topical agent available today which eliminates axillary sweating in the "hyperhidrotic individual" '. They reconsidered the failure of aluminium salts, particularly the chlorhydrate, to act as effectively in the axilla as they did on other areas of skin and, by a patient series of experiments, showed that aluminium chloride hexahydrate or zirconium tetrachloride were the most effective agents, if applied under certain conditions, which they called the 'trinary system'. First, the salt had to be in a concentrated, highly ionised alcohol solution with a high acid pH. Secondly, the application had to be occluded for 2 to 8 h under a Saran or similar wrap or occlusive pad. And finally, it had to be applied when the sweat glands were relatively inactive, e.g. at night. They postulate logical reasons for the success of this approach to axillary hyperhidrosis which, if repeated weekly, ensures comparative freedom from sweating throughout this period. These authors (and Lansdown, 1973) have shown that the strength of aluminium chloride must be 15 per cent or more to achieve these effects and that the pH must be in the region of 2.4 or less. This degree of acidity is very important in depositing the aluminium in the epidermis, possibly reversing the negative change of the keratin. It is too early yet to assess the practical application of this approach to a difficult dermatological problem. At present, the best solution remains the technique of axillary dome resection.

Miscellaneous Formulations

Aluminium chloride

Aluminium salts are effective against a number of organisms, according to Leyden and Kligman (1975). Using a number of different salts, these authors found that a 10 to 20 per cent solution of the chlorhydrate and acetate was better than aluminium acetate alone and that a 30 per cent solution of aluminium chloride (chlorhydrate) was the most effective and equal to Castellani's paint in the control of odour, maceration and toe cracks. Cream and powder formulations were less effective. Marples and Kligman (1974) point out the difficulty of evaluating topical antibacterial agents and stress the mixed nature of infection in areas of maceration where the presence of mycelia can often be regarded as opportunist. It is in this situation that aluminium chloride was found to be effective, as Castellani's paint has been in the past. That it is colourless too, often offers a considerable advantage, particularly since a colourless Castellani's paint was shown to have a feeble action.

Glutaraldehyde

This has been advocated for 'recurrent bullous eruptions of the hands and feet' (pompholyx). Des Groscillers and Brisson (1974) used it as a 10 per cent solution buffered with 5 per cent sodium bicarbonate in water. It was useful in two cases but causes a brown discoloration. It must be refrigerated and is an irritant and sensitiser. We feel that potassium permanganate is equally useful in this condition and less troublesome in several respects.

Silver salts

These have returned to favour recently, partly no doubt because of their low sensitising capacity and simplicity in use. Their tendency to cause a brown discoloration has been their main disadvantage. 'Black wash', an acqueous silver nitrate solution of 0.5 to 2 per cent, is a safe and useful application for leg ulcers and does as much as most other, more 'selective' agents, to reduce the bacterial population. Silver sulphadiazine (Flamazine) has achieved great popularity in the treatment of burns and we have used it with reasonable success in infected leg ulcers. Patch test checks have not so far revealed any sensitisation. In a comparison of silver compounds and combinations in the treatment of burns Lowbury et al (1976) found that all were effective in protecting against infections in the early stage but that, as with other preparations, their effectiveness became less marked with continued use. Sulphonamide-resistant Gram-negative bacilli became predominant, especially with plain silver nitrate. Nevertheless, these agents offer dermatologists an alternative to other, more potentially sensitising agents.

Bufexamac (p-butoxyphenylacethydroxamic acid)

This non-steroid anti-inflammatory agent, introduced in 1965, has been the subject of several reports (Vassant-Thys and Robas, 1970; Grigoriu, 1972; Achten et al, 1973). It was found to have an activity comparable to 0.025 per cent fluocinolone and 0.1 per cent betamethasone. But many of the cases treated had atopic or contact eczema, to which concomitant avoidance or extraneous factors might well play a part in inducing an equal remission. Certainly it has been nowhere as effective, in our hands, in patients with more persistent forms of eczema, though we believe that it does have some anti-inflammatory activity. Since this drug is also given orally and rectally, the absence of sensitisation is important. Smeenk (1973) was the first to demonstrate an allergic reaction. Four further cases have been described. Two of these (Lachapelle, 1975) occurred during treatment of 'superficial phlebitis'. Though still few in relation to its use, they sound a warning note.

α-Hydroxy acids

In a study of more than 60 substances chosen for possible antikeratinogenic properties, Van Scott and Yu (1974) found that the most effective belong to the group of α-hydroxy acids or closely related substances. A thrice daily application of citric, glycolic, lactic, malic, pyruvic and glucuronic acid, for instance, gave excellent results in all forms of ichthyosis except epidermolytic hyperkeratosis. The substances were applied at 5 per cent strength in hydrophilic ointment, though the base was a matter of the patient's preference. Sustained remission was obtained as long as treatment continued.

The use of these agents has been extended to other hyperkeratotic conditions. Five per cent 2-hydroxy-butyric acid abolished the palmar and plantar hyperkeratosis of pityriasis rubra pilaris and a mixture of pyruvic acid and methyl and ethyl pyruvate the lesions of spiny hyperkeratosis.

We have used 5 per cent citric acid in both paraffin and hydrophilic bases (emulsifying ointment B.P.) in a variety of hyperkeratotic conditions. It is certainly a useful adjunct to current therapy but we were seldom able to improve greatly the performance of the traditional salicylic acid ointment. However, we have found that 3 per cent lactic acid in emulsifying (hydrophilic) ointment has been of considerable value to patients suffering from ichthyosis and 'dry-skin' syndromes.

Selenium disulphide

Despite some reservations about the long-term effects of absorption, this continues to be used successfully for the treatment of pityriasis versicolor. Kirby and Borrie (1975) have reported good results in treating confluent and recticulate papillomatosis (Gougerot).

Zinc salts

The use of zinc pyridinium-thiol-*N*-oxide (Zinc Omadine) and of zinc undecylenate has been increasing as antidandruff agents in shampoos, with a high degree of consumer acceptability and a reasonable degree of therapeutic success in mild or moderate cases. Zinc Omadine, a cyclic thiohydroxamic acid, is an active antibacterial and antifungal agent but may owe its success in combating dandruff to other properties, e.g. prevention of aggregation of horny cells into visible flakes (Leyden, McGinley and Kligman, 1975).

Cryotherapy

Although not strictly speaking a form of topical therapy, the revival of interest in this technique of treatment in the last five years and its extension to surgical fields, justify its inclusion in this chapter. Holden and Saunders (1973) reviewed the physical and biological aspects of tissue freezing: rupture of cell membranes, intracellular dehydration and electrolytic disturbance, protein denaturation and cellular hypometabolism as immediate effects; microcirculatory thrombosis and ischaemia as delayed effects; and (possibly) late immunological effects (Shulman, 1968). The reliability of the cell death is enhanced by 'repeat freezing' techniques (Whittaker, 1975), which allow a more rapid effect to take place on the second occasion. For it is the rate of cooling, rather than the level of freezing, that is important. More disruptive crystals were formed in experiments on rodent oral mucosa if 30 min was left between successive freezes (Gill, Fraser and Carter, 1968).

The advantages of liquid nitrogen over carbon dioxide lie in the lower temperature generated and in its ease of application. Its greater availability in the UK in recent years has encouraged dermatologists and surgeons to extend the range of its usefulness. It remains one of the best methods for treating warts; Bunney (1975) believes that it is the treatment of choice for facial warts as it leaves no scarring. We agree with Barr and Coles (1969) that blister formation is not necessary for cure, though the treatment often has to be repeated, especially on hand warts. Leopard (1974) has also treated successfully pseudopyogenic granulomata, some cavernous and capillary haemangiomata (1–3 s; 5 min delay; 10–15 s; refreeze) and premalignant solar keratoses. We have also been impressed with its value in treatment of condylomata within and at the edge of the anal canal. Goldwyn and Rosoff (1969) used it successfully for large haemangiomas in adult patients and Krashen (1970) claimed that it is able to abort an attack of herpes simplex. Lesions in the oral cavity respond particularly well because of the absence of the horny layer, which resist sudden cooling. It is probably the preferred treatment for leukoplakia (vulval as well as oral) and for 'senile' haemangiomas of the mouth. The pain of aphthae is said to be considerably reduced by freezing and some benign cystic conditions may also respond favourably (Poswillo, 1975).

The development of sophisticated cryoprobes and applications and the control of temperature obtained by the use of intradermal thermocouples has extended the range of cryotherapy more securely into the field of malignant tumours. Zacharian (1973) obtained results equivalent to those of ionising radiation. Leopard (1974) had no recurrences in 15 out of 16 patients with basal cell carcinomata treated and followed up for 6 to 24 months.

On a simpler level, liquid nitrogen has been used, as was carbon dioxide before it, for the treatment of nodular and cystic acne. Leyden, Mills and Kligman (1974) applied a cryoprobe to nodular lesions for 20 to 25 s and obtained results equivalent to those from carbon dioxide, nitrous oxide and Freon. Lejman (1971) found a diminution of the cellular infiltrate in rosacea after treatment. No doubt there is a surge of over-enthusiasm, particularly on the part of surgeons, about a form of therapy that has been used, within narrower limits, by dermatologists for many decades. Nevertheless, the refinements added to this technique and the good cosmetic results obtained will encourage the continued use of this effective therapeutic agent.

APPLICATION OF TOPICAL THERAPY

The section that follows brings together various aspects of topical therapy in a few difficult diseases, in which a number of alternative approaches have been described in recent years; and in a few minor but troublesome complaints for which new therapeutic suggestions have been offered.

Psoriasis

For this, the greatest therapeutic problem in dermatology, there is still no specific effective treatment available and no uniformity in management. Many would agree with Coles and Ryan (1975) about the importance of the doctor's psychological approach to the organic problem, but with the numbers involved and the time usually available, most psoriatics fall between the two stools of therapeutic nihilism and over-enthusiastic and potentially harmful treatment.

The use of topical steroids in psoriasis merits special mention. Most would agree that only the fluorinated preparations produce a constant effect in the condition and that they have a valuable and incomparable effect in the treatment of scalp and intertriginous involvement. In other situations their use is permissible, with or without polythene occlusion, to achieve quick control of active and widespread psoriasis before reverting to the more standard tar, dithranol and u.v.l. regimes. It is in the vast number of cases of intermediate severity, however, that one suspects the existence of a gulf between preaching and practice. A tar and salicylic acid ointment is undoubtedly helpful in psoriasis, but the patient will usually be more appreciative of a non-staining corticosteroid, which in most instances will lead to some improvement. The possibility of rebound pustular psoriasis will appear remote to the patient more concerned with some visual and symptomatic relief of his blemishes. Whatever the practitioner's choice of treatment, it must be made in the knowledge of the potential side effects of long-term therapy and there must be an enforceable check on the amount of any corticosteroid prescribed.

The corticosteroids are known inhibitors of epidermal mitosis (Fisher and Maibach, 1971). These authors investigated the effect of a variety of topical antipsoriatic agents on epidermal mitosis and in confirming the antimitotic effect of corticosteroids (and thus giving some rationality to their use) they were unable to demonstrate mitotic inhibition with the other preparations tested (Fisher and Maibach, 1973). Tretinoin increased mitotic activity, while crude coal tar and dithranol had no effect on mitosis in either normal or stripped skin. The very definite therapeutic effect of dithranol must, therefore, be other than through mitotic inhibition. Its uncontroversial usefulness in day to day practice has been extended recently by Seville (1975). In the classical tar bath u.v.l. and dithranol regime, he found that patients often abandoned treatment due to its inconvenience and consumption of time. He omitted u.v.l., talc and dressings and substituted an ordinary bath instead of one containing tar. In place of dithranol paste, this was formulated at 0.5 per cent in a stiff ointment base which the patients found easier to apply and which gave slightly better results than the best paste used previously. The stiff 0.5 per cent dithranol ointment gave quicker results than the paste formulations and so must be applied sparingly initially. This is especially so in areas treated previously with potent fluorinated steroids, if severe irritant reactions are to be avoided. Seville's stiff ointment contains 0.5 per cent dithranol, 0.5 per cent salicylic acid and 2.5 per cent chloroform with hard paraffin B.P. (m.p. 53/55°C) and white soft paraffin, B.P. (m.p. 49°C); equal parts to 100 per cent. The paraffins are heated until part melted, add other substances in chloroform, smooth on slab and store in dark. Studies by Kammereau, Zesch and Schaefer (1975) on the pharmacokinetics of dithranol absorption have given elegant experimental proof of the optimum penetration of dithranol from hydrophobic ointments. Using tritium-labelled dithranol in various bases, they studied biopsies taken from 10 to 100 min after topical application and demonstrated the best penetration of dithranol from vaseline and aqueous woolwax-alcohol ointment and poor penetration from hydrophilic ointments.

Tretinoin is potentially of use in psoriasis, since in low dosage it can induce a well-formed granular layer in the skin (Lawrence and Bern, 1958). Further clinical trials were reported by Peck, Key and Guss (1973), together with a summary of previous reports on vitamin A acid in psoriasis. In general, some improvement seems to occur but on the basis of these reports and our own clinical experience, we agree with Polano in the 1973 edition of this volume that tretinoin offers very little more than the present accepted treatment for psoriasis.

Kaidbey, Petrozzi and Kligman (1975) reported the effect of topical colchicine on stubborn psoriatic plaques. With the reservation that it remains an experimental procedure until more is known of the percutaneous absorption of the antimitotic, the authors found that 1 per cent colchicine in hydrophilic ointment produced substantial resolution of recalcitrant psoriasis, particularly on the trunk. The correspondence on the necessity or otherwise of controls when chronic plaque psoriasis is used as an experimental model makes entertaining reading (Kligman, 1975).

Psoriatic nail dystrophy, a particularly intractable problem, was treated with fluorouracil by Fredriksson (1974). Using a 1 per cent solution, he reported a 75 per cent reduction in the severity of the dystrophy after six months of treatment, the solution being applied daily 'around the margin of the nail, gently massaged into the nail fold and allowed to dry'. Bleeker (1975) reported a longer follow-up on a previous study of intralesional triamcinolone acetonide administered by the Port-o-Jet gun. The matrix was infiltrated three times at intervals of three weeks and 73 per cent of 569 nails in 71 patients showed cure or improvement after an observation period from 5 to 20 months. But there was a recurrence rate of 46 per cent.

The need for a relatively easy, safe and outpatient treatment for psoriasis remains. A ray of black light and hope springs from the technique of photochemotherapy developed at the Massachusetts General Hospital and the subject of a preliminary report by Parrish et al (1974). They report complete clearing in 21 patients with generalised psoriasis after the oral administration of 8-methoxypsoralen and exposure to high intensity longwave ultraviolet light. In 16 of their patients paired comparison showed that methoxsalen and longwave u.v.l. gave better results than methoxy psoralens and conventional u.v.l. In psoriasis, with its accelerated cell cycle, the beneficial effect is thought to result from the inhibition of DNA synthesis by 8-methoxypsoralen and longwave u.v.l. The technique is the subject of trial in many centres and the results are eagerly awaited by all.

Meanwhile, the needs of the patient with this distressing and severely incommoding condition are being met, to some extent, by the increasing membership of the Psoriasis Association, which is doing so much to inform and enlighten patients about the disease and the limitations of wholly effective therapy at the present time. It is currently examining the possible benefits of climatotherapy for patients in the UK, a relaxed and practical form of relief for many patients that is practised widely in other continental countries.

Acne Vulgaris

What is written today, in the unlikely event of its escaping immediate criticism, will almost certainly be the subject of critical comment in the future. It is interesting to note, therefore, that benzoyl peroxide was not mentioned in the topical treatment of acne in the previous edition of this volume and that Polano dismissed it as a useful drug on account of its sensitising capacity. Although sensitisation is a hazard (Poole, Griffith and McMillan, 1970), the drug in cream foundation (sometimes with the addition of hydrocortisone) and in gels containing a concentration of 5 to 10 per cent has earned an undoubted and popular place in the daily topical therapy of acne. Bleaching of the scalp hair (Bleiberg, Brodkin and Abbey, 1973) may occur occasionally and mirrors its industrial use as a bleaching agent for flour. In the main benzoyl peroxide acts as a 'peeling' agent, but Fulton and Pablo (1974) reported its capacity in a gel form to decrease fatty acids in sebum as effectively as systemic tetracycline. The same authors investigated the topical effect of antibiotics in acne on the premise that, when systemically administered, they inhibit *Corynebacterium acnes* and reduce the hydrolysis of triglycerides in sebum. They found that erythromycin, in a concentration of 2 per cent in ethyl alcohol, ethyl glycol monoethyl ether and propylene glycol (ratio 2:2:1), reduced the fatty acid/fatty ester ratio in sebum with corresponding diminution of inflammatory lesions in 10 acne patients. The effect on comedones was negligible and the authors recommend combining the antibiotic therapy with follicular irritants such as tretinoin.

II

Tretinoin (Retin-A) in the form of a 0.025 per cent w/w solution has now an established place in acne therapy, particularly where comedone formation is pronounced. The impression one gains from individual clinicians varies from the enthusiastic to the lukewarm, with reports of either outstanding success or of deep disappointment. Used in cases with the correct morphology, the manufacturers' instructions should be consisely followed. Kligman et al (1973) have explained the management of the preparation's irritancy, the adverse effects from sun exposure and the hypopigmentation which is occasionally produced. Copyright apart, these comments might usefully be supplied with the product. Tretinoin in repeated courses is outstandingly effective in the treatment of senile comedones (Kligman, Plewig and Mills, 1971) and is the treatment of choice in the difficult and otherwise resistant condition of steroid induced acne (Mills, Leyden and Kligman, 1973). It is discussed elsewhere in this chapter.

It is always refreshing to see questioned the standard, routine and time-honoured principles of topical acne therapy. Mills and Kligman (1972) have pointed out the potential comedogenicity of sulphur and, in what they term 'acne detergicans', they question the advisability of obsessional soap cleansing of the skin in acne (Mills and Kligman, 1975). They point out that salts of fatty acids contained in soaps, as well as hexachlorophane contained in some skin cleansers, are mildly comedogenic in the rabbit ear bioassay. They suggest that many acne sufferers are compulsive face washers and that these substances may occasionally be responsible for multitudes of small comedones and papulo-pustules, all at the same stage of development, involving the chin and cheeks.

Warts

Progress in antiviral therapy, however limited, has naturally been adapted to the possible control of this ubiquitous viral disease. Unfortunately, the natural history of viral warts and the unpredictable manner of their disappearance makes the assessment of results extremely difficult. Hursthouse (1975) and Almeida and Concalves (1975) used 5-fluorouracil. The former, using a 5 per cent cream, occluded, obtained a greater response than to a placebo but noted onycholysis as a side-effect. The latter found no effect when used alone but better results when it was incorporated in a 10 per cent salicylic acid varnish. Bunney (1975) obtained a cure rate of 46 to 53 per cent in mosaic warts. 5-Fluorouracil has been more consistently successful in the treatment of condylomata acuminata, particularly when perianal (Haye, 1974; Handojo and Pardjono, 1973; Nels and Fourie, 1973). A high cure rate was obtained.

Other cytotoxic agents have been used. Morison (1975) found that 10/13 patients responded within four weeks to 40 per cent IDU in a cream base (occluded) as opposed to 3/9 who used the same strength of IDU in DMSO over the same period. DNCB was used by Greenberg, Smith and Katz (1973); but a persistent eczematous reaction may follow. Since many children are or become sensitive to colophony in plaster, a selective treatment with colophony paint might be safer. However, it seems unnecessary to go to such lengths in destroying what is essentially a benign self-destroying lesion. Bunney's mixture of salicylic acid, lactic acid and flexible collodion in the ratio 1:1:4 (Bunney et al, 1971) gave as good results in her hands as liquid nitrogen and was particularly effective in plantar warts. However, all forms of treatment are assisted by spontaneous remission and most results are influenced by it. The use of antiviral and cytotoxic agents mentioned merely touches the fringe of the problem but may provide a stimulus for further studies. Wart cures have come and gone from time immemorial and the cold facts of Barr and Coles' survey of 1969 still stand as a reminder that many non-specific remedies all tend to give about the same cure rate.

Mycosis Fungoides

Although rare, this form of malignant lymphoma, with an origin in multiple foci in the skin, poses formidable management problems in its cutaneous and extracutaneous forms. Fuks, Bagshaw and Farber (1974) have suggested a new four-staging classification based on clinical, histopathological, radiological and surgical staging (laparotomy) procedures, and a cooperative study sponsored in the United States by the National Cancer Institute and the National Program for Dermatology is investigating the pathology of the disease and its treatment by chemotherapy, radiotherapy and immunotherapy.

When the disease involves the skin only, long periods of remission can be induced by total body radiation with electron beams (Fuks, Bagshaw and Farber, 1973) or by the topical application of nitrogen mustard (HN2). HN2 is an effective and relatively easily available remedy and Van Scott and Kalmanson (1973) have reported on its use in 76 patients with mycosis fungoides limited to the skin with no palpable lymphadenopathy and no evidence of internal dissemination. A fresh solution of 10 mg of the drug dissolved in approximately 60 ml of tap water is applied to the whole body surface, the frequency varying with the extent of the disease but varying from twice weekly to twice daily, with applications once a week following resolution of the cutaneous lesions. Over a four-year treatment period the authors reported 50 per cent to be free of detectable disease, with 13 having remissions extending beyond two years. Our own experience confirms the usefulness of this form of treatment in allaying the signs and symptoms of the cutaneous stage of mycosis fungoides. NH2 is a frequent cause of delayed hypersensitivity reactions and such sensitivity has been observed to induce remissions (Ratner, Waldorf and Van Scott, 1968). The reaction is extremely uncomfortable for the patient, however, and the drug is capable of inducing remissions without the hypersensitivity reaction (Van Scott and Winters,

1970). Van Scott and Kalmanson (1973) report desensitisation of sensitised patients by daily minute intravenous doses of the drug and with the same procedure have achieved a specific immunological tolerance to NH2 prior to topical therapy. Constantine, Fuks and Farber (1975) have reported desensitisation in three of six sensitised patients using extremely weak concentrations for total body application.

Alternative topical therapy for mycosis fungoides is suggested by Zackheim and Epstein (1975) in the form of nitrosourea compounds. These preparations are effective but produced an irritant contact dermatitis in half of the patients treated. They may be useful alternative to NH2, with which there is no cross reaction (see section above).

Corns and Calluses

Two new methods of treatment have been advocated for this common and painful affliction, which receives scant attention in textbooks. The first is somewhat unexpected and will need to be assessed by further experiences. Gunther (1972) obtained excellent results by treating palmar callosities with 0.1 per cent retinoic acid in yellow soft paraffin, comparing this with a placebo. Regression occurred in three weeks and could be maintained by bi-weekly treatment 'and avoidance of friction'. The second method is ingenious, logical and apparently very successful. Balkin (1975) describes a method of injecting a fluid silicone between the corn and the underlying bony prominence. No complications were noted and cure was obtained in two-thirds of the cases.

Corns will continue to occur as long as women wear shoes that cause friction or deform the foot. Severe cases will still require surgical intervention. But this new approach is attractive and deserves further study on a wide scale.

Black Hairy Tongue

Many forms of treatment have been advocated for the persistent form of this condition. Most rely on adjuvant scrubbing with an old toothbrush and patients themselves have usually found this the most satisfactory short-term remedy. But such repeated abrasion may stimulate further hyperkeratosis and an effective keratolytic would provide a more satisfactory form of therapy. The loosening of the hyperkeratotic strands that form the 'hair' should be amenable to agents used for ichthyosis or hyperkeratosis elsewhere.

Pegum (1971) advocated 40 per cent urea in water. Citric acid, 5 per cent in spirit was ineffective in our hands and retinoic acid, 0.025 per cent lotion, was badly tolerated in three recent personal cases; even persistence for six weeks in one case did not achieve a good result. Much of the difficulty lies in the formulation of a base that will allow intimate contact with the tongue in the presence of movement, saliva and eating.

ADVERSE EFFECTS

Enthusiastic reports of trials on new drugs are usually coupled with the observation that 'sensitisation did not occur'. This freedom from a major disadvantage of topical therapy induces a sense of security, sometimes justified after wide-scale use but sometimes requiring modification in the light of experience. Tolnaftate, for instance, continues to carry a very low rate of sensitisation after many years use, despite reports by Gellen, Maibach and Wachs (1972) and Emmett and Davis (1973). Sensitisation to active medicaments, vehicles and preservatives has been dealt with in the previous edition of this book (Cronin and Wilkinson, 1973) and elsewhere (Wilkinson, 1972). No new major sensitisers have emerged subsequently but there have been further reports of sensitivity reactions to established drugs and additives and a few reports concerning relatively new topical agents. It is important that the dermatologist is aware of these but, equally, that such examples are seen in proportion to the extent of use, formulation used and method of application. We shall also include briefly in this section some adverse reactions due to mechanisms other than allergic ones.

Active Agents

The 'caine' mixture, widely used as anaesthetic ointments and creams, continues to provide a major source of sensitisation—8.4 per cent in the North American Contact Dermatitis Group figures for 1972 to 1974 (Rudner et al, 1975). As lignocaine (Xylocaine) is chemically different and carries so much less risk, it is regrettable that this has not been more widely used as a replacement.

Reaction to antimycotic agents are often reported, probably because of their wide use, but seldom in more than one or two patients. Thus, Meneghini and Angelini (1975) report two cases of sensitivity to pyrrolnitrin, a recently introduced antimycotic. This is related to 1-chloro-2,4-dinitrobenzene. Miconazole nitrate has caused a very few reactions (Degref and Verhoeve, 1975; van Ketel, 1974). Five reactions to bufexamac have now been recorded (Lachapelle, 1975).

Irgasan DP 300, a new antibacterial and deodorant agent, showed no sensitivity on monitored testing by ourselves and others until two cases were reported by Roed-Petersen, Auken and Hjorth (1975). It is widely used in toiletries, foot powders, etc., in a strength of 0.12 to 0.2 per cent, and these isolated cases should cause no undue alarm. But more cases may be expected in view of its extensive field of application.

Retinoic acid (vitamin A acid) is a potential irritant but allergic reactions are rare. However, Jordan, Higgins and Dvorak (1975) reported two cases who reacted to as little as 0.00625 per cent and whose sensitivity was confirmed bv leucocyte migration inhibition tests.

A particularly unfortunate side-effect of the use of hydroquinone for depigmentation is the hyperpigmentation that may occur as a result of sensitisation (Bentley-Phillips and Bayles, 1974).

A warning against the use of podophyllin application for venereal warts in pregnancy was sounded by Chamberlain, Reynolds and Yeoman (1972). Severe peripheral neuropathy and interuterine death occurred in a young woman whose florid vulval warts were treated with 25 per cent podophyllin resin. It is fair to add that 7.5 ml (equivalent to 1.88 g podophyllin) was used in one application. Nevertheless, this drug is capable of being absorbed rapidly and is certainly teratogenic in rats (Kreybig, Preussman and Kreybig, 1970). Care should be exercised, therefore, in treating vulval condylomata in young women, who should always be asked about possible early pregnancy.

The pattern of sensitivity to topical agents obviously differs from country to country. Topical sulphonamides and chloramphenicol are quite frequently used in Germany and East Europe but rarely in Great Britain. Medicament-induced photosensitisation is more prevalent in equatorial countries and may seldom be seen in temperate zones. Even within the same country, local preferences dictate the choice of steroid or other application. Thus, ethylene-diamine is a common sensitiser where Mycolog cream is widely used but far less frequently seen in the UK where Triadcortyl is less popular.

Leg ulcer and eczema

Patients with leg ulcers, with or without eczema, give a very high figure of patch test reactions, especially to medicaments. There have been a number of reports illustrating this in recent years (Malten, Kniper and van der Staak, 1973; Angelini, Mantuccio and Meneghini, 1975). Our own series confirms the frequency of sensitivity to neomycin, soframycin and other medicaments used for the treatment of leg ulcers. The incidence of sensitivity to lanolin is far higher than that found in other dermatoses; the reason is not clear but some of the reactions may be due to a heightened instability of the skin and perhaps not truly allergic. Further work is needed to elucidate this problem.

Pressure sores

Walshe (1975) patch tested 122 patients in a spinal injuries centre. 40.1 per cent of patients gave positive reactions to medicaments or topically applied agents. Of the 69 positive results obtained in 49 patients, mercaptobenzthiazole accounted for 8, neomycin for 7, and colophony for 6. Fucidin, lanolin and Vioform contributed another 9 cases and the remainder were almost all related to therapeutic agents. The pattern was similar to that found in leg ulcers in our series in the same cultural environment. If colophony-based plaster, neomycin (and soframycin) and lanolin-based products were avoided, the incidence of contact sensitivity would be very much lower in these patients. None of these is irreplaceable and there is no reason why this latrogenic disease should continue to occur.

Vehicles and Preservatives

The situation in regard to these has changed little. Parabens, despite their very wide use, do not seem to us to be important sensitisers when the concentration remains low. Chlorocresol, giving less than 1 per cent positive reactions on all patients tested, is not a major sensitiser but must not be overlooked as it is a preservative in many steroid preparations and in Aqueous Cream, B.P. Burry et al (1975) found cross-sensitisation with chloroxylenol. It may be responsible, therefore, for an unexpected resistance to conventional therapy in common therapeutic situations (Burry, et al, 1975). A girl of 12 years with atopic dermatitis had been treated with very moderate success with steroid cream and Aqueous Cream for cleaning. On admission, patch testing revealed chlorocresol sensitivity (2+). A change of prescription, with no increase of steroid strength, brought about a very considerable improvement. Chloroacetamide was incriminated by Smeenk and Prins (1972) as a preservative in Hirudoid ointment; parachlorometaxylenol by Storrs (1975); propyl gallate by Liden (1975). But these must be seen in the context of the wide use of the agents in which they are presented. Rudzki and Zakrawski (1975) related the incidence of reactions to medicaments to the frequency of their use (in Poland) and found an unusually high rate to mercurials and balsam of Peru; chloramphenicol rated surprisingly low in view of the widespread use in that country. In the German Democratic Republic it has been possible to exclude certain substances from official lists on account of their sensitivity properties, e.g. turpentine, balsam of Peru, benzocaine and diphenyldramine in various products (Beerbohm, 1975).

An unusual reaction of acute pharyngeal obstruction was presumed to be due to a first-aid spray containing approximately 1/1000 thiomersal (Maibach, 1975). Contact urticaria to cephalosporin was reported by Tuft (1975), adding yet another agent to several producing this immediate-type reaction (ammonium persulphate, cobalt chloride, penicillin, aspirin, alcohol, etc.). This is presumed to be non-immunological.

Finally, we should mention the interesting observation of Mobacken and his colleagues concerning triphenylmethane dyes. They demonstrated an interference with tissue regeneration in skin wounds (Mobacken, Zelderfeldt and Ahrén, 1973; Mobacken and Zelderfeldt, 1973) and related this to a delayed onset of collagen formation. Further studies of crystal violet on rabbits showed an impaired metabolism of connective tissue cells in vitro and a reduction in oxygen consumption rates at a strength of $10\,\mu g/ml$ (Mobacken, Ahonen and Zelderfeldt, 1974). This work arose from earlier observation of delayed healing in clinical use of triphenylmethane dyes. These dyes have been used for several decades, usually most satisfactorily. But in a recent trial of a crystal violet gel preparation we have also noted an apparent inhibition of healing in a minority of cases in which it was used in leg ulcers. This is an idiosyncratic reaction, reminiscent of the necrotic reactions to dequalinium chloride and seems to us to warrant observation and further study rather than discontinuance of a useful and effective local antibacterial agent.

REFERENCES

INTRODUCTION

Polano, M. K. (1973) Topical therapy. In *Recent Advances in Dermatology*, ed. Rook, A., Edinburgh and London: Churchill Livingstone.

BASES AND EMOLLIENTS

Almeya, J. & Burt, B. W. (1974) Double blind controlled study of treatment of atopic eczema with a preparation of hydrocortisone in a new drug delivery system versus betamethasone 17-valerate. *British Journal of Dermatology*, **91**, 579.

Beare, J. M. (1971) Advance in the treatment of diseases of the skin. *Practitioner*, **207**, 450.

Christophers, E. (1970) Die Wanderungskinetik postmitotischer Epidermiszellen. Autoradiographische Untersuchungen. *Archiv für klinische und experimentelle Dermatologie*, **236**, 161.

Delacrétaz, J., Etter, J. C. & Emah, M. (1971) Étude comparative du comportement de le peau du cobayé en présence d'un ether ou d'un ester de polyéthylene glycol. *Dermatologica*, **143**, 345.

Gaylarde, P. M. & Sarkany, I. (1973) Advantages of measuring epidermal thickness as an index of response to stimulation. *Transactions of the St John's Hospital Dermatological Society*, **59**, 235.

Kligman, A. L. & Mills, O. H. (1972) Acne cosmetica. *Archives of Dermatology*, **106**, 843.

Pope, F. M., Krees, J., Wells, R. S. & Lewis, R. G. S. (1972) Out-patient treatment of ichthyosis: a double blind trial of ointments. *British Journal of Dermatology*, **86**, 291.

Sarkany, I. & Gaylarde, P. M. (1973) Thickening of guinea-pig epidermis due to application of commonly used ointment bases. *Transactions of St John's Hospital Dermatological Society*, **59**, 241.

KERATOLYTICS

Baden, H. P. & Alper, J. C. (1973) A keratolytic gel containing salicylic acid in propylene glycol. *Journal of Investigative Dermatology*, **61**, 330.

Baden, H. P. & Goldsmith, L. A. (1972) Propylene glycol with occlusion for treatment of ichthyosis. *Journal of the American Medical Association*, **220** (4), 579.

Baden, H. P. (1974) Treatment of hyperkeratotic dermatitis of the palms. *Archives of Dermatology*, **110**, 737.

Marks, R., Davies, M. & Catell, A. (1975) An explanation for the keratolytic effect of salicylic acid. *Journal of Investigative Dermatology*, **64**, 283.

RETINOIC ACID

Jordan, Jr W. P., Higgins, M. & Dvorak, J. (1975) Allergic dermatitis to all-trans-retinoic acid; cutaneous and leucocyte migration inhibition testing. *Contact Dermatitis*, **5**, 306.

Polano, M. K. (1973) Topical therapy. In *Recent Advances in Dermatology*, ed. Rook, A., p. 397. Edinburgh and London: Churchill Livingstone.

Symposium (1975) The therapeutic use of vitamin A acid. International Symposium, Flims, Switzerland, January 1975. *Acta dermato-venereologica*, **55**, Suppl. 74, 145–185.

ANTIBACTERIALS AND GERMICIDES

Abbott, L. M., Buckfield, P. M., Ferry, D. G., Malcolm, D. S. & McQueen, E. G. (1972) Blood levels of hexachlorophane in neonates. *Australia Paediatric Journal*, **8**, 246.

Boroda, C. & Monzas, G. J. (1974) The protection of the skin of fracture patients immobilised in plaster of Paris. *Surgery, St Louis*, **75**, 638.

Butcher, H. R., Ballinger, W. F., Gravens, D. L., Dewar, N. E., Ledlie, E. F. & Barthell, W. F. (1973) Hexachlorophane concentration in the blood of operating room personnel. *Archives of Surgery*, **107**, 70.

Bye, P. G. T., Morison, W. & Rhodes, E. L. (1975) The absorption of hexachlorophane from Ultralanum ointment. *British Journal of Dermatology*, **93**, 209.

Curley, A., Hawk, R. E., Kimbrough, R. D., Natherson, G. & Finberg, L. (1971) Dermal absorption of hexachlorophane in infants. *Lancet*, 2, 296.

Frank, L. (1959) Povidone-iodine shampoo for seborrhoeic dermatitis and pyodermas. *New York State Journal of Medicine*, 59, 2892.

Georgiade, N. G. & Harris, W. A. (1972) Medical and surgical antisepsis with Betadine microbicides. *Proceedings of a Symposium in Miami*, p. 113. Fredk. Purdue Co.

Gilmore, O. J. A. & Martin, T. D. M. (1974) The aetiology and prevention of wound infection in appendicectomy. *British Journal of Surgery*, 61, 281.

Gilmore, O. J. A. & Sanderson, P. J. (1975) Prophylactic inter-parietal povidone-iodine in abdominal surgery. *British Journal of Surgery*, 62, 792.

Greenberg, L. (1961) Comparative laboratory evaluation of antiseborroeic dermatological preparations. *Journal of the Pharmaceutical Society*, 50, 480.

Hudson, A. L. (1973) Betadine skin cleanser in acne vulgaris. *Clinical Trials Journal*, 1, 1973.

Hjorth, N. (1974) Personal communication.

Konopka, E. A., Kimble, E. F., Zogonas, H. C. & Heyman, H. (1975) Antimicrobial effectiveness of Locacorten-Vioform cream in secondary infection of common dermatoses. *Dermatologica*, 151, 1.

Kopelman, A. E. (1973) Cutaneous absorption of hexachlorophane in low birth-weight infants. *Journal of Paediatrics*, 82, 972.

Larson, D. L. (1968) Studies show hexachlorophane causes burn syndrome. *Hospitals*, 42, 63.

Leyden, J. J., Marples, R. R. & Kligman, A. M. (1974) *Staphylococcus aureus* in the lesions of atopic dermatitis. *British Journal of Dermatology*, 90, 525.

Lilly, H. A. & Lowbury, E. J. L. (1971) Disinfection of the skin: an assessment of some new preparations. *British Medical Journal*, 3, 674.

Lockhart, J. D. (1972) How toxic is hexachlorophane? *Paediatrics*, 50, 229.

Lowbury, E. J. L. & Lilly, H. A. (1973) Use of 4% chlorhexidine detergent solution (Hibiscrub) and other methods of skin disinfection. *British Medical Journal*, 1, 510.

Lowbury, E. J. L., Lilly, H. A. & Ayliffe, G. A. J. (1974) Pre-operative disinfection of surgeon's hands: use of alcoholic solutions and effects of gloves on skin flora. *British Medical Journal*, 4, 369.

Noble, W. C., Valkenburg, H. A. & Wolters, C. H. (1967) Carriage of *Staphylococcus aureus* in the lesions of atopic dermatitis. *British Journal of Dermatology*, 90, 525.

Pietsch, J. & Meakins, J. L. (1976) Complications of Povidone-iodine absorption of topically treated burn patients. *Lancet*, 1, 280.

Powell, H. A., Swarner, O., Gluck, L. & Lampert, P. (1973) Hexachlorophane myclinopathy in premature infants. *Journal of Paediatrics*, 82, 976.

Shelanski, M. & Shelanski, H. (1956) Polyvinyl-pyrrolidine iodine: history, toxicity and therapeutic uses. *Journal of the International College of Surgeons*, 25, 727.

Zaynoun, S. T., Matta, M. T. & Uwayda, M. M. (1974) Topical antibiotics in pyodermas. *British Journal of Dermatology*, 90, 331.

TOPICAL ANTIVIRALS AND PHOTO-INACTIVATION

Baringer, J. R. & Swoveland, P. (1973) Recovery of herpes simplex virus from human trigeminal ganglions. *New England Journal of Medicine*, 288, 648.

Cheng, T.-W., Fiumara, N. & Weinstein, L. (1975) Methylene blue and light therapy for herpes simplex. *Archives of Dermatology*, 111, 265.

Cheng, T.-W. & Weinstein, L. (1975) Eczema herpeticum. Treatment with methylene blue and light. *Archives of Dermatology*, 111, 1175.

Dawber, R. (1974) Idoxurine in herpes zoster. Further evaluation of intermittent topical therapy. *British Medical Journal*, 2, 526.

Felber, T. D., Smith, E. B., Knox, J. M., Wllis, C. & Melnick, L. (1973) Photodynamic inactivation of herpes simplex. *Journal of the American Medical Association*, 223, 289.

Hall-Smith, S. P., Corrigan, M. J. & Gilkes, M. J. (1962) Treatment of herpes simplex with 5-iodo-2-dioxyuridine. *British Medical Journal*, 2, 1515.

Herrman, E. C. (1961) Plaque inhibition test for detection of specific inhibitors of DNA containing viruses. *Proceeding of the Society for Experimental Biology and Medicine*, 107, 142.

Jarratt, M. T. & Felber, T. (1975) More on neutral red fluorescence. *Archives of Dermatology*, 111, 657.

Juel-Jensen, B. E. (1970) Herpetic whitlows: results of treatment with idoxuridine. *Journal of American College Health Association*, **18**, 227.

Juel-Jensen, B. E. (1973) Herpes simplex and zoster. *British Medical Journal*, **1**, 406.

Juel-Jensen, B. E. (1974) Virus disease. *Practitioner*, **213**, 508.

Juel-Jensen, B. E. & MacCallum, F. O. (1964) Treatment of herpes simplex lesions of the face with idoxuridine. *British Medical Journal*, **2**, 987.

Juel-Jensen, B. E. & MacCallum, F. O. (1972) *Herpes Simplex, Varicella and Zoster*. London: Heinemann.

Juel-Jensen, B. E. & MacCallum, F. O. (1974) Idoxuridine in herpes zoster. *British Medical Journal*, **3**, 41.

Juel-Jensen, B. E., MacCallum, F. O., Mackenzie, A. M. R. & Pike, M. D. (1970) Treatment of zoster with idoxuridine in dimethyl-sulphoxide. Results of two double-blind controlled trials. *British Medical Journal*, **4**, 776.

Kaufman, M. E. (1962) Clinical care of herpes simplex keratitis by 5-iodo-2-dioxyonidine. *Proceedings of the Society for Experimental Biology and Medicine*, **109**, 251.

Kibrick, S. & Katz, A. S. (1970) Topical idoxuridine in recurrent herpes simplex. *Annals of New York Academy of Sciences*, **173**, 83.

Kligman, A. M. (1965) Topical pharmacology and toxicology of dimethylsulphoxide, Parts 1 and 2. *Journal of the American Medical Association*, **193**, 796, 923.

Lynfield, Y. L., Farhangi, M. & Runnels, J. L. (1969) Herpes simplex skin infection in men treated with idoxuridine in dimethylsulphoxide. *British Medical Journal*, **2**, 805.

MacCallum, F. O & Juel-Jensen, B. E. (1966) Herpes simplex skin infection in men treated with idoxuridine in dimethylsulphoxide. *British Medical Journal*, **2**, 805.

Montgomerie, J. Z., Becroft, D. M. O., Crozson, M. C. & Doak, P. B. (1969) Herpes simplex virus infection after renal transplantation. *Lancet*, **2**, 867.

Wallis, C. & Melnick, J. L. (1964) Irreversible photosensitisation of viruses. *Virology*, **23**, 520.

Wallis, C. & Melnick, J. L. (1965) Photodynamic inactivation of animal viruses: a review. *Photochemistry and Photobiology*, **4**, 159.

ANTIFUNGAL PREPARATIONS

Battistini, F., Zaias, N., Sierra, R. & Rebell, E. (1974) Clinical antifungal activity of thiaben dazole. *Archives of Dermatology*, **109**, 695.

Botter, A. A. (1972) Further experiences with miconazole nitrate; a broad spectrum antimycotic with antibacterial activity. *Mycosen*, **14**, 187.

British Medical Journal Today's Drugs (1967) Tolnaftate. *British Medical Journal*, **3**, 785.

Carr, J. F. & Lewis, C. W. (1975) Tinea nigra palmaris. Treatment with thiabendazole topically. *Archives of Dermatology*, **111**, 904.

Clayton, Y. M. & Connor, B. L. (1973) Comparison of clotrimazole cream, Whitfield's ointment and nystatin ointment for the topical treatment of ringworm infections, pityriasis versicolor, erythrasma and candidiasis. *British Journal of Dermatology*, **89**, 297.

Emmett, E. A. & Marrs, J. M. (1973) Allergic contact dermatitis from tolnaftate. *Archives of Dermatology*, **108**, 98.

Epstein, W. L., Shah, V. P., Jones, H. E. & Riegelman, S. (1975) Topically applied griseofulvin in prevention and treatment of Trichophyton mentagrophytes. *Archives of Dermatology*, **111**, 1293.

Gellin, G. A., Maibach, H. I. & Wachs, G. N. (1972) Contact allergy to tolnaftate. *Archives of Dermatology*, **106**, 715.

Gentles, J. C., Evans, E. G. V. & Jones, G. A. (1974) Control of tinea pedis in a swimming bath. *British Medical Journal*, **2**, 577.

Kligman, A. M. & Marples, R. (1974) Methods for evaluating topical antibacterial agents on human skin. *Antimicrobe Chemotherapy*, **5**, 322.

Knight, A. G. (1973) Human models for in vivo and in vitro assessment of topical antifungal compounds. *British Journal of Dermatology*, **89**, 505.

Kunicki, A. (1974) Ergebrisse der Clotrimazol-Therapie bei Candida und Trichomonas Infektionea. *Azneimittel-Forschung*, **24**, 534.

Marger, W. & Adam, D. (1971) Bayer 5097, a new orally applicable antifungal substance with broad spectum activity. *Acta paediatrica*, **60**, 341.

Risold, J. C. & Peguegnot, F. (1969) Étude en dermatologie d'un nouvel antimycosique de contact à large spectre. *Journal Medical de Lyon*, **50**, 233.

Robinson, H. J., Silber, R. H. & Graessia, O. E. (1969) Thiabendazole: toxicological, pharmacological and antifungal properties. *Texas Reports on Biological Medicine*, **27**, 537.

CORTICOSTEROIDS

Abell, E. (1972) Treatment of psoriatic nail dystrophy. *British Journal of Dermatology*, **86**, 79.

Alexander, S. & Lyne, C. (1973) A preliminary clinical trial of hydrocortisone 17-butyrate. *British Journal of Clinical Practice*, **27**, 177.

Almeyda, J. & Burt, B. W. (1974) Double blind controlled study of treatment of atopic eczema with a preparation of hydrocortisone in a new drug delivery system versus betamethasone 17-valerate. *British Journal of Dermatology*, **91**, 579.

Ashurst, P. J. (1972) Hydrocortisone 17-butyrate, a new synthetic topical corticosteroid. *British Journal of Clinical Practice*, **26**, 269.

Bazex, A., Dupré, A., Christol, B. & Labrousse, Cl. (1972) Le Granulome Glutéal Infantile (Tappeiner et Pfleger). Faut-il conçevoir comme des 'fluorides vegentantes de contact' ou des 'halogenides du bourrisson'? *Annales de Dermatologie et de Syphiligraphie*, **99**, 121.

Bleeker, J. J. (1974) Intralesional triamcinolone acetonide using the Port-o-Jet and needle injection in localised dermatoses. *British Journal of Dermatology*, **91**, 97.

Boxley, J. D., Dawber, R. P. R. & Summerley, R. (1975) Generalised pustular psoriasis on withdrawal of clobetasol propionate ointment. *British Medical Journal*, **2**, 255.

Burrows, D. (1969) Flurandrenolone tape. *Transactions of St John's Hospital Dermatological Society*, **55**, 103.

Dupré, A. & Fournié, A. (1973) Leucodermies secondaires à des injections de corticoides. *Bulletin de la Société française de dermatologie et de syphiligraphie*, **80**, 616.

du Vivier, A. & Staughton, R. N. (1975) Tachyphylaxis to the action of topically applied corticosteroids. *Archives of Dermatology*, **111**, 581.

Eaglstein, W. H., Farzad, A. & Caplan, L. (1974) Topical corticosteroid therapy: efficacy of frequent applications. *Archives of Dermatology*, **110**, 995.

Feiwel, M., Munro, D. D. & James, V. H. T. (1967) Effect of topically applied 0.1 per cent betamethasone 17-valerate (Betnovate) ointment on the adrenal function of children. *XIII Congressus Internationalis Dermatologica*, p. 202. Berlin: Springer-Verlag.

Feldman, R. J. & Maibach, H. I. (1974) Percutaneous penetration of hydrocortisone with urea. *Archives of Dermatology*, **109**, 58.

Fry, L. & Wight, D. G. P. (1965) Plasma cortisol levels after topical use of fluocinolone acetonide. *British Journal of Dermatology*, **77**, 582.

Ive, F. A. & Marks, R. (1968) Tinea incognita. *British Medical Journal*, **3**, 149.

Jacoby, R. H. & Gilkes, J. J. H. (1974) A new urea/hydrocortisone powder-cream compared with other topical corticosteroid preparations. *Current Medical Research Opinion*, **2**, 474.

James, V. H. T., Munro, D. D. & Feiwel, M. (1967) Pituitary-adrenal function after occlusive topical therapy with betamethasone 17-valerate. *Lancet*, **2**, 1059.

Kestel, J. L. (1971) Hypopigmentation following the use of Cordran tape. *Archives of Dermatology*, **103**, 460.

Leydon, J. J. & Kligman, A. M. (1974) Steroid rosacea. *Archives of Dermatology*, **110**, 619.

Macmillan, A. L. (1972) Unusual features of scabies associated with topical fluorinated steroids. *British Journal of Dermatology*, **87**, 496.

Maleville, J., Grosshans, A. E., Wassmer, A., Beauvais, A. & Heid, A. (1973) Granulome Gluteal Infantile apparu après application locale prolongeé d'un corticoide fluore. *Bulletin de la Société française de dermatologie et de syphiligraphie*, **80**, 15.

Malone, T., Haleblian, J. K., Poulsen, B. J. & Burdick, K. H. (1974) Development and evaluation of ointment and cream vehicles for a new topical steroid, fluclorolone acetonide. *British Journal of Dermatology*, **90**, 187.

Mooney, A. F. (1974) Dilution of topical corticosteroid preparations. *British Journal of Dermatology*, **90**, 109.

Munro, D. D. & Clift, D. C. (1973) Pituitary–adrenal function after prolonged use of topical corticosteroids. *British Journal of Dermatology*, **88**, 381.

Munro, D. D. & Wilson, L. (1975) Clobetasone butyrate, a new topical corticosteroid. Clinical activity and effect on pituitary-adrenal axis function and model of epidermal atrophy. *British Medical Journal*, **3**, 626.

Polano, M. K. (1973) Topical therapy. In *Recent Advances in Dermatology*, ed. Rook, A., p. 372. Edinburgh and London: Churchill Livingstone.

Polano, M. K. & Kanaar, P. (1973) A clinical trial with hydrocortisone butyrate cream in eczema. *British Journal of Dermatology*, **88**, 83.

Scoggins, E. B. (1962) Decrease of urinary corticosteroids following application of fluocinolone acetonide under an occlusive dressing. *Journal of Investigative Dermatology*, **39**, 473.

Sneddon, I. B. (1969) Adverse effects of topical fluorinated corticosteroids in rosacea. *British Medical Journal*, **1**, 671.

Sneddon, I. B. (1972) Perioral dermatitis. *British Journal of Dermatology*, **87**, 430.

Sneddon, I. B. (1973) A trial of hydrocortisone butyrate in the treatment of rosacea and perioral dermatitis. *British Journal of Dermatology*, **89**, 505.

Sparkes, C. G. & Wilson, L. (1974) The clinical evaluation of a new topical steroid, clobetasol propionate. *British Journal of Dermatology*, **90**, 197.

Sparrow, G. & Abell, E. (1975) Granuloma annulare and necrobiosis lipoidica treated by jet injector. *British Journal of Dermatology*, **93**, 85.

Staughten, R. C. D. & August, P. J. (1975) Cushing's syndrome and pituitary adrenal suppression due to clobetasol propionate. *British Medical Journal*, **2**, 419.

Tan, R. S.-H., & Samman, P. D. (1974) Pustular psoriasis with adrenal suppression following topical corticosteroids. *Proceedings of the Royal Society of Medicine*, **67**, 719.

Verbov, J. L. & Abell, E. (1970) Jet gun intralesional therapy. *Transactions of St John's Hospital Dermatological Society*, **56**, 49.

Walker, S. R., Wilson, L., Fry, L. & James, V. H. T. (1974) The effect on plasma corticosteroid levels of the short-term topical application of clobetasol propionate. *British Journal of Dermatology*, **91**, 339.

Weber, G. (1972) Contra-indication or intolerance reaction to strong steroids. *British Journal of Dermatology*, **86**, 253.

Whitfield, M. & McKenzie, A. W. (1975) A new formulation of 0.1 per cent hydrocortisone cream with vasoconstrictor activity and clinical effectiveness. *British Journal of Dermatology*, **92**, 585.

Wilson, L., Williams, D. I. T Marsh, S. D. (1973) Plasma corticosteroid levels in out-patients treated with topical steroids. *British Journal of Dermatology*, **88**, 373.

DITHRANOL

Braun-Falco, O., Bury, G. & Schoefinius, H. H. (1971) Uber Wirking von Dithranol (Cignolin) bei Psoriasis vulgaris. *Archiv für Dermatologische Forschung*, **241**, 217.

Cox, A. J. & Watson, W. (1972) Histological variation in lesions of psoriasis. *Archives of Dermatology*, **106**, 503.

Diezel, W., Meffert, H. & Sonnichsen, N. (1975) Untersuchungen zum Wirkungsmechanismus von Dithranol: Erhöhte Lipidperoxydation und Enzymhemmung. *Dermatologica*, **150**, 154.

Fisher, L. B. & Maibach, H. I. (1975) The effect of anthralin and its derivatives on epidermal cell kinetics. *Journal of Investigative Dermatology*, **64**, 338.

Liden, S. & Michalesson, G. (1974) Dithranol (anthralin) in psoriasis. The effect on DNA synthesis, granular layer and parakeratosis. *British Journal of Dermatology*, **91**, 447.

Luckacs, S. & Braun-Falco, O. (1973) Uber daes Verhalten von Dithranol (Cignolin) in Pasten und Losungen und seine Beeinflussbarkeirt durch Salicylsaure. *Hautartz*, **24**, 304.

Panec-Waelsch, M. & Hulsebosch, H. J. (1974) Further studies on the interaction between anthralin, salicylic acid and zinc oxides in pastes. *Archiv für Dermatologische Forschung*, **249**, 141.

Raab, W. & Gmeiner, B. (1974) The inhibition of glucose-6-phosphate dehydrogenase activity by dithranol (anthralin), zinc ions and/salicylic acid. *Archiv für Dermatologische Forschung*, **251**, 87.

Seville, R. H. (1975) Simplified dithranol treatment for psoriasis. *British Journal of Dermatology*, **93**, 205.

Wrench, R. & Britten, A. Z. (1975) Evaluation of dithranol and a 'synthetic tar' as antipsoriasis treatment using the mouse tail test. *British Journal of Dermatology*, **93**, 75.

CYTOSTATIC AGENTS

Almeida Concalves, J. C. (1975) 5-Fluorouracil in the treatment of common warts of the hands. *British Journal of Dermatology*, **92**, 89.

Burnett, J. W. (1975) Two unusual complications of topical fluorouracil therapy. *Archives of Dermatology*, **111**, 398.
Constantine, V. S., Fuks, Z. Y. & Farber, E. M. (1975) Mechlorethamine desensitisation in therapy for mycosis fungoides. *Archives of Dermatology*, **111**, 484.
Eaglstein, W. H., Weinstein, G. D. & Frost, P. (1970) Fluorouracil: mechanism of action in human skin and actinic keratoses. *Archives of Dermatology*, **101**, 132.
Goette, D. K. (1974) Erythroplasia of Querat. Treatment with topically administered fluorouracil. *Archives of Dermatology*, **110**, 271.
Polano, M. K. (1973) Topical therapy. In *Recent Advances in Dermatology*, ed. Rook, A., p. 372. Edinburgh and London: Churchill Livingstone.
Shelley, W. B. (1972) Onycholysis due to topical 5-fluorouracil. *Acta dermato-venercologica (Stockholm)*, **52**, 320.
Van Scott, E. J. & Kalmanson, J. D. (1973) Complete remissions of mycosis fungoides lymphoma induced by topical nitrogen mustard (HN2). *Cancer*, **32**, 18.
Zackheim, H. S. (1972) Treatment of mycosis fungoides with topical nitrosourea compounds. *Archives of Dermatology*, **106**, 177.
Zackheim, H. S. & Epstein, E. H., Jr (1975) Treatment of mycosis fungoides with topical nitrosourea compounds. Further studies. *Archives of Dermatology*, **111**, 1564.
Zelickson, A. S., Mottaz, J. & Weiss, L. W. (1975) Effects of topical fluorouracil on normal skin. *Archives of Dermatology*, **111**, 1301.

COAL TAR

Muller, S. A. & Kierland, R. R. (1964) Crude coal tar in dermatologic therapy. *Proceedings of the Mayo Clinic*, **39**, 275.
Tanenbaum, L., Parrish, J. A., Pathka, M. A., Anderson, R. R. & Fitzpatrick, T. B. (1975) Tar phototoxicity and phototherapy for psoriasis. *Archives of Dermatology*, **111**, 467.
Tring, F. C. (1973) Skin colour changes in psoriasis. Effect of UV light irradiation. *Dermatologica*, **147**, 309.
Wrench, R. & Britten, A. Z. (1975a) Evaluation of coal tar fractions for use in psoriaform diseases using the mouse tail test. 1. High and low temperatures and their constituents. *British Journal of Dermatology*, **92**, 569.
Wrench, R. & Britten, A. Z. (1975b) Evaluation of coal tar fractions for use in psoriasiform diseases using the mouse tail test. III. High boiling tar acids. *British Journal of Dermatology*, **93**, 67.
Wrench, R. & Britten, A. Z. (1975c) Evaluation of dithranol and a synthetic tar as antipsoriatic treatments using the mouse tail test. *British Journal of Dermatology*, **93**, 75.
Young, E. (1970) The external treatment of psoriasis: a controlled investigation of the effects of coal tar. *British Journal of Dermatology*, **82**, 510.

DINITROCHLORBENZENE

Heid, E., Grosshans, E. & Basset, A. (1975) Sensibilisation au DNCB. Usage thérapeutique. *Bulletin de la Société française de dermatologie et de syphiligraphie*, **82**, 132.
Helm, F. (1974) Cancer immunology. Possible mechanism. *Cutis*, **14**, 525.
Malek-Mansour, S., Castermans-Elias, S. S. & Lapière, Ch. M. (1973) Régression de méstastases de mélanome après thérapeutique immunologique. *Dermatologica*, **146**, 156.
Remy, W & Stuttgen, G. (1972) Die experimentelle Austosung der Spatreektion als immunologisches Indikatur. *Allergie und Immunologie*, **18**, 97.
Sanderson, K. W. (1975) In discussion. *Proceedings of the Royal Society of Medicine*, **68**, 346.

DEPIGMENTING AGENTS

Arndt, K. A. & Fitzpatrick, T. B. (1965) Topical use of hydroquinone as a depigmenting agent. *Journal of the American Medical Association*, **194**, 117.
Becker, J. W., Jr & Spencer, M. C. (1962) Evaluation of monobenzone. *Journal of the American Medical Association*, **180**, 279.
Bleehen, S. S., Pathak, M. A., Hori, Y. & Fitzpatrick, T. B. (1968) Depigmentation skin with 4-isopropyl catechol, mercaptoamines and other compounds. *Journal of Investigative Dermatology*, **50**, 103.
Cahn, B. I. (1972) Leukoderma acquisitum: secondary to intralesional steroid injection. *Cutis*, **9**, 509.

Jimbow, K., Obata, O., Pathak, M. A. & Fitzpatrick, T. B. (1974) Mechanism of depigmentation by hydroquinone. *Journal of Investigative Dermatology*, **62**, 436.

Kligman, A. M. & Willis, I. (1975) A new formula for depigmenting human skin. *Archives of Dermatology*, **111**, 40.

Malten, K. E., Seutter, E., Hara, I. & Nakajima, T. (1971) Occupational vitiligo due to paratertiary butylphenol and homologues. *Transactions of St John's Hospital Dermatological Society*, **57**, 115.

Riley, P. A. (1969) Hydroxyanisole depigmentation; in vitro studies. *Journal of Pathology*, **97**, 193.

Riley, P. A. (1970) The mechanism of hydrocyanisole depigmentation. *Journal of Pathology*, **101**, 163.

Spencer, M. C. (1965) Topical use of hydroquinone for depigmentation. *Journal of the American Medical Association*, **194**, 962.

LIGHT BARRIERS AND SCREENS

Fusaro, R. M. & Dunge, W. J. (1970) Erythropoietic protoporphyria. IV. Protections from sulphur. *British Medical Journal*, **1**, 730.

Fusaro, R. M. & Johnson, T. A. (1975) Protection against long ultraviolet and/or visible light with topical dihydroxyacetone. *Dermatologica*, **159**, 346.

Johnson, J. A. & Fusaro, R. W. (1972) Dihydroxyacetone-naphthoquinone sunscreens. *Journal of the American Medical Association*, **222**, 1651.

Joó, I. & Simon, N. (1974) Die Benzotriazolderivate als UV-Absorber. *Archiv für Dermatologische Forschung*, **249**, 13.

Katz, S. I. (1970) Relative effectiveness of selected sunscreens. *Archives of Dermatology*, **101**, 466.

Langner, A. & Kligman, A. M. (1972) Further suncreen studies of aminobenzoic acid. *Archives of Dermatology*, **105**, 851.

MacLeod, T. M. & Frain-Bell, W. (1971) The study of the efficacy of some agents used for the protection of the skin from exposure to light. *British Journal of Dermatology*, **84**, 266.

MacLeod, T. M. & Frain-Bell, W. (1975) A study of chemical light screening agents. *British Journal of Dermatology*, **92**, 417.

Pothak, M. A., Fitzpatrick, T. B. & Frenk, E. (1969) Evaluation of topical agents that prevent sunburn—superiority of para-aminobenzoic acid and its ester in ethyl alcohol. *New England Journal of Medicine*, **280**, 1459.

Willis, I. & Kligman, A. M. (1970) Aminobenzoic acid and its esters. *Archives of Dermatology*, **102**, 405.

INSECT REPELLANTS

Feldman, R. J. & Maibach, H. I. (1970) Percutaneous penetration of some organic compounds in man. *Journal of Investigative Dermatology*, **54**, 399.

Khan, A. A., Maibach, H. I. & Skidmore, D. L. (1969) Increased attractiveness of man to mosquitoes with induced eccrine sweating. *Nature*, **223**, 859.

Khan, A. A., Maibach, H. I. & Skidmore, D. L. (1973) A study of insect repellants. II. Effect of temperature on protection time. *Journal of Ecology and Entomology*, **66**, 433.

Maibach, H. I., Khan, A. A. & Akers, W. (1974) Use of insect repellants for maximum efficacy. *Archives of Dermatology*, **109**, 32.

ANTIPERSPIRANTS

Abell, E. & Morgan, K. (1974) Treatment of idiopathic hyperhidrosis by glycopyrronium bromide and tap water iontophoresis. *British Journal of Dermatology*, **91**, 87.

Cronin, H. J. (1924) Hexamethylene amine poisoning in the rubber industry. *Journal of the American Medical Association*, **88**, 250.

Cullen, S. I. (1975) Topical methenamine therapy for hyperhidrosis. *Archives of Dermatology*, **111**, 1158.

Cunliffe, W. J., Johnson, C. E. & Williamson, D. M. (1972) Localised unilateral hyperhidrosis —a clinical and laboratory study. *British Journal of Dermatology*, **86**, 374.

Lansdown, A. B. G. (1973) Production of eipdermal damage in mammalian skin by some simple aluminium compounds. *British Journal of Dermatology*, **89**, 67.

Polano, M. K. (1973) Topical therapy. In *Recent Advances in Dermatology*, ed. Rook, A., p. 399. Edinbrugh and London: Churchill Livingstone.
Shelley, W. B. & Hurley, H. J., Jr (1975) Studies on topical antiperspirant control of axillary hyperhidrosis. *Acta dermato-venereolojica (Stockholm)*, **55**, 241.

MISCELLANEOUS FORMULATIONS
Achten, G., Bowload, A., Haven, E., Lapière, Ch. M., Pierard, J. & Reyhaers, H. (1973) Étude du bufexamac onguent dans le traitment de diverses dermatoses. *Dermatologica*, **146**, 1.
Des Groseillers, J. P. & Brisson, P. (1974) Localised epidermolysis bullosa. A report on two cases and evaluation of therapy. *Archives of Dermatology*, **109**, 70.
Grigoriu, D. (1972) Comparative study of the effects of *p*-butoxyphenylacethydroxamic acid and of the betamethasone 17-valerate applied topically in various inflammatory dermatoses. *Médecine et Hygiène (Genève)*, **1004**, 491.
Hasan, N. & Majid, A. (1972) The treatment of burn wounds with silver nitrate. A study of 42 patients. *Pakistan Journal of Medical Research*, **11**, 12.
Kirby, J. D. & Borrie, P. F. (1975) Confluent and reticulate papillomatosis (two cases). *Proceedings of the Royal Society of Medicine*, **68**, 532.
Lachapelle, I. M. (1975) Contact sensitivity to bufexamac. *Contact Dermatitis*, **1**, 261.
Leyden, J. J. & Kligman, A. M. (1975) Aluminium chloride in the treatment of symptomatic athlete's foot. *Archives of Dermatology*, **111**, 1004.
Leyden, J. J., McGinley, J. & Kligman, A. M. (1975) Shorter methods for evaluating antidandruff agents. *Journal of the Society of Cosmetic Chemists*, **26**, 573.
Lowbury, E. J. L., Babb, J. R., Bridges, K. & Jackson, D. M. (1976) Topical chemoprophylaxis with silver sulphadazine and silver-nitrate chlorhexidine creams: emergence of sulphonamide-resistant Gram-negative bacilli. *British Medical Journal*, **1**, 493.
Marples, R. R. & Kligman, A. M. (1974) Methods for evaluating topical antibacterial agents on human skin, *Antimicrobe Therapy*, **5**, 322.
Smeenk, G. (1973) Contact allergy to bufexamac. *Dermatologica*, **147**, 334.
Van Scott, E. J. & Yu, R. J. (1974) Control of keratinisation with α-hydroxy acids and related compounds. I. Topical treatment of ichthyotic disorders. *Archives of Dermatology*, **110**, 586.
Vassant-Thys, D. & Robas, J. (1970) Pharmacological studies of bufexamac topically applied on the skin. *Pharmacodyn*, **187**, 401.

CRYOTHERAPY
Barr, A. & Coles, R. B. (1969) Warts on the hands. A statistical survey. *Transactions of St John's Hospital Dermatological Society*, **52**, 69.
Bunney, M. H. (1975) Warts. *British Journal of Hospital Medicine*, **13**, 567.
Gill, W., Fraser, J. & Carter, D. C. (1968) Repeated freeze-thaw cycles in cryosurgery. *Nature*, **219**, 410.
Goldwyn, R. M. & Rosoff, C. B. (1969) Cryosurgery for large haemangiomas in adults. *Plastic and Reconstructive Surgery*, **43**, 605.
Holden, H. B. & Saunders, S. (1973) Cryosurgery: its scientific basis and clinical application. *Practitioner*, **210**, 543.
Krashen, A. J. (1970) Cryotherapy of herpes of the mouth. *Journal of American Dental Association*, **81**, 1163.
Lejman, K. (1971) L'evaluation de la cryotherapie comme d'une methode auxiliaire dans letraitment de l'acne rosacee. *Giornale Italiano Dermatologia Minerva Dermatologica*, **46**, 141.
Leopard, P. J. (1974) Cryosurgery for facial skin lesions. *Proceedings of the Royal Society of Medicine*, **68**, 606.
Leyden, J., Mills, O. & Kligman, A. M. (1974) Cryoprobe treatment of acne conglobata. *British Journal of Dermatology*, **90**, 335.
Poswillo, D. E. (1975) Cryosurgery of the oral mucous membrane. *Proceedings of the Royal Society of Medicine*, **68**, 608.
Shulman, S. (1968) In *Cryosurgery*, ed. Rand, R. W., Rinfret, A. P. & Von Leden, H. Springfield, Illinois: Charles C. Thomas.

Whittaker, D. K. (1975) Ultrastructural changes in microvasculature following cryosurgery of oral mucosa. *Journal of Periodontal Research*, **10** (3), 148.
Zacharina, S. A. (1973) *Cryosurgery of Tumours of the Skin and Oral Cavity*. Springfield, Illinois: Charles C. Thomas.

APPLICATION OF TOPICAL THERAPY
Almeida Concalves, J. C. (1975) 5-Fluorouracil in the treatment of common warts of the hands. *British Journal of Dermatology*, **92**, 89.
Balkin, S. S. (1975) Treatment of corns by injectable silicone. *Archives of Dermatology*, **111** 143.
Barr, A. & Coles, R. B. (1969) Warts on the hands. A statistical survey. *Transactions of St John's Hotpisal Dermatological Society*, **52**, 69.
Bleeker, J. J. (1975) Intradermal triamcinolone acetonide treatment of psoriatic nail dystrophy with Port-o-Jet. *British Journal of Dermatology*, **92**, 479.
Bleiberg, J., Brodkin, R. H. & Abbey, A. A. (1973) Bleaching of hair after use of benzoyl peroxide acne lotion. *Archives of Dermatology*, **108**, 583.
Bunney, M. H., Hunter, A. A., Ogilvie, M. M. & Williams, D. A. (1971) The treatment of plantar warts in the home. *Practitioner*, **207**, 197.
Bunney, M. H. (1975) Warts. *British Journal of Hospital Medicine*, **13**, 566.
Coles, R. B. & Ryan, T. J. (1975) The psoriasis sufferer in the community. *British Journal of Dermatology*, **93**, 111.
Constantine, V. S., Fuks, Z. Y. & Farber, E. M. (1975) Mechlorethamine desensitisation in therapy for mycosis fungoides. *Archives of Dermatology*, **111**, 484.
Fisher, L. B. & Maibach, H. I. (1971) The effect of corticosteroids on human epidermal mitotic activity. *Archives of Dermatology*, **103**, 39.
Fisher, L. B. & Maibach, H. I. (1973) Topical antipsoriatic agents and epidermal mitosis in man. *Archives of Dermatology*, **108**, 375.
Fredricksson, T. (1974) Topically applied fluorouracil in the treatment of psoriatic nails. *Archives of Dermatology*, **110**, 735.
Fuks, Z., Bagshaw, M. A. & Farber, E. M. (1973) Prognostic signs and the management of mycosis fungoides. *Cancer*, **32**, 1385.
Fuks, Z., Bagshaw, M. A. & Farber, E. M. (1974) New concepts in the management of mycosis fungoides. *British Journal of Dermatology*, **90**, 355.
Fulton, J. E. & Pablo, G. (1974) Topical antibacterial therapy for acne. *Archives of Dermatology*, **110**, 83.
Greenberg, J. H., Smith, L. & Katz, R. M. (1973) Verrucae vulgaris rejection. *Archives of Dermatology*, **107**, 580.
Gunther, S. (1972) Topical administration of vitamin A acid (Retin A) in palmar keratoses—callosities, hyperkeratotic eczema, hypertrophic lichen planus, pityriasis rubra pilaris. *Dermatologica*, **145**, 344.
Handojo, I. & Pardjono (1973) Treatment of condyloma acuminata with 5 per cent 5-fluorouracil ointment. *Asian Journal of Medicine*, **9** (5), 162.
Haye, K. R. (1974) Treatment of condyloma acuminata with 5 per cent 5-fluorouracil (5 FU cream). *British Journal of Venereal Diseases*, **50**, 466.
Hursthouse, M. W. (1975) A controlled trial in the use of topical 5-fluorouracil on viral warts. *British Journal of Dermatology*, **92**, 93.
Kaidbey, K. H., Petrozzi, J. W. & Kligman, A. M. (1975) Topical colchicine therapy for recalcitrant psoriasis. *Archives of Dermatology*, **111**, 33.
Kammereau, B., Zesch, A. & Schaefer, H. (1975) Absolute concentrations of dithranol and triacetyl dithranol in the skin layers after local treatment. In vivo investigations with four different types of pharmaceutical vehicles. *Journal of Investigative Dermatology*, **64**, 145.
Kligman, A. M., Plewig, G. & Mills, O. H. (1971) Topical applied tretinion for senile (solar) comedones. *Archives of Dermatology*, **104**, 420.
Kligman, A. M., Mills, O. H., Leyden, J. J. & Fulton, J. E. (1973) Postscript to vitamin A acid therapy for acne vulgaris. *Archives of Dermatology*, **107**, 296.
Kligman, A. M. (1975) Letter. *Archives of Dermatology*, **111**, 1213.
Lawrence, D. I. & Bern, H. A. (1958) On the response of mouse epidermis to vitamin A. *Journal of Investigative Dermatology*, **31**, 313.

Mills, O. H. & Kligman, A. M. (1972) Is sulphur helpful or harmful in acne vulgaris? *British Journal of Dermatology*, **86**, 620.

Mills, O. H. & Kligman, A. M. (1975) Acne detergicans. *Archives of Dermatology*, **111**, 65.

Mills, O. H., Leyden, J. J. & Kligman, A. M. (1973) Tretinoin treatment of steroid acne. *Archives of Dermatology*, **108**, 381.

Morison, W. L. (1975) Anti-viral treatment of warts. *British Journal of Dermatology*, **92**, 97.

Nels, W. S. & Fourie, E. D. (1973) Immunotherapy and 5 per cent topical 5-fluorouracil ointment in the treatment of condylomata acuminata. *South African Medical Journal*, **47**, 45.

Parrish, A. J., Fitzpatrick, T. B., Tanenbaum, L. & Parhak, M. A. (1974) Photochemotherapy of psoriasis with oral methoxsalen and longwave ultraviolet light. *New England Journal of Medicine*, **291**, 1207.

Peck, G. L., Key, D. J. & Guss, S. B. (1973) Topical vitamin A acid in the treatment of psoriasis. *Archives of Dermatology*, **107**, 245.

Pegum, J. (1971) Urea in the treatment of black hairy tongue. *British Journal of Dermatology*, **84**, 602.

Poole, R. L., Griffith, J. F. & McMillan, F. S. K. (1970) Experimental contact sensitisation with benzyl peroxide. *Archives of Dermatology*, **102**, 635.

Ratner, A. C., Waldorf, D. S. & Van Scott, E. J. (1968) Alteration of lesions of mycosis fungoides lymphoma by direct imposition of delayed hypersensitivity reactions. *Cancer*, **21**, 83.

Seville, R. H. (1975) Simplified dithranol treatment for psoriasis. *British Journal of Dermatology*, **93**, 205.

Van Scott, E. J. & Winters, P. L. (1970) Responses of mycosis fungoides to intensive external treatment with nitrogen mustard. *Archives of Dermatology*, **102**, 507.

Van Scott, E. J. & Kalmanson, J. D. (1973) Complete remissions of mycosis fungoides lymphoma induced by topical nitrogen mustard. *Cancer*, **32**, 18.

Zackheim, H. S. & Epstein, E. H. (1975) Treatment of mycosis fungoides with topical nitrosourea compounds. *Archives of Dermatology*, **111**, 1564.

ADVERSE EFFECTS

Angelini, G., Mantuccio, F. & Meneghini, C. L. (1975) Contact dermatitis in patients with leg ulcers. *Contact Dermatitis*, **1**, 81.

Beerbohm, P. (1975) Legislation on prevention of occupational dermatoses. *Contact Dermatitis*, **1**, 207.

Bentley-Phillips, B. & Bayles, M. A. H. (1974) Acquired hypomelanosis: hyperpigmentation following reaction to hydroquinone. *British Journal of Dermatology*, **90**, 232.

Burry, J. N., Kirk, R., Reid, J. G. & Turner, T. (1975) Chlorocresol sensitivity. *Contact Dermatitis*, **1**, 41.

Chamberlain, M. J., Reynolds, A. L. & Yeoman, W. B. (1972) Toxic effect of podophyllin application in pregnancy. *British Medical Journal*, **3**, 391.

Cronin, E. & Wilkinson, D. S. (1973) Contact dermatitis. In *Recent Advances in Dermatology*, 3rd end, ed. Rook, A. J., p. 170. Edinburgh and London: Churchill Livingstone.

Degref, H. & Verhoeve, L. (1975) Contact dermatitis to miconazole nitrate. *Contact Dermatitis*, **1**, 269.

Emmett, E. A. & Davis, J. M. (1973) Allergic contact dermatitis from Tolnaftate. *Archives of Dermatology*, **108**, 98.

Gellen, G. A., Maibach, H. I. & Wachs, G. N. (1972) Contact allergy to tolnaftate. *Archives of Dermatology*, **106**, 715.

Jordan, W. P., Jr, Higgins, M. & Dvorak, J. (1975) Allergic contact dermatitis to all-trans-retinoic acid; epicutaneous and leucocyte migration inhibition testing. *Contact Dermatitis*, **1**, 306.

Kreybig, T. von, Preussman, R. & Kreybig, I. von (1970) Chemische Konstitution und keratogene wirking bei der Ratte. 3N-alkylcarbonhydrazide, noeitere hydrazint derivate. *Arzeimittel-Forschung*, **20**, 363.

Lachapelle, J. M. (1975) Contact sensitivity to bufexamac. *Contact Dermatitis*, **1**, 261.

Liden, S. (1975) Alpholysyl sensitivity and propyl gallate. *Contact Dermatitis*, **1**, 257.

Maibach, H. I. (1975) Acute laryngeal obstruction presumed secondary to thiomerial (metholate) delayed hypersensitivity. *Contact Dermatitis*, **1**, 221.

Malten, K. E., Kniper, J. P. & van der Staak, W. B. J. M. (1973) Contact allergies investigations in 100 patients with ulcis cruris. *Dermatologica*, **147**, 241.
Meneghini, C. L. & Angelini, G. (1975) Contact dermatitis from pyrriolnitrin (an actinycotic agent). *Contact Dermatitis*, **1**, 288.
Mobacken, H., Zelderfeldt, B. & Åhrén, C. (1973) Effects of two cationic tryphenylmethane dyes on the healing of skin incisions. *Acta dermato-venereologica (Stockholm)*, **53**, 161.
Mobacken, H. & Zelderfeldt, B. (1973) Influence of a cationic triphenylmethane dye on granular tissue growth in vivo. An experimental study in rats. *Acta dermato-venereologica (Stockholm)*, **53**, 167.
Mobacken, H., Ahonen, J. & Zelderfeldt, B. (1974) The effect of a cationic triphenylmethane dye (crystal violet) on rabbit granulation tissue. *Acta dermato-venereologica (Stockholm)*, **54**, 343.
Roed-Petersen, J., Auken, G. & Hjorth, N. (1975) Contact sensitivity to Irgasan, DP300. *Contact Dermatitis*, **1**, 293.
Rudner, E. J., Clendenning, W. E., Epstein, E., Fisher, A. A., Jillson, O. F., Jordan, W. P., Kanof, N., Larson, W., Maibach, H., Mitchell, J. C., O'Quinn, S. E., Schorr, W. F. & Sulzberger, M. B. (1975) The frequency of contact sensitivity in North America 1972–74. *Contact Dermatitis*, **1**, 277.
Rudzki, E. & Zakrawski, Z. (1975) Incidence of contact sensitivity to topically applied drugs as compared with the frequency of their prescription. *Contact Dermatitis*, **1**, 249.
Smeenk, G. & Prins, F. J. (1972) Allergic contact eczema due to chloracetamide. *Dermatologica*, **144**, 108.
Storrs, F. J. (1975) Parachlor-meta-xylenol. Allergic contact dermatitis in seven individuals. *Contact Dermatitis*, **1**, 211.
Tuft, E. H. (1975) Contact urticaria to cephalosporins. *Archives of Dermatology*, **111**, 1609.
Van Ketel, W. G. (1974) Allergy to micronazole nitrate (Daktarin). *Contact Dermatitis Newsletter*, **16**, 517.
Walshe, M. M. (1975) Contact dermatitis in a spinal injuries centre. *Contact Dermatitis*, **1**, 3.
Wilkinson, D. S. (1972) Sensitivity to pharmaceutical additives. In *Mechanisms in Drug Allergy*, ed. Dash, C. H. & Jones, H. E. H., p. 75. Edinburgh and London: Churchill Livingstone.

10

IONISING RADIATION IN BENIGN DERMATOSES

Neville Rowell

It may seem strange in a book of recent advances that a chapter should be devoted to a form of treatment which has tended to be used less frequently in the past 20 years. This is not a chapter on recent developments but a short review of the present place of ionising radiation in the treatment of benign disorders in dermatology. In the early 1950s there was considerable interest in the use of this form of treatment and many papers were published. However, a search of the *Index Medicus* between 1960 and 1974 reveals only about a score of references. Nevertheless, it may well be that there is a revival of interest because many dermatologists feel that the reaction against radiotherapy for benign conditions has been overdone.

In this article the treatment of neoplasms will not be dealt with as, in the United Kingdom, this is almost exclusively the province of departments of radiotherapy. This is not so in other countries. In the United States of America (Goldschmidt, 1975) 80 per cent or more dermatologists, using superficial x-ray therapy, treat basal cell or squamous cell carcinomata. This is also the case in Germany and other European countries. The reader is referred to several extensive monographs available in the literature (Cipollaro and Crossland, 1967; Storck, 1972; Braun-Falco and Lukacs, 1973).

The decrease in the use of radiotherapy for benign disorders in the United Kingdom and elsewhere in recent years has occurred mainly because of the introduction and increasing effectiveness of other forms of therapy, such as corticosteroids. There has also been an excessive reaction to the hazards of radiotherapy. Because of the lack of suitable facilities and dermatologists conversant in radiotherapeutic techniques, there has been a lack of training of the younger dermatologists in the use of superficial radiotherapy. In the United Kingdom some dermatologists have even gone as far as to advocate that superficial radiotherapy should be abandoned altogether except for the treatment of malignant lesions in the skin (Sweet, 1968). In some areas it is now impossible to obtain superficial radiotherapy even in the teaching hospitals. This reaction, which some believe to be unwarranted, has not occurred to the same extent in the United States and Canada. A recent questionnaire, returned by 2444 dermatologists in these countries, showed that more than half the dermatological offices were equipped with superficial x-ray machines and/or Grenz-ray units and that 44.3 per cent of dermatologists used conventional superficial x-ray or Grenz ray regularly (Goldschmidt, 1975). It was interesting that, in this survey, superficial radiotherapy was used by younger dermatologists as much as by older ones.

The purpose of the present chapter is to put the matter in perspective and to try to define the indications for therapy and the precautions required for the protection of the patient. The mechanism of actions of ionising radiation, the design of apparatus and the methods of calibration of sources of ionising radiation are fully covered in the monograph by Cipollaro and Crossland (1967).

Types of Superficial Radiotherapy

There are two main types of superficial radiotherapy:

1. Conventional superficial x-radiation at 50 to 100 kV with a half value layer (HVL) of 0.5 to 1.0 mm Al.
2. Grenz (Bucky) rays at 8 to 15 kV with an HVL of 0.018 to 0.036 mm Al.

Contact low voltage therapy at 29 to 45 kV and 'intermediate' x-radiation using a beryllium window modification will not be considered, nor will treatment with Thorium X, which is now hardly ever used.

The effect of ionising radiation on the tissues depends upon the quantity and penetrating power of the rays used. The factors which must be considered in any radiation therapy of the skin include the kilovoltage, milleamperage, time, distance from the tube to the skin, the size of the area to be treated and its site, the type and depth of the lesion, the quality of the radiation, the dose, the interval between doses and the total dose to be given. It is important to remember that the tissue dose, i.e. the amount of radiation absorbed by the tissue, includes the secondary radiation, or back scatter, from tissue. The increase in skin surface dose over the air dose is approximately 1 per cent for areas 1 cm in diameter, 4 per cent for areas 2 cm in diameter, 7 per cent for areas 3 cm in diameter, 10 per cent for areas 4 cm in diameter and 12 per cent for areas 5 cm in diameter. For lesions less than 1 cm in diameter, the air dose and the skin dose are approximately the same (Baer and Witten, 1955). The HVL is the thickness of aluminium that reduces the intensity of the radiation to half when inserted in the path of the rays. Aluminium removes the softer rays giving rise to a more penetrating beam. Some lesions deeper in the skin, such as lesions of hidradenitis or deep acne cysts, require greater penetration than very superficial lesions. The tendency nowadays is to use the softest rays whenever possible—Grenz rays—by the use of machines containing beryllium windows which allow the softer rays to pass through. Fifty per cent of such Grenz radiation is absorbed in the first 0.5 mm of the skin whereas the harder radiation of conventional superficial x-ray produced by 50 kV or more, is only absorbed by 4 mm of skin.

It has already been pointed out that the amount of radiation must be kept to the minimum. Wherever possible the use of Grenz ray should be considered. However, conventional x-ray may have a better and longer-lasting effect than Grenz ray. Dosage schedules vary. Even as early as 1953 the accent was on small doses. Miescher (1953) noted that 60 rad doses were as effective as those of 100 rad in eczema and lichen simplex. Many authors use weekly doses of 75 rad to a total dosage of 600 to 750 rad. For many years at Leeds we have used 100 rad at three-weekly intervals for three doses with satisfactory results. This allows three or four courses of 300 rad in a lifetime and this has been found to be a safe total dosage (Rowell, 1973).

Radiosensitivity

The sensitivity of tissues depends on the rate of mitosis and the degree of differentiation of the tissue. Rapidly dividing non-differentiating cells are the most sensitive. Areas of normal skin vary in their radiosensitivity (Kalz, 1941) and this is a practical point which must be borne in mind in therapy. The following parts of the body are listed in order of decreasing sensitivity:

Anterior aspect of neck, antecubital and popliteal fossae
Flexural surfaces of the extremities, chest and abdomen
Face—not pigmented
Back and extensor surfaces of extremities
Face—pigmented
Nape of neck
Scalp
Palms and soles

The ability of the skin to repair after radiation decreases with age, so children's skin tolerates radiation well. Chu et al (1960) and Glicksman et al (1960) showed that there was no statistical difference in the erythema response to radiation of fair skinned patients, those of medium complexion and Negro patients. It has been said that light skinned patients tolerate radiation less well than dark skinned persons and that pigmentation is greater in the dark skinned after irradiation than in the light skinned. There is, in fact, no evidence of any such correlation between intensity of the skin reaction and the colour of the skin. The biological and histopathological changes of radiation are well reviewed by Rubin and Casarett (1968).

CONVENTIONAL X-RAY THERAPY

Adverse Effects of Conventional Superficial X-ray Therapy

Acute radiodermatitis

Acute radiodermatitis is a localised inflammatory reaction which usually results from some error in technique such as the use of the wrong filter, overlapping fields of irradiation or an error in the timing of the dose. There is particular danger of giving an excessive amount of irradiation when combined units delivering both conventional superficial x-ray therapy at 50 kV or more and Grenz ray at about 10 kV, are used. These combined machines have been condemned by many writers in the past but modern machines have built-in safety devices which tend to cut down the risk of human error. Sweet (1962) reported a very unfortunate incident in which 11 patients were accidentally exposed to over 6000 rad. Acute radiation damage occurred when a soft x-ray unit was incorrectly operated so that, instead of patients receiving Grenz ray at 10 kV, they received x-rays generated at 50 kV, through an 0.05 mm aluminium filter for a time appropriate for the delivery to the skin surface of 100 rad at 10 kV. The dose delivered at the skin surface was 6450 rad instead of 100 rad.

There are four distinct phases in acute radiodermatitis. Initial erythema and oedema with blanching of areas exposed to the greatest amount of radiation reaches a peak at about 48 h and is followed by a relatively quiet phase. On the third to the sixth day secondary erythema is sometimes accompanied by extravasation of blood into the skin and the development of vesicles and bullae. After about three weeks the bullae dry up and, during the fourth phase, the skin heals although ulceration may persist for some time.

Chronic radiodermatitis

This results from the cumulative effect of repeated small doses of x-rays rather than from an acute overdose. The clinical features include telangiectasia due to poorly supported dilated vessels, hypopigmentation and patchy hyperpigmentation, decreased sebaceous gland activity and the development of keratoses. The skin is usually thin but occasionally thickening or tethering may occur with ulceration in areas of trauma. The effects of chronic irradiation are increased by exposure to ultraviolet light (Sulzberger, Baehr and Borotra, 1952) and the process of ageing.

A follow-up study of 100 patients who had received 1600 rad or more to the face, 1500 rad or more to the hands, 1600 rad or more to the fingernails or 1600 rad or more to the feet for benign dermatoses over the preceding 34 years has recently been reported (Rowell, 1973). The lowest total dose of superficial radiotherapy to produce keratoses, atrophy, pigmentation and telangiectasia is shown in Table 10.1. This indicates that postradiation changes generally occur at a lower dosage on the face than on the hands, confirming that the facial skin is more liable to be damaged by radiation, probably due to the additive effect of sunlight. Atrophy of the skin occurred in nearly half of those irradiated with more than 1600 rad to the face, but this was usually mild. Keratoses and telangiectasia were more common in those who had had 2000 rad to the hands than in age and sex matched controls who had not had any irradiation, but these features had not usually been noted by the patients.

It is not inevitable that a high total dose of radiation causes visible sequelae.

One patient who had had 2750 rad to the face had an apparently normal skin. Miescher and Böhm (1948) noted that mild sequelae could occur with over 1600 to 1800 rad in a series of 192 patients examined 1 to 22 years after irradiation for hyperhidrosis of the hands, feet and axillae. Borak, Eller and Eller (1949), however, did not find any sequelae in 122 patients with hyperhidrosis who had had less than 1600 rad through 2 to 4 mm Al. Sulzberger et al (1952) concluded that there is no evidence that fractionated doses of superficial irradiation totalling 1000 rad or less would cause any sequelae and that when total doses of more than 1000 rad were given, it could be expected that 1.5 per cent of patients would show relatively mild sequelae of only cosmetic importance.

X-ray induced tumours

These are more likely to occur in areas subjected to many small doses administered at intervals over a long period (Ryan, 1972). Many authors

Table 10.1 The lowest total dose of conventional superficial radiotherapy to produce changes (Rowell, 1973)

	Hands (rad)	Face and neck (rad)
Carcinoma	3170	2090
Keratoses	1800	2090
Atrophy	2175	1600
Pigmentation	2175	1600
Telangiectasia	2050	1600

have reported on the additive effect of sunlight (Sulzberger et al, 1952). The latent period between exposure and the development of carcinoma varies inversely with the dose (Mole, 1972) and intervals of between 3 and 64 years have been noted (Martin, Strong and Spiro, 1970). The long-term cumulative effect of irradiation depends on the total dose given to an area of skin regardless of the time over which the dose is given. Martin et al (1970) noted that almost 19 per cent of 192 patients with skin cancer of the head and neck had had a previous history of radiation for benign conditions, compared with only 5 per cent 357 patients without skin cancer. There is doubt about these findings because almost nothing was known of the dosage that had been given. Many patients had been irradiated before 1928 and some had been treated in lay institutes or beauty parlours for hirsuties. More noteworthy is the report by Wilson et al (1958) of 12 patients who developed carcinoma of the thyroid under the age of 35 years. In six of these there was a history of irradiation of the neck region for benign cutaneous lesions by radium or x-rays in early childhood. The dose given ranged from 130 to 2700 rad and the latent period was between 5 and 18 years. Carcinoma developed in the part of the thyroid exposed to the greatest radiation. Albright and Allday (1967) described five patients treated with radiotherapy for adolescent acne in middle to late adolescence who developed a thyroid cancer after several years. The causal relationship between the two events could not be disproved. DeLawter and Winship (1963) found no cases of malignancy in a period of 20 years follow-up of 222 patients who had had thyroid irradiation after the age of 20 years. This seems to show the relative resistance of the thyroid gland to carcinogenesis in adult life. The younger the patient is irradiated, the greater the risk of later development of thyroid carcinoma. Nowadays, the neck of children would not be irradiated and the thyroid area would be screened in patients of all ages, so these tragedies should not occur.

Basal cell carcinomata are more liable to occur on the face, scalp and trunk, and squamous cell carcinoma on the backs of the hands after radiotherapy for benign conditions (Ridley, 1962; Sarkany et al, 1968; Albert and Omran, 1968; Kozlova, 1969). Basal cell carcinomata have been reported after radiation treatment of lupus vulgaris (Pegum, 1972) and on the scalps of children after epilation (Ridley, 1962). Several other types of tumour have also been reported after radiation and these include fibrosarcoma after irradiation for lupus vulgaris and hirsutes (Russell, 1959), melanoma (Traenkle, 1963) and dermal cylindroma after epilation of the scalp (Black and Jones, 1971). There may be an increased risk of leukaemia as well as cancer after epilation (Albert et al, 1966).

Rowell (1973) noted that four patients had developed basal cell carcinoma out of 25 patients who had had 1600 rad or more to the face in the preceding 34 years. The lowest total dose to cause carcinoma on the face was 2090 rad, but six other patients had had 2000 rad or more to the face without any sign of carcinoma. The only patient to develop a carcinoma (squamous) out of 41 patients who had had more than 2000 rad to the hands, had had a total dose of 3170 rad. Five other patients who had had more than 3000 rad to the hands showed no evidence of carcinoma. The evidence in this follow-up study suggests that a total lifetime dose to any area of skin should not exceed 1200 rad. This agrees with Crossland's experience (1957) of re-examining 1000 patients at the New York Skin and Cancer Unit 5 to 23 years after treatment. No sequelae had been seen with total dosages of 1000 rad.

Other side effects of superficial radiotherapy

Hypoplasia of the growing breast after superficial radiotherapy was reported by Kolar, Bek and Vrabec (1967) who found 33 cases in the medical literature and reported 14 cases of their own. These patients had been irradiated in infancy for haemangiomata or lymphangiomata. Only when the dose was less than 3000 rad were there no signs of hypoplasia. Hypoplasia of the breast has also been reported after radium treatment for haemangioma in two patients (Weidman, Zimany and Kopf, 1966).

Safety Precautions

Most sequelae of superficial radiotherapy occurred in the early days of such therapy and were mainly due to inadequate knowledge of the danger of radiation and also of the techniques involved. Superficial radiotherapy should only be given by dermatologists or radiographers trained in the techniques and aware of the dangers. The minimum dose should be used and Grenz radiation should be considered if at all feasible. Patients must be questioned about previous therapy and this is particularly important with the increased mobility of the population and, particularly, if there is more than one dermatological centre in a city. Good records must be maintained and it is advisable to keep separate radiation record cards in addition to the usual case notes. These should be retained indefinitely. The machines must be regularly calibrated by skilled personnel, preferably in association with a Radiation Physics Department. In the United Kingdom there is usually an Area Radiological Protection Adviser who should be consulted about safety precautions. The staff should have regular blood counts and wear a monitoring film badge at all times. Domonkos and Cameron (1957) drew attention to the amount of stray radiation from superficial radiotherapy machines. This point should be checked by the Radiological Protection Adviser. Only the part to be treated should be exposed to radiation and the patient should be shielded by lead sheeting or an apron. Particular attention should be paid to protection of the eyes, thyroid area, pelvis and genitalia. Witten, Sulzberger and Stewart (1957) studied the dose to the gonads in dermatological x-ray therapy. Important factors were the distance of the tube head from the gonads, the tilt of the tube in relation to the gonads, the position of the patient, scattered radiation from various sources and leakage of radiation from the tube head. Stewart, Witten and Sulzberger (1958) gave methods for cutting down the dose to the gonads. They advocated the use of lead rubber sheet $\frac{1}{16}$ in. thick over the lower two-thirds of the body. This reduces the gonadal dose by 50 per cent. It is even better to shield the whole of the body not being irradiated. Reducing the kilovoltage from 90 to 52 reduced the amount of radiation to about 20 per cent of that at the higher dosage. Three-quarters of the gonadal dose in a seated subject comes from scatter from the table and adjacent structures and one-quarter from the tube head and peripheral portion of the primary beam. The former can be largely eliminated by lead sheeting under the table and the latter by the use of suitable cones. The field should be kept as small as possible. The use of all these measures reduces the gonadal dose by about 97 per cent.

There have been no reports of any genetic damage from superficial x-ray therapy.

Uses of Conventional X-ray Therapy

Eczema

Superficial radiotherapy may be useful in lichenified areas of constitutional eczema and for lesions of localised lichen simplex. Brown (1958) reviewed 773 patients treated for eczema with superficial x-rays. He obtained good results with 60 rad at 70 kV. It was claimed that the results were considerably better than with 100 rad at 100 kV. Our experience indicates that three doses of 100 rad at 50 kV at three-weekly intervals is often very helpful. Controlled trials are required to compare the results of conventional x-ray therapy with Grenz-ray therapy and with patients not treated with any form of radiation. It is our impression that the effect is better and longer lasting than with Grenz-ray therapy.

Psoriasis

The indications for superficial radiotherapy in psoriasis include small areas resistant to treatment with Dithranol especially if lichenified, persistent pustular psoriasis of the palms and soles (palmoplantar pustulosis, persistent pustular pomphlyx) and psoriasis of the nails. Braun-Falco and Lukacs (1973) also use it for anogenital psoriasis in patients over the age of 60 years. Harber (1958) compared the effectiveness of conventional superficial radiotherapy and Grenz-ray therapy in patients with psoriasis. He noticed a marked difference between patients who had been irradiated compared with patients who had not. Improvement was less marked in very scaly lesions compared with those with little scale. Improvement occurred in 50 per cent after only one treatment but the maximum improvement occurred after two- to three-weekly doses. In over 70 per cent of patients there was no difference between conventional superficial therapy and Grenz-ray therapy. He also did not notice any difference in the duration of improvement between patients treated with both types of radiation. Baer and Witten (1958) considered that the effect of superficial x-ray treatment is longer lasting than with Grenz ray, and this is my experience. Nevertheless, the safety of Grenz-ray therapy and the possibility of repeating courses is very important.

Lichen planus

The only indication for superficial x-ray therapy in lichen planus is for the lichenified lesions of hypertrophic lichen planus, particularly those on the legs. This should be as an adjunct to other forms of therapy such as occlusion with coal-tar preparations, topical corticosteroids or intralesional corticosteroids.

Keloids and hypertrophic scars

The majority of keloids and hypertrophic scars occur after surgical incisions, accidental wounds and burns. The injury may be trivial. They may also occur after infections such as chickenpox and in patients with acne. They represent a hyperplastic repair state in which abnormal tissue overgrowth occurs, despite restoration of surface continuity. Prognosis is difficult to assess because of the tendency to spontaneous regression. Some surgeons and dermatologists have advocated treatment with radiation alone. Others have favoured surgery with radiation either before or after, or both before and after. Many authors have failed to recognise the fact that many spontaneously regress, and others have advocated small fractionated doses which would be incapable of reducing the size of an established keloid.

Fischer and Storck (1957) advocated radiotherapy alone. In a 20-year follow-up of 316 patients they found that keloids responded best in the first six months after their development. They claimed that 75 per cent regressed with x-ray alone and only 5 per cent had changes which could be attributed to radiation 5 to 10 years afterwards. The total dose they used was between 800 and 2400 rad in divided doses over two to five months. They noted results were best with keloids following injury, operation or infection rather than those resulting from burns, scalds or caustics.

Van den Brank and Minty (1960) were more critical in a study of 140 patients treated either by primary irradiation without surgery or by excision associated with pre- or postoperative radiotherapy, or both. A good response to radiation was defined as 'complete flattening, softening and paling of the lesion within six months of the first irradiation treatment'. The results of this study, together with pathological and experimental studies, gave the following conclusions. Primary irradiation of very recent keloids which are still cellular, well vascularised and growing, may cause some resolution if more than 1000 rad is given. There is no merit in fractionating the dose. On the other hand, when dealing with established keloids, primary radiation alone failed to cause resolution, although it relieved symptoms such as pruritus. If 1000 rad or more is used as a single dose, atrophy of the irradiated area may mask the volume of the keloid. Higher doses can cause radionecrosis leading to further keloid formation. They found that preoperative radiation was unsatisfactory, as the area irradiated must be large enough to take in the excision wound with an adequate margin and there may be rapid recovery from radiation giving rise to superregeneration. They found that postoperative radiation within 48 h of surgery is the most efficient technique, but the dose must be between 1000 and 1500 rad. This dose inevitably causes atrophy of subcutaneous tissues which is unsightly and potentially dangerous. There should be a margin of 0.5 cm of normal skin. Growth of bones in young children may be retarded by even single doses of less than 400 rad, so irradiation is contraindicated where the metaphysis of a growing bone may be in the field of radiation.

Arnold (1975) advocated the use of a putty containing bismuth as a shield for the surrounding skin when giving radiotherapy postoperatively. He recommends 500 rad every five days for four doses starting on the post operative day when the stitches are removed. He reminds us that good operative techniques are essential. There should be no tension on the suture line, the incision should be made if possible along the lines of Langer, and burns should be grafted early. Belisario (1957) advocates a combined technique of intralesional injections of hydrocortisone and hyaluronidase followed by surgery and radiotherapy.

Braun-Falco and Lukacs (1973) also prefer radiation in association with intralesional steroids after surgical excision, particularly when the lesions are large. They also consider that radiotherapy is best for small lesions of less than six months duration.

My own opinion is that, although radiation is probably best when given early, time should be allowed for spontaneous resolution to occur, and intralesional corticosteroids should be used at this stage. If spontaneous resolution does not start within six months to a year, then excision followed by radiotherapy is indicated.

Acne

There has been a strong reaction to the treatment of acne with superficial radiotherapy since Baer and Witten (1955) said: 'x-rays still are probably the best single form of treatment for this common disorder'. Many now feel it should be abandoned altogether (Milne, 1972). Strauss and Kligman (1960) noted temporary suppression of sebum production and of the size of sebaceous glands following superficial radiotherapy. Biopsy specimens 10 to 12 weeks after exposure showed the sebaceous glands had returned to normal size. The same authors noted that superficial radiotherapy with 75 rad for seven to eight doses, or 150 rad for four doses, suppressed sebaceous gland activity and helped acne. They thought the benefit was temporary and that relapse was common. Baer and Witten (1960), however, claimed that superficial radiotherapy, used as an adjunct to other forms of therapy, had an effect for some years. Maggiora, Bujard and Jadassohn (1965) found that fractionation of 300 rad, into three-weekly doses of 100 rad, had a stronger inhibitory effect on sebum excretion than when 300 rad was given in a single dose. Jelliffe, Soutter and Meara (1969), in the first reported controlled trial, noted that there was only slight benefit from 50 kV.

Cunliffe and Cotterill (1975) consider that superficial x-ray therapy can be useful in some patients with acne. It should be reserved for patients over 17 years of age with severe acne not responding to conventional topical and oral antibiotic therapy. This view is also held by Reisner (1975). It seems to be particularly helpful in cystic acne and acne conglobata. Braun-Falco and Lukacs (1973) also use superficial x-ray therapy in severe cases of acne in patients over 17 years of age.

It is very important to shield the patient thoroughly, especially the area of the thyroid and gonads. It would seem reasonable not to treat acne of the front of the chest because of the potential danger from the scattering of rays.

The introduction of a 2 mm aluminium filter may be helpful in treating cystic acne in order to get the maximum effect on deep lesions.

Rosacea

Although small doses of superficial radiotherapy (70 rad at three-weekly intervals for three doses) is helpful in rosacea, this form of treatment has been mainly supplanted by oral tetracycline therapy.

Hidradenitis suppurativa

This inflammatory disorder of apocrine sweat glands can be either acute or chronic. It involves particularly the axillae but also can occur under the breasts, around the umbilicus, or in the inguinal, genital, perianal and perineal areas. In the chronic form nodules, abscesses and sinuses develop and healing occurs with bridge-type scars. The chronic form is very difficult to treat. It does not always respond to local or systemic antibiotics and may require surgical drainage or excision. Zeligman (1965) reviewed treatment with superficial x-ray therapy and described satisfactory results with single doses of 450 to 500 rad at 100 kV, without a filter. This produced temporary epilation. There was no recurrence in his series during the period of nine months to six years follow-up. This treatment was also effective in peri-folliculitis capitis abscedens et suffodiens (McMullan and Zeligman, 1956). Cipallaro and Crossland (1967) have used 75 to 100 rad, filtered through 3 mm Al, weekly for four to six doses, but other authors have advocated larger doses in chronic cases, e.g. a total of 1000 to 2000 rad. This does not appear to be justified and, in my experience, if conventional superficial x-ray therapy is thought to be indicated, a dosage schedule of 100 rad three times at three-week intervals produces good results. The lesions are usually too deep for Grenz-ray therapy to be effective.

Warts

Radiotherapy for warts is now almost universally condemned in view of the risk of radiation damage. Kopp and Reymann (1967) described a high incidence of sequelae after an interval of 10 to 15 years following destructive doses of x-ray. Scarring occurred in three-quarters of the cases and there was a considerable incidence of epidermal atrophy, subcutaneous atrophy (often deep), hyperkeratosis, telangiectasia and ulceration.

Haemangiomata

The recognition that 90 per cent or more haemangiomatous naevi resolve spontaneously without blemish (Rook, 1972) has led to a very great decrease in the use of x-rays and radium in the treatment of these lesions. Although a few cases of carcinoma of the thyroid resulted from the treatment of haem-angiomatous naevi of the neck with superficial radiotherapy, when the danger was unrecognised (Wilson et al, 1958), it is fortunate that Li, Cassady and

Barnett (1974) have found that there was no significant excess of cancer deaths in a series of 4746 patients treated with irradiation in infancy for haemangioma of the skin between 1946 and 1968. Eighty-five per cent of these had been irradiated in the first year of life, usually with between 300 and 600 rad at 50 kV. Although Oeser, Krokowski and Schondorf (1964) considered that radiation provides a stimulus for regression, and recommended treatment as early as possible, Nordberg and Sundberg (1963), in reviewing 830 children treated with radium or x-ray, sounded a note of caution. They considered that radiation was not generally indicated, but early treatment may be required for rapidly growing lesions on the face and on the perineum. Nowadays extensive naevi, especially those affecting the eyelids and orbit and those causing difficulty in feeding, are treated with steroids (Fost and Esterly, 1968). Ten to 30 mg of prednisone is given daily for three weeks. Regression starts within two weeks and the dose can be reduced fairly rapidly. The mechanism of action is unknown. Only those patients not responding satisfactorily are considered for radiotherapy. Cipollaro and Crossland (1967) recommend 150 rad monthly for a total of four treatments. Port-wine stains are better treated with Grenz ray (see later).

Angiomata with thrombocytopenia and haemorrhagic manifestations are now increasingly recognised. These haemangiomata are usually cavernous in type and are present at birth, or develop in the first few months. Rapid enlargement may occur within a few weeks. Although oral corticosteroids are the treatment of choice, radiotherapy may be required for the local lesion. Up to 400 rad in divided doses is given (Atkins, Wolff and Sitarz, 1963).

Recurrent herpes simplex

Recurrent herpes simplex is a very annoying problem. Although topical idoxiuridine probably increases the rate of healing in individual episodes, it does not always prevent recurrences. Superficial radiotherapy is then well worth trying. Robert (1940) used single doses of 250 rad or two doses of 155 rad. Nineteen patients were followed up two years later and eight had cleared, eight improved and three had failed to improve. Frankl (1949) used one or two doses of 130 rad. Ten out of 12 patients given this treatment were clear at follow-up after two years. Our dosage schedule is 100 rad on three occasions at three-week intervals.

Lymphocytoma cutis

This is a benign hyperplasia of the reticuloendothelial tissues of the skin usually occurring in late teenage or early adult life. The condition presents as single or multiple papules or nodules, often on the face and ear lobes. Circumscribed and disseminated forms are described (Beare, 1972). Histologically the lymphocytic infiltration often takes a follicular arrangement. The circumscribed form responds better than the disseminated form to radiotherapy (Bäfverstedt, 1962), and 500 to 1500 rad are given either as a single dose or fractionated over several weeks. Bluefarb (1975) uses 75 to 100 rad weekly for five to seven doses.

Chronic perionychia

The cause of chronic perionychia is often multifactorial. Despite treatment of any *Candida* infection with nystatin, bacterial infection with genticin cream and advice about keeping the fingers dry and avoiding trauma to the cuticles, it can be very intractable and cause considerable pain and discomfort. For such cases some relief may be obtained by giving doses of x-ray of 100 rad at three-week intervals for three doses. Controlled trials are needed to establish the efficacy of this treatment. No sequelae were found on follow-up of 11 patients treated with a total of over 1600 rad to the nailfolds (Rowell, 1973).

Cheilitis exfoliativa

This is another intractable condition for which there is often no effective treatment. Several cases seem to have been helped by superficial radiotherapy.

Pruritus ani

When all organic causes of pruritus ani have been eliminated and, if possible, treated, there remain a number of patients who have an intractable itch–scratch–itch habit. Superficial radiotherapy is sometimes a very useful adjunct to topical applications and oral tranquillisers.

Hyperhidrosis

Superficial radiotherapy has been used in the past for the treatment of hyperhidrosis but is no longer recommended. Sedatives, anticholinergic preparations and localised excision of the sweat-bearing area helps axillary hyperhidrosis, and cervical sympathectomy may be very effective for excessive sweating of the hands.

GRENZ RAY

Grenz rays are very soft x-rays. The physical effects are qualitatively identical to conventional x-rays but the penetration is considerably less. The Grenz-ray machine, with an output between 6 and 15 kV, differs from conventional superficial radiotherapy equipment in several ways. The tube window is of beryllium which allows the emission of soft rays. Fluctuation in output can occur at low energy levels so that voltage line stabilisers are incorporated in the machine and regular calibration is of particular importance. The HVL is 0.018 to 0.033 mm of Al. Ninety to 95 per cent of the dose is absorbed by the upper 1 mm of the skin.

To compare Grenz ray with conventional superficial radiation, it can be said that 50 per cent of Grenz radiation is absorbed by 0.5 mm of skin whereas the same amount of hard radiation, produced at 60 to 100 kV, is only absorbed in 4 or more millimetres of skin. Grenz-ray machines, working up to 12 kV, are 30 to 50 times softer than conventional superficial radiation.

The scatter is very small indeed and there is very little hazard to the patient, operator or to others in the building. Fractionation produces less reaction than does a single dose. Bucky and Combes (1954) state that treatment can be given daily and consider that 100 rad daily for five days has a prompter and better effect than 500 rad in a single dose. Brauer (1975) advocates a course of treatment of 200 rad weekly for five weeks. Subsequent courses can be given after a rest period of four to five months. We have had satisfactory results with 300 rad given at three-weekly intervals for three doses.

Close shielding should be avoided in order to reduce the sharp line of pigmentation which may result from therapy. This occurs within one to two weeks of radiation and persists for several weeks, although is never permanent. Pigmentation is minimal with 300 rad or less and varies with race, age and body region, e.g. the scrotum. The patient should be warned about the possibility of temporary pigmentation. The eyes should be closed when the face is treated.

Grenz-ray therapy and carcinoma

Although Grenz-ray therapy has been claimed to be without danger and Bucky and Combes (1954) considered that epithelial proliferation, hypoplasia or neoplasia do not result from Grenz-ray therapy, this is not true. The development of squamous cell carcinoma after Grenz radiation has been reported by Kalz (1959), Ohkido and Horiuchi (1965) and Cipollaro and Crossland (1967). Brodkin and Bleiberg (1968) described a patient with psoriasis who was given 13 000 rad of Grenz ray to the buttocks over 21 months. She had not had any other local or internal medication nor was she known to have had any arsenic previously. Seven years later she was noted to have extensive areas of chronic radiodermatitis with marked atrophy, telangiectasia, depigmentation and hyperpigmentation in the area of irradiation. A squamous cell carcinoma was excised from one area. Abe, Sugai and Saito (1969) reported an unusual erythematous, purpuric and telangiectatic rash on the scrotum of a Korean man given 4200 rad in divided doses for lichen simplex about a year previously. Four sessile dark red tumours developed and one of these had the histology of an angiokeratoma with unusual and unexplained acantholysis.

These reports of carcinomata after Grenz-ray therapy must be put in perspective. Obviously the incidence of carcinoma after Grenz-ray therapy is very small.

Other side effects of Grenz-ray therapy

Radiodermatitis has been reported in two cases (Tsukinogi, 1963; Urano and Kanda, 1964). Pigmentation is the main side effect which is seen in patients after Grenz-ray therapy. This occurs frequently and may be quite disfiguring. It is not permanent but may take many months to clear. There is no evidence that it is more marked in patients on the contraceptive pill. It can be particularly embarrassing in Negroes. To reduce the amount of cosmetic disturbance it is usual to avoid screening off the area of irradiation.

Uses of Grenz-ray Therapy

The possibility of using Grenz-ray therapy instead of conventional superficial radiotherapy should always be considered because it is much safer. This is especially so when repeated courses may have to be given. In the main the indications for Grenz-ray therapy are those for conventional therapy, but there are some differences because of the poor penetration of Grenz rays. For a full account of Grenz-ray therapy the monographs of Bucky and Combes (1954) and Hollander (1968) should be consulted.

Eczema

Grenz ray, given in a dosage of 200 rad weekly for four doses, is useful for isolated patches of eczema (Sulzberger, 1975) and also for lichen simplex (Lynne-Davies, 1975). It has also been advocated in resistant cases of otitis externa (Stewart, 1975b).

Psoriasis

Although, in my experience, pustular psoriasis of the palms is more likely to respond to conventional superficial radiotherapy, 200 rad weekly of Grenz ray for five doses repeated, if necessary, after six months, is advocated by Stewart (1975a). Single doses of 300 rad are also helpful for plaques of psoriasis resistant to treatment with dithranol preparations. Grenz-ray therapy probably has no influence on psoriasis of the nails.

Lichen planus

Although there is little indication for radiotherapy in lichen planus, apart from areas of hypertrophic lichen planus, which respond better to conventional superficial radiotherapy, it is interesting to note that Kopp and Reymann (1956) gave three doses of 200 rad of Grenz ray at weekly intervals to 20 patients with lichen planus. They treated only one side of the body and gave simulated treatment, without actual administration of any radiation, to the other side. After three weeks the lesions were better on the treated side compared with the untreated side. Three weeks treatment was then given to the other side alone and after six weeks the results on both sides were equal. At that time 12 out of the 20 patients were clear of lichen planus and four others were greatly improved.

Brodkin and Bleiberg (1965), however, report a patient with acute eruptive lichen planus who developed an acute flare of lichen planus in the irradiated area on the back, one week after the fourth dose of 100 rad of Grenz ray when other areas were spontaneously clearing.

Garretts (1975) treats intractable lichen planus of the mouth with Grenz ray and claims remissions of between two and seven years. He gives 200 rad for three doses at fortnightly intervals. Bucky and Combes (1954) also found that lichen planus of the oral mucosa responded well, but they gave 800 to 1000 rad every two or three weeks.

Port wine stains

Several authors (Cipollaro and Crossland, 1967; Hollander, 1968; Rook, 1972) find Grenz ray disappointing in the treatment of port wine stains. However, Bucky and Combes (1954) show a picture of blanching of a port wine stain after 4000 rad in divided doses and quote other treatment schedules which have given good results. Braun-Falco and Lukacs (1973) advocate 100 to 150 rad on two consecutive treatments and this regime may be repeated later. Maresova (1957) gave 6000 to 8000 rad over 6 to 18 months and noted, in a series of 91 patients, complete clearing without side effects in 31, diminution with a few telangiectases and pigmentation in 35, diminution with considerable telangiectases and pigmentation in 10, and no improvement in 6 patients. The dosage schedule seems too high. Up to one year 500 rad, between one and two years 600 rad, and older patients 700 rad, was given every three to four weeks. Results were better with younger patients.

My own experience indicates that 800 rad every four to six months, starting at about 18 months of age, to a total of about 10 000 rad, is safe and pales the lesions to some extent. This may not seem very dramatic improvement but many patients and parents are very pleased with the results, because the camouflaging with covering creams is more effective. The treatment is safe. Rowell (1973) found no sequelae in five patients who had been given a total of 6400 to 12 800 rad for this purpose.

Darier's disease

There are several reports of improvement or complete clearance of lesions of Darier's disease after Grenz-ray therapy (Hollander, 1968). Sometimes there is no recurrence.

Hailey–Hailey disease

Familial benign chronic pemphigus is particularly suitable for Grenz-ray therapy in view of the superficial nature of the lesions, the regions affected (neck, flexures, scrotum) and chronicity. Grenz rays, 200 to 300 rad, at three-weekly intervals for three doses caused remissions of several months in six patients with Hailey–Hailey disease (Sarkany, 1959). This regime was better than a single dose of 400 rad.

Pruritus scroti, ani and vulvae

Grenz-ray therapy may be helpful in these intractable conditions. Cipollaro and Crossland (1967) claim that Grenz ray should not have any effect on sperm production.

Recurrent herpes simplex

Grenz ray has been effectively used to prevent recurrent episodes of herpes simplex. Knight (1972) used 200 rad at fortnightly intervals for four doses in 35 patients. Fifty-five per cent of irradiated patients were clear of episodes on follow-up at six months and 50 per cent were clear at one year and two years. A control group of 10 patients on no treatment at all remained unchanged over two years. The only criticism is that a fairer comparison could have been made if the control patients had been exposed to the Grenz-ray machine in the same way as the patients, except for the absence of radiation, and had been assessed by an observer without this knowledge.

Acne

Grenz ray is not effective in acne. Although Jelliffe et al (1969) found in a preliminary study that six out of seven patients had improved after Grenz-ray therapy, a subsequent controlled trial showed that there was no benefit from Grenz ray.

Wright (1964) treated 95 patients with up to 1200 rad of Grenz ray in divided doses and found no significant improvement after six months follow-up. He noted the hazard of increased pigmentation which took up to six months to clear. A similar opinion is held by DeGroot et al (1963). Pigmentation may be very disfiguring.

Keloids

Grenz ray is not suitable for the treatment of keloids.

CONVENTIONAL VERSUS GRENZ-RAY TREATMENT

Uses and limitations of conventional superficial x-ray therapy

Although in the past a considerable amount of emotion has been engendered by the use of superficial radiotherapy for benign disorders because of doubts about its safety, it can now be stated that this form of treatment is a safe procedure, as an adjunct to other forms of therapy, provided the following recommendations are accepted.

1. No area of skin should be subjected to more than 1200 rad in a lifetime.
2. The dose should be fractionated. A reasonable schedule is 100 rad, at 50 kV, at intervals of three to four weeks for three doses. At least two years should elapse between such courses. If further radiation is required after 900 rad have been given, Grenz ray, although less effective, should be considered as an alternative.

3. The face is more susceptible to radiation changes and care should be taken in irradiating the face, especially in patients liable to excessive exposure to sunlight.
4. Conventional superficial radiotherapy should not be given to children under 17 years of age unless absolutely necessary.
5. All areas of the body, other than the area to be irradiated, should be shielded, with particular attention being paid to shielding the eyes, the thyroid and the gonads.
6. Adequate records of all radiation should be kept.
7. All patients should be questioned about previous radiation at other clinics.
8. Superficial radiotherapy of the skin should only be given by staff who understand these recommendations.

Conventional superficial radiotherapy is useful in lichenified areas of eczema, resistant patches of psoriasis, pustular psoriasis of the palms and soles, hypertrophic lesions of lichen planus, severe cases of acne, hidradenitis suppurativa, areas involved by recurrent herpes simplex, chronic perionychia, pruritus ani, lymphocytoma cutis, and after excision of keloids if spontaneous resolution has not occurred.

Uses and limitations of Grenz-ray therapy

Although chronic radiodermatitis and carcinomata have been described after Grenz-ray therapy (see p. 342), the incidence is very rare indeed. It is likely that a total dose of 10 000 rad is safe although much larger total doses have been given. A dosage regime of 300 rad for three doses at three to four weekly intervals can be repeated on several occasions to a single area of the skin. Pigmentation may be disfiguring but is only temporary. The possibility of using Grenz ray should be considered first when conventional superficial x-ray therapy is indicated. It is particularly useful for port wine stains, Hailey–Hailey disease, and for the treatment of lesions in certain radio-sensitive areas such as the face, flexures, perineum and scrotum.

Conclusions

Radiotherapy is still a useful adjunct to other forms of treatment for certain non-malignant skin diseases. The safety of properly administered therapy has now been established. There is still a need, however, for controlled trials to evaluate the benefits of radiotherapy in most of the conditions for which it is currently used. The dose should be kept to a minimum and the softest possible radiation used. Dermatologists and radiotherapists should be trained in the use of conventional superficial x-ray and Grenz-ray therapy for benign disorders of the skin, and facilities for giving such radiotherapy should be available in all major dermatological centres.

REFERENCES

Abe, Y., Sugai, T. & Saito, T. (1969) Radiation angiokeratoma following Grenz radiation. *Archives of Dermatology*, **100**, 294.

Albert, R. E. & Omran, A. R. (1968) Follow-up study of patients treated by x-ray epilation for tinea capitis. I. Population characteristics, post-treatment illnesses, and mortality experience. *Archives of Environmental Health*, **17**, 899.

Albert, R. E., Omran, A. R., Brauer, E. W., Dove, D. C., Cohen, N. C., Schmidt, H., Baumring, R., Morrill, S., Schulz, R. & Baer, R. L. (1966) Follow-up study of patients treated by x-ray for tinea capitis. *American Journal of Public Health*, **56**, 2114.

Albright, E. C. & Allday, R. W. (1967) Thyroid carcinoma after radiation therapy for adolescent acne. *Journal of the American Medical Association*, **199**, 280.

Arnold, H. L. (1975) Keloids. In *Current Medical Management*, 2nd edn, ed. Madden, S., p. 194. St Louis: C. V. Mosby.

Atkins, H. L., Wolff, J. A. & Sitarz, A. (1963) Giant hemangioma in infancy with secondary thrombocytopenic purpura. *American Journal of Roentgenology*, **89**, 1062.

Baer, R. L. & Witten, V. H. (1955) Selected aspects of dermatologic therapy with superficial x-ray and Grenz ray. *Year Book of Dermatology and Syphilology*, 1955–56, p. 7. Chicago: Year Book Medical Publishers.

Baer, R. L. & Witten, V. H. (1958) Comment in *Year Book of Dermatology*, 1958–59 series, p. 96.

Baer, R. L. & Witten, V. H. (1960) Acne vulgaris. *Year Book of Dermatology*, 1959–60. Chicago: Year Book Medical Publishers.

Bäfverstedt, B. (1962) Unusual forms of lymphadenosis benigna cutis (LABC). *Acta deramato-venereologica (Stockholm)*, **42**, 3.

Beare, M. (1972) In *Textbook of Dermatology*, 2nd edn, ed. Rook, A., Ebling, J. & Wilkinson, D. S., p. 1379. Oxford: Blackwell.

Belisario, J. C. (1957) Treatment of keloids. *Acta dermato-venereologica*, **37**, 165.

Black, M. M. & Jones, E. W. (1971) Dermal cylindroma following x-ray epilation of the scalp. *British Journal of Dermatology*, **85**, 70.

Bluefarb, S. M. (1975) In *Current Medical Management*, 2nd edn, ed. Madden, S., p. 274. St Louis: C. V. Mosby.

Borak, J., Eller, J. J. & Eller, W. D. (1949) Roentgen therapy for hyperhidrosis: observation of 122 patients. *Archives of Dermatology and Syphilology*, **59**, 644.

Brauer, E. W. (1975) Grenz ray therapy. In *Current Medical Management*, 2nd edn, ed. Madden, S., p. 25. St Louis: C. V. Mosby.

Braun-Falco, O. & Lukacs, S. (1973) Dermatologische Röntgen-therapie. Berlin, Heidelberg, New York: Springer-Verlag.

Brodkin, R. H. & Bleiberg, J. (1965) Grenz rays and lichen planus: case report of isomorphic phenomenon following Grenz-ray therapy. *Archives of Dermatology*, **91**, 149.

Brodkin, R. H. & Bleiberg, J. (1968) Neoplasia resulting from Grenz radiation. *Archives of Dermatology*, **97**, 307.

Brown, R. H. (1958) Comparative statistical studies on influence of hardness of radiation and size of dose on results of x-ray treatment of eczema. *Dermatologica*, **117**, 215.

Bucky, G. & Combes, F. C. (1954) *Grenz-ray Therapy*. Springer Publishing Co. Inc.

Chu, F. C. H., Conrad, J. T., Bane, H. N., Glicksman, A. S. & Nickson, J. J. (1960) Quantitative and qualitative evaluation of skin erythema. I. Technique of measurement and description of the reaction. *Radiology*, **75**, 406.

Cipollaro, A. C. & Crossland, P. M. (1967) *X-rays and Radium in the Treatment of Diseases of the Skin*, p. 394. Philadelphia: Lea and Febiger.

Code of Practice for the protection of persons against ionising radiations arising from medical and dental use, published by Her Majesty's Station Office, 1972.

Crossland, P. M. (1957) Dermatologic radiation therapy in this nuclear age. *Journal of the American Medical Association*, **165**, 647.

Cunliffe, W. J. & Cotterill, J. A. (1975) *The Acnes. Clinical Features, Pathogenesis and Treatment*, London, Philadelphia, Toronto: W. B. Saunders Co. Ltd. p. 233.

DeGroot, W. P., Prakken, J. R., Verbeek, A. M. J. A. & Woerdeman, M. J. (1963) The value of Grenz-ray therapy for acne vulgaris. *Dermatologica*, **126**, 319.

DeLawter, D. S. & Winship, T. (1963) Follow-up study of adults treated with roentgen rays for thyroid disease. *Cancer, N.Y.*, **16**, 1028.

Domonkos, A. & Cameron, S. H. (1957) Radiation protection in dermatology. *Archives of Dermatology*, **76**, 694.

Fischer, E. & Storck, H. (1957) X-ray treatment of keloids. *Schweizerische medizenische Wochenschrift*, **87**, 1281.

Fost, N. C. & Esterley, N. B. (1968) Successful treatment of juvenile hemangiomas with prednisone. *Journal of Pediatrics*, **72**, 351.

Frankl, J. (1949) Nouvelles données sur la radiotherapie de l'herpès récidivant. *Annals of Dermatology and Syphilology*, **9**, 168.

Garretts, M. (1975) Personal communication.

Glicksman, A. S., Chu, F. C. H., Bane, H. N. & Nickson, J. J. (1960) Quantitative and qualitative evaluation of skin erythema. II. Clinical study in patients on a standardised irradiation schedule. *Radiology*, **75**, 411.

Goldschmidt, H. (1975) Ionising radiation therapy in dermatology. Current use in the United States and Canada. *Archives of Dermatology*, **111**, 1511.

Harber, L. C. (1958) Clinical evaluation of radiation therapy in psoriasis. *Archives of Dermatology*, **77**, 554.

Hollander, M. B. (1968) *Ultrasoft X-rays: an Historical and Critical Review of the World Experience with Grenz Rays and Other X-rays of Long Wavelength.* Baltimore: Williams and Wilkins.

Jelliffe, A. M., Soutter, C. & Meara, R. H. (1969) An investigation into the treatment of acne vulgaris with Grenz rays. *British Journal of Dermatology*, **81**, 617.

Kalz, F. (1941) Theoretic considerations and clinical use of Grenz rays in dermatology. *Archives of Dermatology*, **43**, 447.

Kalz, F. (1959) Observations of Grenz-ray reactions. I. The response of normal human skin to Grenz rays. II. The effect of overdosage. *Dermatologica*, **118**, 357.

Knight, A. G. (1972) Grenz-ray treatment of recurrent herpes simplex. *British Journal of Dermatology*, **86**, 172.

Kolar, J., Bek, V. & Vrabec, R. (1967) Hypoplasia of growing breast. *Archives of Dermatology*, **96**, 427.

Kopp, H. & Reymann, F. E. (1956) Lichen planus treated with Grenz ray: preliminary report. *Acta dermato-venereologica*, **36**, 477.

Kopp, H. & Reymann, F. (1967) Follow up study of treatment of plantar warts with ultrasoft x-rays. *Acta dermato-venereologica*, **47**, 46.

Kozlova, A. V. (1969) Conditions of the development of radiation cancer (an analysis of 38 observations). *Medical Radiology, Moscow*, **14**, 3.

Li, F. P., Cassady, J. R. & Barnett, E. (1974) Cancer mortality following irradiation in infancy for hemangioma. *Radiology*, **113**, 177.

Lynne-Davies, G. (1975) Lichen simplex chronicus. In *Current Medical Management*, 2nd edn, ed. Madden, S., p. 203. St Louis: C. V. Mosby.

McMullan, F. H. & Zeligman, I. (1956) Perifolliculitis capitis abscedens et suffodiens: its successful treatment with x-ray epilation. *Archives of Dermatology*, **73**, 256.

Maggiora, A., Bujard, E. & Jadassohn, W. (1965) Effect of roentgen radiation on the sebaceous glands of the guinea-pig and of man. *Hautarzt*, **16**, 298.

Maresova, J. (1957) Radiation therapy of nevus flammeus with Bucky rays. *Ceskoslovenská Dermatologie*, **32**, 156.

Martin, H., Strong, E. & Spiro, R. H. (1970) Radiation-induced skin cancer of the head and neck. *Cancer*, **25**, 61.

Miescher, G. (1953) Recent advances in dermatologic x-ray therapy. *Dermatologica*, **107**, 225.

Miescher, G. & Böhm, C. (1948) Roentgen therapy for hyperhidrosis: follow-up of 192 treated patients. *Schweizerische medizenische Wochenschrift*, **78**, 14.

Milne, J. A. (1972) Acne vulgaris. In *Recent Trends in Dermatology*, No. 3, ed. Rook, A. Edinburgh: Churchill-Livingstone.

Mole, R. H. (1972) Radiation-induced tumours—human experience. *British Journal of Radiology*, **45**, 613.

Nordberg, U.-B. & Sundberg, J. (1963) Indications and methods for radiotherapy of cavernous haemangiomas. Study of 1191 haemangiomas following radiotherapy. *Acta radiologica (Therapy)*, **1**, 257.

Oeser, H., Krokowski, E. & Schondorf, K. W. (1964) Rationale of irradiation of cutaneous angiomas. *Radiologie*, **4**, 204.

Ohkido, M. & Horiuchi, Y. (1965) A case of squamous cell carcinoma caused by Grenz-ray irradiation. *Japanese Journal of Clinical Dermatology*, **19**, 315.

Pegum, J. S. (1972) Radiation-induced skin cancer. *British Journal of Radiology*, **45**, 613.

Reisner, R. M. (1975) Acne vulgaris. In *Current Medical Management*, 2nd edn, ed. Madden, S., p. 62. St Louis: C. V. Mosby.

Ridley, C. M. (1962) Basal cell carcinoma following x-ray epilation of the scalp. *British Journal of Dermatology*, **74**, 222.

Robert, P. (1940) The treatment of recurrent herpes with radiotherapy. *Dermatologica*, **82**, 108.

Rook, A. (1972) Telangiectatic naevi. In *Textbook of Dermatology*, 2nd edn, ed. Rook, A., Ebling, J. & Wilkinson, D. S., p. 139. Oxford: Blackwell.

Rowell, N. R. (1973) A follow-up study of superficial radiotherapy for benign dermatoses: recommendations for the use of x-rays in dermatology. *British Journal of Dermatology*, **88**, 583.

Rubin, P. & Casarett, G. W. (1968) *Clinical Radiation Pathology*, Vol. 1. Philadelphia: Saunders.

Russell, B. (1959) Fibrosarcomata of the skin and subcutaneous tissues. *Transactions and Annual Report of the St John's Hospital Dermatological Society*, **42**, 15.

Ryan, T. (1972) Ionising radiation. In *Textbook of Dermatology*, 2nd edn, ed. Rook, A., Ebling, J. & Wilkinson, D. S., p. 469. Oxford: Blackwell.

Sarkany, I. (1959) Grenz-ray treatment of familial benign chronic pemphigus. *British Journal of Dermatology*, **71**, 247.

Sarkany, I., Fountain, R. B., Evans, C. D., Morrison, R. & Szur, L. (1968) Multiple basal cell epitheliomata following radiotherapy of the spine. *British Journal of Dermatology*, **80**, 90.

Stewart, W. D. (1975a) Eczema. In *Current Medical Management*, 2nd edn, ed. Madden, S., p. 144. St Louis: C. V. Mosby.

Stewart, W. D. (1975b) Otitis externa. In *Current Medical Management*, 2nd edn, ed. Madden, S., p. 234. St Louis: C. V. Mosby.

Stewart, W. D., Witten, V. H. & Sulzberger, M. B. (1958) Studies on the quantity of radiation reaching the gonadal areas during dermatologic x-ray therapy. III. Shielding technics and other precautions for reducing the gonad dose. *Journal of Investigative Dermatology*, **30**, 237.

Storck, H. (1972) Superficial radiotherapy of the skin. In *Handbuch der Medizinischen Radiologie*, Vol. XII, p. 17. Springer-Verlag.

Strauss, J. S. & Kligman, A. M. (1960) Effect of x-rays on sebaceous glands of human face: radiation effect of acne. *Journal of Clinical Investigation*, **33**, 347.

Sulzberger, M. B. (1975) Atopic dermatitis. In *Current Medical Management*, 2nd edn, ed. Madden, S., p. 109. St Louis: C. V. Mosby.

Sulzberger, M. B., Baehr, R. L. & Borotra, A. (1952) Do roentgen-ray treatments as given by skin specialists produce cancers or other sequelae? *Archives of Dermatology*, **65**, 639.

Sweet, R. D. (1962) Acute accidental superficial x-ray burns. An interim report of 11 cases. *British Journal of Dermatology*, **74**, 392.

Sweet, R. D. (1968) Radiation for conditions other than cancer. *British Journal of Dermatology*, **80**, 265.

Traenkle, H. L. (1963) X-ray induced cancer in man. *National Cancer Institute Monograph*, **10**, 423. Department of Health, Education and Welfare.

Tsukinogi, K. (1963) A case of radiodermatitis with calcinosis following Grenz-rays treatment. *Clinical Dermatology*, **5**, 165.

Urano, K. & Kanda, Y. (1964) Skin disturbance due to overdoses of Grenz radiation. *Japanese Journal of Clinical Dermatology*, **18**, 897.

Van den Brank, H. A. & Minty, C. C. (1960) Radiation in the management of keloids and hypertrophic scars. *British Journal of Surgery*, **47**, 595.

Weidman, A. I., Zimany, A. & Kopf, A. W. (1966) Underdevelopment of the human breast after radiotherapy. *Archives of Dermatology*, **93**, 708.

Wilson, G. M., Kilpatrick, R., Eckert, H., Curran, R. C., Jepson, R. P., Blomfield, G. W. & Miller, H. (1958) Thyroid neoplasms following irradiation. *British Medical Journal*, **2**, 929.

Witten, V. H., Sulzberger, M. B. & Stewart, W. D. (1957) Studies on the quantity of radiation reacting the gonadal areas during dermatologic x-ray therapy. II. Methods, quantitative measurements, and analysis of some important factors influencing gonad dose. *Archives of Dermatology*, **76**, 683.

Wright, W. L. (1964) Grenz ray in the treatment of acne vulgaris. *Archives of Dermatology*, **89**, 417.

Zeligman, I. (1965) Temporary x-ray epilation therapy of chronic axillary hidradenitis suppurativa. *Archives of Dermatology*, **92**, 690.

11
DRUG REACTIONS

Ashley Levantine   John Almeyda

With the ever-increasing use of drugs in the treatment of disease more adverse reactions are noted each year. These are manifest predominantly as cutaneous reactions.

In view of the magnitude of this subject, this chapter is restricted to general considerations of classification and mechanisms, with a more detailed report on four selected reactions.

CLASSIFICATION AND MECHANISM OF DRUG REACTIONS

The mechanism of most drug reactions is unknown. However, we have good evidence that untoward responses to drugs can arise in several ways. It is important to note that drug allergy (or hypersensitivity) is often said to be the cause of a reaction on insufficient evidence.

Overdosage. The resulting reaction is directly related to the total amount of drug in the body. Overdosage may be absolute, due to deliberate over-ingestion or overprescribing, or relative, due to an underlying abnormality in the patient such as renal failure which diminishes drug excretion.

Intolerance. When this occurs there is a low threshold to the normal pharmacological action of a drug. Thus an abnormally small dose produces the characteristic effects of the drug. Both excretion defects and pharmaco-genetic mechanisms (see below) may predispose an individual to drug intolerance.

Idiosyncrasy. An uncharacteristic response to a drug which is not due to an immunological mechanism. Pharmacogenetic mechanisms often play a part.

Pharmacogenetics

Very few drugs are eliminated from the body unchanged. They may be metabolised by oxidation, reduction, hydrolysis or conjugation. More than one of these reactions may be involved either simultaneously or consecutively. The various enzymes involved are subject to variations on a hereditary basis, so that there may be differences in the way in which individuals metabolise drugs. These differences depend on polymorphism in specific enzymes.

Acetylation defects. The hepatic enzyme, acetyl transferase, acetylates certain drugs, including isoniazid, dapsone, phenelzine and hydralazine.

Slow acetylation is inherited as an autosomal recessive trait (Evans, Manley and McKusick, 1960). The slow acetylator phenotype occurs with variable frequency in populations of different racial origin. Slow acetylators accumulate high levels of isoniazid on normal doses of the drug and, after prolonged ingestion, they tend to develop signs of toxicity such as peripheral neuropathy. Slow acetylators are more likely to develop haematological effects from dapsone (Peters et al, 1970) and subjective side effects from phenelzine (Evans, Davidson and Pratt, 1965).

Slow acetylation may also result in hydralazine toxicity. Both hydralazine and isoniazid have a potential for inducing a disseminated lupus erythematosus-like syndrome (Alarćon-Segovia, 1969). Perry, Sakamato and Tan (1967) have shown that prolonged ingestion of hydralazine, in a group of hypertensive patients, resulted in the production of an unusually high incidence of antinuclear antibodies, and toxic symptoms in the slow acetylators of the group. The mechanism of the antinuclear antibody production is not well understood. Patients with hydralazine-induced lupus erythematosus have antibodies to diazotised hydralazine, and their lymphocytes transform in the presence of the drug, suggesting that hydralazine allergy is present (Hahn et al, 1972).

Glucose-6-phosphate dehydrogenase deficiency is inherited as a sex-linked dominant character, and has been observed most frequently in Negroes. Affected individuals develop acute haemolysis when exposed to certain drugs. These include primaquine, phenacetin, nitrofurantoin, dapsone, aspirin and a number of sulphonamides. Ingestion of, or exposure to, the pollen of the fava bean may result in haemolytic anaemia in enzyme-deficient subjects.

Suxamethonium. In a few patients, neuromuscular blockade due to suxamethonium is very much prolonged, because their plasma pseudocholinesterase is atypical and cannot hydrolyse the drug.

Acute toxicity

This may result from overdosage, or an abnormally fast or great absorption of the drug. Certain drugs have predictable toxic effects by virtue of their pharmacological nature. In view of its widespread use and high incidence of allergic reactions, penicillin has a surprisingly low incidence of toxicity.

Chronic toxicity

This results from the chronic accumulation of drugs and their metabolites. This may be a simple deposition of the drug in the phagocytic cells of the skin and mucous membranes. Argyria, for example, is due to deposition of silver, and may result from absorption after prolonged application of silver salts to the mucous membranes. Continued administration of gold may result in a faint purple gingival discoloration (Dummett, 1965). Repeated applications of mercury-containing ointments or cosmetics may give rise to grey-brown pigmentation, limited to areas of application, with accentuation in the skin folds (Jeghers, 1944). Burge and Winkelmann (1970), using the electron microscope, demonstrated that melanin pigmentation increased secondary to the presence of the metal.

The accumulation of melanin, or melanin plus chlorpromazine or its metabolites, is thought to cause the purple skin discoloration in patients receiving chlorpromazine for long periods. Perry et al (1964) suggested that hydroxychlorpromazine, or a metabolite of this compound, is converted to a purple compound on exposure to ultraviolet light.

Chronic arsenical accumulation produces a wide variety of adverse reactions. The most noted of these include both cutaneous and internal malignancies, keratoses and the classical 'rain-drop' pigmentation. The mechanism of arsenical pigmentation is thought to be related to its chemical binding with sulphydryl groups, thus freeing copper and activating tyrosinase.

Acute intermittent porphyria. It is widely accepted that the administration of certain drugs to patients with acute intermittent porphyria can worsen the course of the disease and also precipitate attacks in subjects with latent porphyria. Barbiturates are the most notable drugs to produce this effect, but chlorpropamide, griseofulvin, phenytoin and oral contraceptives may also precipitate this form of porphyria. The possible mechanism has been discussed fully by De Matteis (1967).

Secondary or facultative effects

These are indirect effects mainly due to a disturbance caused by the drug in homeostatic and other control mechanisms. Candidiasis of the anogenital region and oral mucous membranes after the administration of broad-spectrum antibiotics is a common example. The most likely mechanism is the suppression of natural competitors, thus allowing *Candida albicans* to multiply at an increased rate. Corticosteroids and immunosuppressive drugs may also favour the multiplication of *Candida.*

The Jarisch–Herxheimer reaction

This reaction is the focal exacerbation of lesions of infective origin when specific antibiotic therapy is initiated. The reaction is thought to be due to sudden release of pharmacologically active substances from dying micro-organisms or damaged tissue. The classical example is observed in the treatment of early syphilis with penicillin.

Hypersensitivity

Hypersensitivity reactions develop from an allergic sensitisation to a drug, resulting from previous exposure to that drug or to a chemically related substance. The reactions are of two main types depending on whether sensitisation produces humoral antibody or a cell-mediated response. The subject of allergic drug reactions has recently been covered in detail by Amos (1976).

It is generally accepted that drugs of low molecular weight, or the degradation products of drugs, must bind covalently to a carrier molecule in order to become immunogenic. However, recent work on the immunogenicity of small molecules, such as nucleic acids or hapten-oligopeptides, have also indicated that binding through non-covalent bonds to an immunogenic protein may suffice to induce an immune response against the haptenic group (De Weck, 1972). In sensitisation to small molecular weight chemicals in vivo, the role of the carrier molecule is assumed to be played by autologous proteins. Haptens which bind reversibly to proteins do not become immunogenic (Ackroyd, 1975). Those haptens which are not combined with a carrier molecule cannot stimulate an immunological reaction even in a highly sensitised person, but they may block the reaction of hapten–macromolecular complex with antibody by combining reversibly with the antigen-combining sites of the antibody (Ackroyd, 1975; Parker et al, 1962; Locher, Schneider and De Weck, 1969). A well-recognised fact is that conjugates carrying several antigenic determinants (multivalent) are most efficient in eliciting immediate-type allergy reactions due to specific immunoglobulins and in forming antigen–antibody complexes (De Weck, 1972). Univalent haptens, as free drugs or unconjugated drug metabolites, not only fail to elicit allergic responses but compete with multivalent antigens for antibody. This action helps to explain why the incidence of anaphylactic or serum sickness to drugs is low (Parker et al, 1962). When drug-induced anaphylaxis occurs, the drug has a high degree of chemical reactivity that allows it to react rapidly with serum and tissue proteins to form multivalent conjugates. Penicillin possesses this property and thus has a tendency to produce anaphylaxis (Parker, 1975a).

There is still little known about the mechanisms of cell-mediated drug sensitivity. De Weck (1972) felt that exanthematic drug eruptions are a manifestation of cellular immunity and delayed-type hypersensitivity. Of course, exanthematic reactions account for a large number of drug reactions.

As well as immediate-type reactions, drugs may also induce reactions involving the formation of immune complexes (serum-sickness type; Arthus type) and delayed type hypersensitivity. Most of the research has been performed on penicillin allergy.

Immediate reactions

These reactions occur within seconds or minutes after the offending drug is administered. The severest cases develop anaphylactic shock. Injected soluble penicillin is the most common drug to produce this reaction.

The penicillins contain a number of antigenic determinants with high sensitising potential. The major haptenic determinant in penicillin allergy is the penicilloyl group (Ackroyd, 1975). Penicilloyl is formed either by direct reaction between penicillin and amino acid carriers or by degradation of penicillin to penicillanic acid, which then forms penicilloyl amino acid conjugates. Penicillin also contains several other antigens, collectively referred to as the minor determinants. These include penicillin breakdown products and protein impurities. Recent studies show that immediate type reactions to penicillin are largely mediated by IgE antibodies (Juhlin and Wide, 1972).

Accelerated urticarial and late urticarial reactions

These reactions are probably associated with skin sensitising antibodies and IgG antibodies of benzylpenicilloyl specificity. Levine (1966) found that any loss of urticaria as penicillin therapy continued appeared to be due to the spontaneous rise in titre of benzylpenicilloyl-specific IgG antibodies acting as 'blocking' antibodies. The difference between accelerated and late reactors is that the former have benzylpenicilloyl-specific antibodies before penicillin therapy, whereas in late reactors these antibodies develop during the course of therapy.

Serum sickness type reactions

Serum sickness is a systemic allergic reaction produced by circulating immune complexes. It is characterised by fever, rash, arthritis, lymphadenopathy, nephritis and oedema. Urticarial and maculopapular eruptions are particularly common. Many cases of drug sensitivity, in particular penicillin and sulphonamides, are examples of this type of reaction. The manifestations are produced by antigens that remain in the circulation for prolonged periods so that at the time antibody is first formed, intravascular antigen is still present, thus allowing the formation of circulating antigen–antibody complexes (Parker, 1975a). Symptoms develop after a latent period of six days or more, and the delay is due to the time needed to synthesise appreciable amounts of antibody.

Levine (1966) investigated 16 patients with this type of reaction. Three patients had skin sensitising antibodies to the minor determinants and IgM, or IgG and IgM antibodies of penicilloyl specificity. Fellner (1968) biopsied urticarial lesions in a patient with serum sickness due to penicillin. Using fluoresceinated antipenicilloyl antibody, penicillin was demonstrated in mononuclear cells and eosinophils. This suggested that, as in classical serum sickness, the lesions are due to immune complexes (Ackroyd, 1975).

Arthus type reactions

These reactions depend on the formation of complement activating immune complexes as a result of interaction of antigen with antibody in antigen excess (Coombs and Gell, 1968). As mentioned above this type of complex is only formed in response to antigens that are multivalent (De Weck, 1972). Investigation of the sera for immune precipitate formation in patients with drug hypersensitivity has largely been inconclusive (Ackroyd, 1975). In penicillamine-induced nephrotic syndrome, electronmicroscopic studies have shown glomerular subepithelial deposits virtually identical with those seen in immune-complex nephritis (Jaffe, 1968).

Delayed hypersensitivity to drugs

As mentioned above, it has been thought that many exanthematic drug eruptions are due to delayed type hypersensitivity (De Weck, 1972). Redmond and Levine (1968) found that the lesions of delayed hypersensitivity to penicillin, produced by intradermal injection of the drug, were identical to those produced by tuberculin. They stated that the incidence of delayed type hypersensitivity, as demonstrated by skin testing, is about 10 times higher than the incidence of actual sensitivity reactions to penicillin. Therefore, in a considerable number of patients, delayed type skin reactions to penicillin are not associated with drug reactions. This may indicate only that the patient has been exposed to the drug or to an immunochemically related compound and has developed an immunological, but not necessarily a clinical reaction to it (Ackroyd, 1975).

Factors influencing the development of hypersensitivity

The effect of age is difficult to assess, but it has been said that allergic reactions to drugs occur less commonly in children. It may be due to a less vigorous antibody response in children or to less previous drug exposure, but the exact mechanism is unknown (Parker, 1975b). The atopic constitution has been regarded as being associated with an increased risk of developing reactions to drugs such as penicillin. There is, however, no statistically significant difference in penicillin reactivity in atopic and non-atopic individuals (Rytel et al, 1963). Juhlin and Wide (1972) found that none of 15 patients with a positive radio-allergosorbant test to penicilloyl had any history of atopic disease.

Patients who have suffered an allergic reaction to one drug occasionally seem to react to other drugs. The reason for this observation is certainly not clear but in some cases the history of drug allergy may have been based solely on the patient's understanding of this phenomenon (Parker, 1975b). Other cases may be due to cross-sensitivity.

In general, the larger the dose and the longer that a drug is administered, the greater is the possibility of developing hypersensitivity. On the other hand, minute doses may elicit severe, even fatal reactions, in a sensitised subject.

Any route of administration can result in hypersensitivity. It has been said that anaphylaxis is less common with oral than with parenterally administered drugs (Spark, 1971). However, the incidence of hypersensitivity does not appear to be influenced very much by the way in which a drug is given.

Cross-sensitisation

This reaction occurs when allergic symptoms induced by one compound are subsequently produced in the same patient by one or more related substances.

The drug which originally resulted in sensitivity is referred to as the primary allergen, and other drugs to which the patient reacts are called secondary allergens. Not all subjects sensitised to the same primary allergen show the same range of cross-sensitisation. A knowledge of cross-sensitivity is important, for the failure to recognise a chemical relationship between different drugs, may lead to the inadvertent substitution of a secondary allergen in a patient who has had had a severe reaction. Therefore the possibility of cross-sensitisation must be borne in mind when a reaction persists.

The association of cross-sensitivity between drugs causing contact dermatitis and drugs given systemically is mentioned below.

Hyposensitisation

The natural duration of hypersensitivity varies from a few days to several years, so that apparently successful hyposensitisation is difficult to evaluate.

The procedure of hyposensitisation usually consists of the administration, at short intervals of initially minute, but gradually increasing doses. In view of the risks involved hyposensitisation should only be carried out if the offending drug is essential for the patient's life or health. It is important to take rigorous precautions so that one is prepared to deal with a life-threatening anaphylactic reactions. Hyposensitisation has been accomplished with isoniazid, diphenylhydantoin, penicillamine, tetracycline, nitrogen mustard and streptomycin usually on a slowly increasing dosage programme extending over a period of several days to a week (Parker, 1975c).

It is thought that the mechanism of hyposensitisation involves the development of non-reaginic antibodies, which combine preferentially with the allergen and so prevent its combination with anaphylactic antibody, which would lead to histamine release (Lowell, 1965). Levene (1972) reported on hyposensitisation to streptomycin in one patient (Levene and Withers, 1969) and to platinum in another (Levene and Calnan, 1971). He commented that, during the procedure both patients developed lesions which resembled type III reactions (Coombs and Gell, 1968). This was consistent with the view that non-reaginic antibodies were induced during hyposensitisation, and that these antibodies could be connected with the patient's improved ability to handle the allergen without anaphylactic reactions.

The practical use of monovalent haptens to inhibit allergic reactions to drugs and particularly to penicillin has made an encouraging start (De Weck, 1972). The parenteral administration of a penicilloyl hapten already conjugated to an amino acid, and thus non-immunogenic, has shown marked inhibitory activity in penicillin-sensitive patients (De Weck and Schneider, 1972; De Weck and Girard, 1972). In such patients penicillin treatment could be continued under cover of the hapten.

THE DIAGNOSIS OF DRUG ERUPTIONS

The clinical manifestations of drug reactions are so varied that, with the exception of a few distinctive reaction patterns, it is seldom possible to incriminate any one drug. Skin rashes are probably the commonest manifestations of drug reactions and may also be accompanied by visceral reactions. The clinical appearances of most drug eruptions are non-specific. Uncommonly, as with carbromal, the eruption is almost pathognomonic. Certain reactions, such as fixed drug eruptions may allow the range of suspects to be narrowed. Difficulties are encountered, in that identical eruptions may be seen from completely unrelated drugs, and different types of eruption may be seen with any one drug (Copeman, 1972). In fact, most drugs have been reported as causing an eruption, although the high risk group includes antibiotics (particularly penicillin), sulphonamide and barbiturates.

The basic disease of the patient should always be taken into account, for the tissue reaction may have been caused by the disease rather than the drug therapy. For example, when an antibiotic is given for an infection, any eruption which develops might be associated with the properties of the organism itself or its breakdown products. An adequate history should be taken of recent operative and diagnostic procedures and of other treatments such as radiotherapy.

Polypharmacy is very common so that once a reaction has developed it is essential to enquire about all drugs that the patient is receiving. A detailed history should also include the date on which each drug was first administered in relation to the date of onset of the reaction. It is important to know whether the patient has taken the same or related drugs before and whether he has ever suffered from a drug reaction. One difficulty often experienced is that the patient may deny taking any drugs at all. Drugs popularly regarded as harmless, such as those bought without prescription, are often forgotten and not regarded as drugs. The history should also include details of diet and of any chemical exposures at home or at work.

The timing of a drug reaction depends, to a large extent, on the mechanism. Thus an anaphylactic reaction occurs within minutes of re-exposure to the drug. A reaction may not develop until after the drug administration has ceased. Serum sickness symptoms appear 7 to 10 days after the effective sensitising dose. Long-acting depôt preparations will modify the timing and duration of reaction. Of course the effects of inorganic arsenic may not become apparent for many years.

In Vivo Tests

Discontinuation of the drug

Whenever a drug reaction is suspected, all therapy should, if possible, be stopped. When a drug is essential for the patient, the commonest offenders should be withdrawn first. If the reaction subsides, this strengthens one's suspicions of a drug reaction, but does not confirm them, for the reaction may have been a naturally occurring self-limiting event unrelated to the therapy. As mentioned above, slow excretion or depôt preparations may result in prolonged reactions, as also will the inadvertent substitution of the drug with a chemically related drug. Cross-sensitisation to chemicals in food and drinks, e.g. quinine in bitter drinks, may complicate the situation thus prolonging the reaction. Penicillin may be present in sufficient quantity in milk and its products to sustain a hypersensitivity reaction.

Readministration

A test dose administered, after recovery from the reaction, may reliably incriminate a drug. In hypersensitivity, fatal reactions to minimal amounts of drugs have been recorded, particularly with penicillin (Rose, 1953). Readministration may be justified in a patient dependent on a drug for which no chemically unrelated alternative is available. Even then it is safer to use other methods of establishing drug allergy first and all means to combat an anaphylactic reaction should be close at hand. It must be realised that readministration of the responsible drug does not always result in a positive reaction. Hypersensitivity to the drug may disappear or the test dose may be too small.

Skin tests

In general, skin tests are of limited value in the diagnosis of drug eruptions. A positive reaction on intradermal, scratch or prick testing, merely indicates cutaneous hypersensitivity to the substance. Therefore a patient who gives a positive skin test to a drug may tolerate its administration by any but the percutaneous route. Also, negative skin tests are not infrequently recorded in patients who have subsequently experienced systemic reactions. Severe, even fatal reactions, following intradermal testing to penicillin have been reported (Boger et al, 1953), so that skin testing should be not carried out in patients with a history of anaphylactic hypersensitivity.

The use of skin tests is limited by lack of knowledge of the actual allergen. A derivative of the drug, rather than the drug itself, may be the effective antigenic determinant, and the type of sensitivity demonstrated by the test may not be identical with the type of sensitivity responsible for the allergic reaction.

Intradermal testing

Knowledge of the antigenic determinants of penicillin has led to the development of skin tests of increasing reliability. As mentioned above, the major haptenic determinant in penicillin allergy is the penicilloyl group. Penicilloyl-polylysine, which is a conjugated form of the penicilloyl group, has been found to be most suitable for skin testing (Brown, Price and Moore, 1964).

The correlation between immediate type hypersensitivity reactions to penicillin and a positive skin test with penicilloyl-polylysine has varied from 17 to 91 per cent, according to different investigators (Idsøe et al, 1968). Brown et al (1964) used this test for the detection of penicillin hypersensitivity in 16 239 patients. In 1003 patients with a history of penicillin sensitivity, 396 had a positive skin test compared to a positive test in 775 of 12 559 patients with a negative history. They observed reactions to penicillin treatment in 63 of 13 530 patients with negative tests. Of 212 patients with a moderately positive, and 206 with a strongly positive skin test who were subsequently given penicillin, only 9 and 21 respectively developed reactions.

Since the antigenic specificities of the skin-sensitising antibodies in patients with immediate type reactions are not necessarily only due to the penicilloyl group, it is important to test to the minor antigenic determinants. This can be done using benzyl penicillin, although other minor determinants may be used (Levine, 1966).

In practice, penicilloyl-polylysine is usually tested first, and if this is negative benzylpenicillin is tried. To avoid dangerous reactions it is safer to perform prick tests first, and if these are negative the reagents are injected intradermally. In testing with penicilloyl-polylysine it is usually safe to begin with the intradermal injection of a 10^{-5} M solution (with respect to the penicilloyl concentration) followed by a 50×10^{-5} M solution. If the history does not suggest severe sensitivity, testing can be initiated with a scratch test using 100 to 200 units/ml followed by the successive intradermal injection of solutions containing 20, 400, and 5000 units/ml at intervals of about 10 min (Parker, 1975c).

Interpretation of intradermal tests may be difficult (Green and Rosenblum, 1971). Positive reactions are indicated by the development of a wheal and erythema response. The significance of minimal reactions, particularly erythema without oedema, has not been established. Therefore measurement error may be significant.

Green and Rosenblum (1971) reported that skin testing to penicilloyl-polylysine and benzylpenicillin was safe, and that there was a significant correlation with a history of clinical penicillin hypersensitivity. They found that the reaction rate was highest in patients who experienced immediate type hypersensitivity: 46.5 per cent of patients gave positive tests to penicilloyl-polylysine while 30.4 per cent were positive to benzylpenicillin. A total of 55.5 per cent were positive to one or the other or both reagents. Of those patients with immediate hypersensitivity, 84 per cent were positive to penicilloyl-polylysine and 55 per cent were positive to benzylpenicillin. They emphasised the importance of using both reagents for testing.

Juhlin and Wide (1972) showed a close correlation between penicilloyl-specific IgE antibodies in the patient's serum and positive skin tests with phenoxymethyl penicilloyl-polylysine or benzylpenicillin.

On similar lines aspiryl-polylysine has been used in the investigation of allergic-type responses to aspirin. Phills and Perelmutter (1974) investigated 18 such patients. Eight patients gave a history of anaphylaxis and 10 exhibited the frequently observed triad of asthma, nasal polyps and aspirin sensitivity. To determine the participation of IgE reagins in these reactions they performed skin tests with aspiryl-polylysine, and the rat mast cell test to aspirin (Schwartz et al, 1965) on all sera. They also studied IgE immunoglobulin adsorption of four sera giving both positive rat mast cell test responses and positive direct skin tests to aspiryl-polylysine, and repeated the rat mast cell test after adsorption. The findings suggested that the aspirin triad patients' symptoms were mediated by a non-reaginic pathway, as both direct skin tests and rat mast cell tests were negative. Patients with a history of anaphylaxis has positive skin tests and positive rat mast cell tests. Removal of IgE from the sera of four of these patients abolished the positive rat mast cell test responses to aspirin. The results therefore suggested a participation of IgE-type reagins in anaphylactic-type reactions to aspirin.

The skin window technique

This is a method of studying the inflammatory reaction induced by the abrasion of normal skin over an area of a few millimetres. Drugs as antigens are applied to this surface and the cellular response harvested on coverslips (Sarkany, 1968). The test is rather difficult to perform and the results are not always reliable.

Passive transfer tests

This involves the injection of reaginic serum into the skin of a normal subject and forms the basis of the Prausnitz–Kustner reaction. Reaginic antibody has a high affinity for human skin. Subsequent challenge of skin by drug antigen, in skin injected with specifically sensitised serum, gives a wheal and flare reaction. This test is limited by the risk of developing serum hapatitis.

Patch tests

The value of patch testing in the diagnosis of hypersensitivity to drugs given systemically is very limited. Patch tests are, however, extremely useful in the diagnosis of allergic eczematous contact dermatitis (Agrup, 1972).

Patch testing has been used in fixed drug eruptions. In some cases a patch test with the drug applied to the previously involved skin may become positive (Schultz and Schmidt, 1967).

Uncommonly, patch-testing with a solution of carbromal induces a local purpura, particularly if the venous return is briefly occluded at the test site (Ackroyd, 1962). This type of reaction might be due to allergy to a complete antigen formed by the drug and the endothelial cells of the small vessels (Agrup, 1972).

In patients with eruptions of an eczematous type provoked by drugs to which they have been sensitised by previous epidermal contact, patch testing may reveal the sensitiser and establish the range of cross-sensitivity. Drugs which may cause such eczematous reactions include, sulphonamides, penicillin, neomycin and phenothiazines. Application of a drug to the skin involves a much greater risk of sensitisation than if the drug is used systemically (Agrup, 1972). This is particularly so with highly sensitising compounds such as chlorpromazine, and the risk is aggravated if the patch test is combined with exposure to ultraviolet light, (Epstein, 1968). The risk of sensitisation to penicillin when used topically is roughly 100 times greater than when the drug is given orally (Schultz, 1964).

In summary, the value of skin tests in drug hypersensitivity other than penicillin is questionable. Current intradermal tests for penicillin sensitivity show promising results but are far from being routine procedures. For this reason and because of the possible dangers of skin testing, much research has been done on in vitro tests.

In Vitro Tests

Most laboratory investigations have been concerned with drug hypersensitivity with particular reference to penicillin. Estimation of blood and tissue levels of a drug is usually not helpful in identifying a responsible agent, since the levels are not usually in the toxic range. However, quantitative toxicological studies are the basis of a more accurate diagnosis in the case of overdose.

General investigations
Eosinophilia may suggest that an eruption is due to a drug, but it is non-specific and inconsistent.

Histopathology
In most drug eruptions the histological changes are non-specific and will only be indicative of the clinical features, e.g. erythema multiforme and urticaria. In lichenoid eruptions the changes may closely resemble lichen planus although the cellular infiltrate tends to be more pleomorphic and less dense. Such a picture would allow one to narrow the field to drugs which are known to cause lichenoid eruptions.

Laboratory procedures for the detection of reaginic antibody (IgE)
For several years the Prausnitz–Kustner test was used as a measure of reaginic activity. This test is not used very much today because of the dangers of transferring serum hepatitis. There are now several in vitro procedures for measuring reaginic antibody. However, most of these methods are costly and require laboratory animals and sophisticated techniques, making them unsuitable for use in every hospital.

Reaginic antibody may be measured by release of mediators after addition of antigen, and by virtue of its cytophilia for basophils and mast cells, and also with a specific anti-IgE antiglobulin reagent after the reaginic antibody attaches itself to the allergen which has previously been coupled to a carrier.

Basophil degranulation tests

These tests depend on the release of histamine from tissue mast cells and basophils in the blood due to a reaction involving antibody and the drug to which the patient is sensitive. The basophils are examined for loss of granules.

The direct basophil degranulation test was devised by Shelley and Juhlin (1961). A solution of the drug is mixed with the patient's heparinised blood. After allowing time for any reaction to occur the blood is fixed, and the white cells concentrated and stained. The basophil granules are then examined, comparing them with controls. A drawback of this test is that basophils are very sparse in human blood, and therefore the indirect test was developed (Shelley, 1962, 1963).

The indirect basophil degranulation test depends on the degranulation of rabbit basophils. One drop of the patient's serum is placed on a slide which has already been stained. A drop of rabbit buffy coat and a drop of a solution of the suspected drug in saline are added and mixed. A coverslip is applied and subsequently the basophil granules are observed.

Technical difficulties make these tests unreliable for the routine use in diagnosis of drug allergy. False positive reactions may occur due to the presence of agglutinating antibodies in the sera, and it is difficult to assess the effects of toxic levels of the drug in solution. Further work needs to be done on the mechanism of degranulation, particularly in relation to the class of sensitising antibody (Amos, 1976).

Release of histamine from sensitised tissues and leucocytes

For some time now, procedures have been available for measuring release of mediators from chopped lung and normal human leucocytes (Schild et al, 1951; Lichtenstein and Osler, 1964). Lung tissue is rich in histamine and therefore sensitisation can easily be detected. Human lung has proved to be more sensitive, and possibly more specific, than monkey lung in testing for natural allergies (Assem and Schild, 1968). Less agreement has been found between results with human and monkey lung in penicillin allergy than in pollen allergy, and Assem (1972) has suggested that monkey lung may be capable of sensitisation by human antibodies other than reagins.

The principle of these tests depends on the passive sensitisation of lung tissue or human leucocytes. Histamine release is estimated by bioassay and is taken to be a measure of reaginic activity. Assem (1972) reported the results of the human lung test in 62 patients with drug allergy. In 40 patients with penicillin allergy, tests with benzylpenicillin and penicilloyl-polylysine were carried out. When penicilloyl-polylysine was used, passive sensitisation of human lung could be shown in 21 patients tested (52.5 per cent). Benzyl-penicillin, however, elicited a response in only 10 of these patients (25 per cent). In other drug allergies the lung test was positive in only 6 out of 22 patients (27 per cent). Skin tests were positive in 55 per cent of patients compared with 44 per cent of positive lung tests.

Normal human leucocyte suspensions have been used in the same way. In this case the mediator cell is the basophil which, like the mast cell, can be sensitised by reaginic antibody. Histamine is released following a reaction between the allergen and reaginic antibody fixed to the basophils. Assem (1972) reported a positive leucocyte test in a higher proportion of drug allergic patients than the human lung test. It was felt, however, that false positives occurred with the leucocyte test.

Rat mast cells have also been passively sensitised to undergo histamine release (Korotzer and Haddad, 1970; Perelmutter, Liakopoulou and Larose, 1970).

Serotonin release

Histamine may be released from platelets both in vivo and in vitro in sensitised animals, and in man during the course of antigen–antibody reactions. Caspary and Comaish (1967) attempted to use this phenomenon for the in vitro diagnosis of hypersensitivity states. Burrows, Bell and Bridges (1968) studied serotonin uptake and release by platelets in the presence of penicillin in 17 patients clinically hypersensitive to penicillin, and in four control subjects. No significant differences could be demonstrated between the patients and the controls. Comaish (1968) reported a disappointing total of positive results in drug allergy, although more positive results were obtained in patients who had reacted to horse antitetanus serum.

The radioallergosorbent test (RAST) for specific IgE antibody (Wide, Bennich and Johansson, 1967)

As mentioned above, the reaginic antibodies involved in the immediate type reactions belong to the IgE class. Serum reaginic IgE antibody is measured by adding the serum to allergen-linked cyanogen bromide-activated dextran (Sephadex). After thorough washing, the adsorbed IgE antibodies are measured by the uptake of isotope labelled purified anti-IgE. The RAST is probably the most accurate and sensitive test available for detection of anaphylactic antibodies.

Juhlin and Wide (1972) demonstrated the value of RAST in drug hypersensitivity. In addition to this test they measured IgE levels and performed skin tests and provocation test. Fifteen patients with a recent history of immediate type hypersensitivity to penicillin showed a positive RAST to phenoxymethylpenicilloyl-polylysine and benzyl penicillin. The RAST values decreased with time after the clinical reaction. Skin tests and RAST reactions were negative for 40 patients with a history of morbilliform and scarlatiniform exanthema. They found no reaginic antibodies to penicilloyl in the sera of 184 patients with asthma, allergic rhinitis and/or atopic eczema. Most the these patients showed increased IgE levels.

The RAST is an extremely promising test for the measurement of immediate type hypersensitivity, but requires somewhat sophisticated laboratory techniques, and is therefore not available for routine use.

Lymphocyte transformation

Peripheral blood lymphocytes, when cultured in vitro for up to a week in the presence of certain substances, may be stimulated to transform into lymphoblastoid cells which subsequently synthesise DNA and undergo mitosis. Phytohaemagglutinin (PHA) is a non-specific mitogen and will cause transformation in a high proportion of peripheral blood lymphocytes from any normal subject. Other agents are antigen specific so that purified protein derivative of tuberculin (PPD) will cause significant transformation in cultures of lymphocytes obtained only from tuberculin-sensitive donors.

The value of the lymphocyte transformation test in drug hypersensitivity is still far from clear, and was reviewed in detail by Levene and Baker (1968). One of the first reports came from Hirschhorn et al (1963). They reported positive transformation with lymphocyte cultures from a penicillin-sensitive patient, when penicillin was the antigen added to the culture. Positive results in single patients have been reported by Holland and Mauer (1964) in a child with phenytoin sensitivity, and Caron and Sarkany (1965) using sulphadiazine in lymphocyte cultures from a patient sensitive to phthalysulphathiazole.

Much of the research has been concerned with penicillin sensitive patients and the results have been conflicting. Ripps and Fellner (1966), found that only 11 of 17 patients giving a history compatible with an allergic reaction to penicillin, had a positive lymphocyte transformation to penicillin. Several members of the control group, having no history of reaction following penicillin therapy, also had a positive response. The one factor common to all persons who had a positive lymphocyte response, was the presence of a positive reaction to intradermal injection of benzylpenicillin or penicilloyl-polylysine. Almost all the subjects whose cells responded to penicillin in vitro gave an immediate wheal and flare response. The others exhibited delayed hypersensitivity. Vischer (1966) obtained only two positive transformation tests in 13 patients with a history of penicillin sensitivity. In five cases of other drug allergies, none was positive. Girard et al (1967) found seven out of nine penicillin-sensitive subjects positive when using benzylpenicillin as the antigen and four out of four when penicilloyl-polylysine was used. Halpern, Ky and Amache (1967) recorded positive lymphocyte transformation in all 30 patients suspected of having penicillin hypersensitivity, and negative findings in 32 of 33 controls. Sarkany (1967) investigated 40 patients with clinically suspected drug reactions. Lymphocyte transformation was shown to occur in seven of these patients. Penicillin, sulphadimidine, streptomycin, sodium amino-salicylate and chlorpropamide induced lymphocyte transformation in vitro conformed to the clinical hypersensitivity reactions and there were no false positives. Karna and Chyrek-Borowska (1975) reported positive results in between 41.7 and 66.6 per cent of patients with penicillin hypersensitivity and in 63.1 to 75 per cent of patients with streptomycin sensitivity, depending on the concentration of these antibiotics used in the tests.

The significance of a positive lymphocyte transformation in terms of correlation with a particular immunological mechanism is unclear, although it has been considered to be a correlate of delayed-type hypersensitivity (Assem, 1972). It is recognised that positive results may be obtained in classical examples of immediate-type hypersensitivity (Girard et al, 1967). Assem (1972) found positive results in the majority of patients with immediate type sensitivity due to drugs. The divergence of results in drug hypersensitivity may be explained by differences in technique. Many workers made smears of the cells at the end of the culture period and counted the percentage of transformed cells. Scintillation counting of cells which have incorporated radioisotope-labelled thymidine into DNA overcomes these difficulties and is entirely objective. More problems arise when it is remembered that the drug used in vitro may not contain the allergenic metabolite formed in vivo, or that the haptenic determinant may be on the wrong carrier. The degree of lymphocyte transformation is known to be dependent on the dose of the drug and therefore optimum concentrations of each drug will have to be established. In the light of these conflicting results and practical difficulties encountered, lymphocyte transformation is not yet established as a test for drug hypersensitivity. It is possible that improvements on technique may make the test more useful in the future.

The leucocyte migration test

This test depends on the release of biologically active proteins (lymphokines) from sensitised lymphocytes in the presence of antigen. The basic method is essentially that of David et al (1964), in which the lymphokines released, including migration inhibition factor, will retard the migration of guinea-pig peritoneal exudate macrophages. A modification of this test, devised by Bendixen and Søborg (1967), involves placing buffy-coat leucocytes in capillaries and allowing them to migrate into chambers which do, or do not contain antigen. Inhibition of migration implies a positive response which is thought to indicate the presence of delayed hypersensitivity.

When drugs are used as allergens in the migration test difficulties are encountered in maintaining the viability of cells in culture when many drugs are only soluble at acid pH (Brostoff, 1972).

Haemagglutination

Haemagglutination tests with penicillin-sensitised red blood cells, primarily measures IgG and IgM antibodies specific for the penicilloyl group (Thiel, Mitchell and Parker, 1964). High antibody titres are commonly associated with symptoms of serum sickness or other types of penicillin allergy, but may be observed in the absence of known allergy (Parker, 1975c).

COMMON DRUG REACTIONS

Nalidixic Acid

Nalidixic acid was introduced in 1962 as an antibacterial agent for treatment of urinary tract infections. Bullous photoreactions following administration of this drug were noted soon afterwards. Women are given this drug more frequently as they have a higher prevalence of urinary tract infection than males. This is reflected in the incidence of bullous photoreactions that are seen with this drug. In children the sex difference is slight, but in adults 20 females are affected for every one male affected and this probably reflects the increase in urinary tract infections in postpubertal women.

Bullae appear within a few days to two weeks after commencing exposure to the sun. They are usually associated with a sharply demarcated erythema (Baes, 1968) but occasionally may appear on normal appearing skin (Brehm and Korting, 1972).

The eruption frequently starts when the patient is on holiday and a high level of ambient sunlight seems to be more important than the length of time that the drug has been taken (Ramsay, 1973). Previous sensitivity to sun exposure is uncommon (Brauner, 1975). The dorsal surfaces of the feet, lower legs and hands are most frequently affected and the face seems to be only rarely involved.

The bullae vary in size from several millimetres to several centimetres, being tense and painful. They may itch but the patient complains more of pain.

The bullae usually heat without scarring, provided no secondary infection has occurred, but bullae continue to appear for many months after the drug has been stopped. Fragility of the skin persists for a similar period, both when exposed to sunlight and also without sunlight, and without measurable nalidixic acid in the blood (Birkett, Garrett and Stevenson, 1969). This clinically suggests a form of porphyria but no abnormality has been found in porphyrin metabolism. Urine, stool and blood porphyrin levels are normal, as are liver function tests and bacteriological examinations. A positive Nikolsky sign has been recorded (Brehm and Korting, 1972) but this does not occur in the majority of patients. Postinflammatory hyperpigmentation followed by hypopigmentation may occur (Luscombe, 1970).

Histological examination of biopsies of bullae shows normal epidermis without spongiosis, a mild perivascular lymphohistiocytic infiltrate, some basophilic degeneration of collagen and separation at the dermoepidermal junction (Birkett et al, 1969). Intra-epidermal separation has been described by Thivolet et al (1970).

Patch tests and photo-patch tests have been performed and found to be negative (Haven and Geerts, 1967). Brehm and Korting (1972) showed direct immunofluorescence in the region of the stratum granulosum and circulating antibodies to dermal extracts, but not to epidermis vessels or thymus. He interpreted the latter findings as suggestive of incomplete antibodies to the dermis and as a possible mechanism for bulla formation.

Phototesting of such patients has produced varying results, which are difficult to interpret. Evidence suggests that, besides nalidixic acid, some metabolic intermediate of it, or a tissue fixed intermediate, or an unknown induced abnormal metabolite may be the effector of the erythema and bullae.

Haven and Geerts (1967) showed a positive lightband (fluorescence of the urine when exposed to 500 nm radiation) during the eruptive phase of the rash. This is the only clue that an unusual possible metabolite not activated in the short wavelength ultraviolet radiation may be responsible for the reaction.

The inability to show a positive photo-patch test adds further evidence that a metabolic step may be necessary before photoactivation by long wavelength ultraviolet radiation.

Ramsay (1973) showed reactions to long wave ultraviolet light in three out of seven patients, but two volunteers, who were given nalidixic acid 4 g daily for one week, also showed an immediate erythematous reaction to long wave ultraviolet radiation.

That nalidixic acid photosensitivity is a photoallergic and not a phototoxic phenomenon is strongly suggested by

1. The low clinical incidence of reactors and the inability to create lesions in controls.
2. There seems to be an incubation period between exposure to sunlight and the eruption.
3. Even though nalidixic acid has been cleared from the circulation reactivity continues.
4. The biological action spectrum is of longer wavelength than the absorption spectrum.

However, the fact that the patients' eruptions are strictly localised to sun-exposed areas without spread is more characteristic of phototoxic reactions, and the histological changes of minimal epidermal destruction can be seen in either photoallergy or phototoxicity.

A definite explanation for nalidixic acid photosensitivity is not yet described. Fortunately the clinical appearance is sufficiently characteristic to incriminate nalidixic acid and lead to cessation of the drug. Short and long wavelength ultraviolet light exposure should be avoided, as possibly should visible light. As there is no acceptable topical screening agent that will achieve this it probably explains the persistent rash. Therefore direct and strong sunlight must be avoided. Ramsay and Obreshkova (1974) state that if this is so nalidixic acid administration can be continued but it is wiser to stop the drug even though the condition is not serious and will slowly, over many months, burn itself out.

Practolol

Drugs which inhibit adrenergic β-receptors have become very popular in treatment of cardiac disorders. The first of these drugs, pronethanol, produced many side effects including light-headedness, incoordination and gastro-intestinal disturbances. This was superseded by propranolol (1-isopropyl-amino-3(1-naphyloxy)-2-propranolol hydrochloride) which is about 10 times more effective in its β-blocking activity. Unfortunately propranolol is an equally effective inhibitor of β-receptors in the bronchial tree and the peripheral circulation, limiting its usefulness in the management of cardiac arrhythmias and angina.

Practolol (4-(2-hydroxy-3-isopropylaminopropoxy)acetanilide) was synthesised in an attempt to minimise these side effects. By substituting an acetamide group in the p-position, lipid solubility is reduced, resulting in low concentration of the drug in the central nervous system and approximately 90 per cent being excreted unchanged in the urine. Practolol is used instead of propranolol where β-blockade is necessary, but respiratory function cannot be impeded. It is a selective β-adrenoceptor blocking agent as opposed to propranolol which is a non-selective β-blocker.

Adverse reactions to practolol were recorded by Wiseman (1971), who noted 7 patients out of 2100 (0.3 per cent) who developed non-specific micropapular, eczematous or urticarial rashes. Raftery and Denman (1973) described patients who, whilst on practolol, developed an LE syndrome consisting of an arthralgia, particularly of the small joints of the hands, a non-specific rash, raised ESR and positive LE cells and antinuclear factor (ANF). Antibody to DNA was not demonstrated, a finding which is typical of drug induced LE (Hughes, 1971).

Assem and Banks (1973) also noted a positive ANF and LE cells in a patient receiving practolol, but the major features of the reaction were that the rash was most marked on the thighs, buttocks, extensor surfaces of elbows, axillae, hands and feet, and that it fluctuated in quality, being at times psoriasiform and at other lichenoid. Forty-eight hours after stopping practolol there was a marked improvement in the rash. Intradermal injection of 10 μg/ml practolol produced irritation and a 10 mm lesion after 48 h.

In vitro tests showed a highly significant lymphocyte transformation test to practolol. Serum collected one year before the patient changed from propranolol to practolol was negative for ANF. Within four weeks of stopping practolol, LE cells could not be detected and the test for ANF became weakly positive; within six weeks no ANF could be detected. Serum samples from the patient containing ANF were tested for anti-DNA antibodies. Results were within normal limits. Hughes (1971) reports that patients with drug-induced lupus, for whom standard ANF and LE cells were positive, did *not* have anti-DNA antibodies. The lymphocyte transformation test provided evidence of a specific immunological response to practolol and was the first reported case with such a response.

These findings suggested that practolol might produce a specific type of rash. Felix, Ive and Dahl (1974), then reported a series of 21 patients with practolol-induced rashes conforming to a clinically recognisable diagnostic pattern.

Clinical features

The rash is psoriasiform in character, most marked over the bony prominences, with guttate lesions on the trunk and erythematous macules with marginated scaling and gyrate patterns. Regularly, there is hyperkeratosis of the palms, fingers and soles which, although frequently preceding the other skin manifestations, may coincide with them. Itching is present and particularly affects the palms and soles. The rash develops slowly over several months and clears gradually on stopping practolol.

Less commonly, in the early stages, the skin may show a pattern similar to exfoliative dermatitis which later develops into a psoriasiform rash. Occasionally, the rash is very diverse, resembling ichthyosis, eczema, lupus erythematosus, lichen planus or mycosis fugoides.

Histological changes (Felix et al, 1974) are unlike psoriasis and consist of patchy swelling and disruption of the basement membrane, with epidermal atrophy and colloid bodies migrating through the epidermis.

Eye changes are a characteristic part of the syndrome. Wright (1975) reported a series of 27 patients who developed damage to the conjunctiva which, on occasions, led to severe visual impairment. The main findings were of a reduction in tear flow followed by corneal changes. Hyperaemia with increased prominence of the papillary tufts and a less ordered pattern of blood vessels developed with some areas of relative avascularity and other areas where vessels actively proliferated. This was followed by a sub-conjunctival sheet of fibrovascular tissue which later contracted to produce the typical scarring, conjunctival shrinkage, and fornix obliteration. In the most severely affected patients unusual corneal changes were seen, consisting of the sudden appearance of yellow or white opacities involving the whole thickness of stroma. Alternatively sudden stromal melting and loss of corneal substance lead to rapid perforation. Most of these patients also had practolol skin rashes at some time. Some patients, most often those with severe ocular effects, also complained of auditory symptoms, mainly impairment of hearing. Otological examination showed sterile secretory otitis media, which on finer testing may be shown to be associated with cochlear damage.

More recently patients have been reported who developed a sclerosing peritonitis. Brown et al (1974) reported three such cases in patients on practolol, and since then further cases have been recorded (Windsor, Kurrein and Dyer, 1975; Hansen, Rhemneo and Oberius Kaptejin, 1975). These patients present with non-specific abdominal pain, subacute small bowel obstruction or an apparent abdominal mass. At laparotomy the peritoneal cavity appears obliterated, with gross thickening and contraction of the parietal and visceral layers. The small bowel is encased in a rigid tube of thickened peritoneum and is considerably shortened. Histology of the peritoneal biopsy shows a non-specific inflammatory reaction. Beneath the attenuated mesothelium is a thick layer of laminated fibrous tissue, with no evidence of giant cells or panniculitis. This condition can develop several months after stopping the drug.

Some of the case reports that have been published have referred to dry eyes and skin lesions apparently preceding the abdominal symptoms but, in the absence of such detail in other reports, it cannot be assumed that this is always the sequence of events.

Other side effects have been recorded which are probably part of the syndrome, namely, dry mouth, nose and non-productive cough, with nasal or oral ulceration (Wright, 1975), pericardial and pleural effusions, and one patient who developed the nephrotic syndrome (Farr, Wingate and Shaw, 1975).

From present evidence propranolol seems to be free from producing this syndrome, and as yet no convincing evidence has been presented to implicate any of the other β-blocking drugs, although a careful watch must be maintained and all suspected cases thoroughly investigated.

The mechanism of the practolol reaction

Raftery and Denman (1973) were unable to show specific immunological sensitisation to practolol by lymphocytes, nor were they able to show antibody receptors for practolol using the rosette technique described by Perrudet-Badoux and Frei (1971). They did, however, claim that a depression in lymphocyte transformation to PHA, Con A, and pokeweed mitogen occurred. They suggested that lymphocyte function may be altered by drugs which have receptor blocking functions, and hypothesised that practolol is capable of suppressing a 'T' cell subpopulation which controls the emergence of 'B' lymphocytes, with autoimmune propensities.

Amos, Brigden and McKerron (1975) investigated patients with the oculo-mucocutaneous syndrome. They described a circulating antibody which binds to the intercellular region of guinea-pig stratified epithelium which appeared similar in its site of binding and in titre to the antibodies seen in pemphigus. They were able to distinguish between the two groups by their binding ability to trypsin-isolated guinea-pig epidermal cells. Pemphigus antibodies bound to the cell membranes whereas practolol antibodies did not.

Sixteen of these patients were investigated using the lymphocyte transformation test (Brigden, Amos and Camps, 1976). They all showed normal transformation to PHA, but only one of nine tested was shown to transform to practolol or a practolol–albumen conjugate.

Felix et al (1974) described IgG, IgM and C_3 deposition in the region of the dermoepidermal junction, though they did not look for circulating antibodies. Van Joost, Crone and Overdijk (1976) reported a patient in whom IgG and complement deposition occurred along the basement membrane of the buccal mucosa.

Gaylande and Sarkany (1975) suggest that the mechanism of the psoriasiform eruption may be due to β-blockade, reducing epidermal cyclic AMP, leading to cell division.

Ampicillin

Ampicillin is a synthetic penicillin derived from the 6-aminopenicillanic acid nucleus. It was introduced into clinical medicine in 1961, since when it has become the most frequently prescribed of the synthetic penicillins.

It was the first of the penicillins to have marked activity against Gram-negative organisms, although it is generally less active against Gram-positive organisms than benzyl penicillin. It is the most widely prescribed antibiotic in general practice for sore throats, even though the majority of these infections are of viral origin and the remainder are due to haemolytic streptococci which are more easily dealt with by ordinary penicillin.

Patients suffering from infectious mononucleosis are often given an antibiotic in the early stages of the illness on the assumption that they are suffering from a bacterial infection. Patel (1967) and Pullen, Wright and Murdoch (1968) independently noted a high incidence of rash in infectious mononucleosis patients who had been given ampicillin, the rash being different from that commonly seen in infectious mononucleosis and also in ampicillin hypersensitivity.

This type of rash has also been reported in patients with cytomegalo-virus mononucleosis treated with ampicillin (Klemola, 1970) and in lymphatic leukaemia patients similarly treated (Cameron and Richmond, 1972). Shapiro et al (1972) and Lee Potter (1972) recorded similar rashes from ampicillin administration in patients already receiving allopurinol, and in a patient with stage 4 reticulosarcoma. It has also been noted that patients with viral infections receiving ampicillin develop a rash more frequently than those being treated for a bacterial infection.

Clinical features of the ampicillin rash

The typical ampicillin rash may appear as early as the first day of treatment but usually is seen between 5 and 14 days. It is often first noticed after ampicillin has been stopped, and this can be a cause of a missed diagnosis.

The rash frequently continues to become more florid and spread after the drug has been withdrawn.

The rash starts most commonly on the extensor aspects of the limbs with accentuation over the bony prominences of the elbows and knees, spreading symmetrically to most parts of the body, frequently being morbilliform or maculopapular before becoming confluent. The colour is dull red, but not infrequently becomes haemorrhagic in severe cases, then taking a week or more to subside before desquamating and staining, in contrast to the mild rash which subsides spontaneously in a few days. Involvement of the mucous membranes, particularly the palate, is common if searched for. Although slight fever may occur the patient is rarely systemically ill, his major concern being fear over the extent of the rash. Itching is not a major symptom in most patients.

Pathogenesis

The cause of the ampicillin rash remains unknown. Certain toxic and allergic aetiologies have been suggested. A proteinaceous impurity in ampicillin preparations was implicated in early studies but purification of the product has not eliminated the incidence of reactions.

The penicilloyl group has been regarded as the major allergic component in penicillin allergy. Being the nucleus common to all synthetic penicillins, it was assumed that ampicillin rashes would also be due to allergy to this component. The clinical observation that high incidence of rash in infectious mononucleosis has not been produced by benzyl or phenoxymethyl penicillin, suggests that ampicillin rashes may not be due to true 6-aminopenicillanic acid nucleus hypersensitivity (Pullen et al, 1968b).

Nazareth (1971) treated 10 patients suffering from infectious mononucleosis with ampicillin, giving them graduated doses of ampicillin some months after they had recovered from ampicillin rashes but whilst they were still affected by infectious mononucleosis; no rash developed in any of these patients. This added clinical support to the views of Knudsen (1969) and Pullen (1969) who concluded that most morbilliform rashes reported during ampicillin therapy were apparently ampicillin-specific and that patients affected in this way should not necessarily be regarded as sensitive to the other penicillins.

Since then many patients have been given penicillin after this type of ampicillin rash without developing any adverse effect.

These findings together with the relatively short incubation period, the infrequency of anaphylaxis, the inability to demonstrate reaginic antibodies (Knudsen, 1969) and negative lymphocyte transformation tests (Sarkany, 1968) suggest that hypersensitivity is not the main cause of the ampicillin rash.

The discovery that spontaneous polymerisation occurred in solution raised the possibility that macromolecular forms of ampicillin could be allergenic (Dewdney, Smith and Wheeler, 1971) and that some of the reactions were due to type 4 allergy (Gell and Coombs, 1963). Webster and Thompson (1964) investigated in vivo and in vitro reactivity to ampicillin polymer in patients with infectious mononucleosis. Peripheral blood leucocytes cultured in the presence of the polymer were found to incorporate radioactively labelled thymidine at a faster rate than control unstimulated cultures. This was accompanied by morphological transformation.

They postulated that this ampicillin polymer-mediated lymphocyte stimulation may play a role in the development of the ampicillin skin rash.

Drug-induced Systemic Lupus Erythematosus (SLE)

Syndromes indistinguishable from SLE have been reported following the administration of a large number of drugs. Four of these, hydrallazine, isoniazid, phenytoin, and procainamide have featured in published reports very much more often than the others, which include penicillin, sulphonamides, D-penicillamine, tetracycline, griseofulvin, methyldopa, oral contraceptives, thiouracil, para-amino salicylic acid, streptomycin, chlorpromazine, methysergide phenylbutazone, practolol, carbamazepine, ethosuximide, primidone and nitrofurantoin (Selroos and Edren, 1975).

Over 300 patients with features of the SLE syndrome developing after drug therapy have been reported.

Definition of drug-induced SLE

Besides the features which are necessary for the diagnosis of SLE, Lee and Chase (1975) suggest that the following features must be added to make a diagnosis of *drug*-induced SLE.

1. A drug must have been administered before the onset of any sign or symptom of SLE.
2. The disease process must reverse itself promptly upon cessation of drug treatment. Clinical signs and symptoms must begin to clear within days, but laboratory findings may not change for months or years.
3. Resumption of drug therapy should result in prompt recrudescence of symptoms and signs.

Clinical features

The main clinical manifestations of the drug-induced SLE syndrome are polyarthralgia, myalgia, pleural and pulmonary involvement, pericarditis, fever, weight loss, hepatosplenomegaly, lymphadenopathy, abdominal pain, Raynaud's phenomenon and rash.

Laboratory findings show LE cells, antinuclear antibodies and antinucleoprotein antibodies. Antibodies to denatured (single strand) deoxribonucleic acid (DNA) may be present, but antibodies to native (double stranded) DNA are only very rarely found (Hahn et al, 1972).

However, it is possible that such apparent demonstration has resulted from technical errors in the assay methods (Winfield and Davis, 1974).

Leucopenia and thrombocytopenia occur infrequently and occasionally false positive serological tests for syphilis are found. Abnormal laboratory findings characteristic of SLE often occur in the absence of any other sign of the disease. This has been noted in patients taking procainamide, half of whom develop antinuclear antibodies during the first six months of treatment. Alpha methyldopa has been shown to induce the formation of antinuclear antibodies in some patients (Feltkamp, Dorhout and Nieuwehnuis, 1970), but no patient has yet been reported to have developed symptomatic SLE from this drug.

There are significant differences between the drug induced and idiopathic forms of SLE. Most authors agree that renal damage with proteinuria casts, microscopic haematuria and azotaemia is uncommon in drug-induced SLE, but it can occur, and that the severity of the disease is less, particularly concerning fever, cutaneous manifestations and lymphadenopathy. The disease is usually reversible on stopping the offending drugs, though some cases of hydraallazine lupus have had more prolonged courses.

Chantler et al (1973) have suggested that a microepidemic of SLE in Nevada may have been due to exposure to gamma radiation. Eosin, an essential ingredient of lipsticks, has been suggested as a cause of SLE by Burry (1960) but further evidence for or against these hypotheses is lacking.

Pathogenetic mechanisms

A number of mechanisms producing drug-induced SLE have been suggested and controversy still exists. A few patients may develop SLE during a course of treatment, the SLE being coincidental. Other patients may have a genetic predisposition for SLE which becomes manifest only after a strong stimulus provided by a drug, as has been shown with hydrallazine and isoniazid, where genetically determined differences in rates of detoxification (acetylation) appear to produce SLE as discussed previously.

The frequent finding of clinical or, more usually, immunological manifestations of SLE in relatives of the patient, and the report of procainamide-induced lupus syndrome in siblings (Novack and Paine, 1975), supports the genetic hypothesis, although the frequent regression of the disease in drug-related cases after withdrawal of the drug is rather against this theory (Harpey, 1973).

Some drugs, e.g. procainamide, hydrallazine, isoniazid and the anti-convulsants (Alarcón-Segovia, 1969), produce the SLE syndrome by some pharmacologic effect, while others operate to produce an immune reaction which has some of the manifestations of SLE. Lee and Chase (1975) suggested that for all drugs the pathogenetic pathway leads through the production of antinuclear antibodies and that these are produced because the drugs in question are able to form complexes with deoxyribonucleoprotein released

13

through normal catabolic processes that the drug–nucleoprotein complexes represent a 'denatured' nucleoprotein.

It is still unknown why some patients who form antinuclear antibodies by this sequence later develop symptoms and signs of complex disease and others do not.

ACKNOWLEDGEMENT

We are most grateful to Dr G. M. Levene for carefully examining the manuscript.

REFERENCES

Ackroyd, J. F. (1962) The immunological basis of purpura due to drug hypersensitivity. *Proceedings of the Royal Society of Medicine*, **55**, 30–36.

Ackroyd, J. F. (1975) Immunological mechanisms in drug hypersensitivity. In *Clinical Aspects of Immunology*, 3rd edn, ed. Gell, P. G. H., Coombs, R. R. A. & Lachmann, P. J., pp. 913–961. Oxford, London, Edinburgh, Melbourne: Blackwell Scientific.

Agrup, G. (1972) Patch testing in drug allergy. In *Mechanisms in Drug Allergy*, a Glaxo Symposium, ed. Dash, C. H. & Jones, H. E. H., pp. 135–138. Edinbrugh and London: Churchill Livingstone.

Alarćon-Segovia, D. (1969) Drug-induced lupus syndrome. *Mayo Clinic Proceedings*, **44**, 664–681.

Amos, H. E. (1976) *Allergic Drug Reactions*, Current Topics in Immunology Series, General Editor, Turk, J. London: Arnold.

Amos, H. E., Brigden, W. D. & McKerron, R. A. (1975) Untoward effects associated with practolol: demonstration of antibody binding to epithelial tissue. *British Medical Journal*, **1**, 598–600.

Assem, E. S. K. (1972) The passive sensitisation of human lung as a test for drug allergy. In *Mechanisms in Drug Allergy*, a Glaxo Symposium, pp. 112–120. ed. by Dash, C. H. & Jones, H. E. H. Edinburgh and London: Churchill Livingstone.

Assem, E. S. K. & Banks, R. A. (1973) Practolol-induced drug eruption. *Proceedings of the Royal Society of Medicine*, **66**, 179–181.

Assem, E. S. K. & Schild, H. O. (1968) Detection of allergy to penicillin and other antigens by in vitro passive sensitisation and histamine release from human and monkey lung. *British Medical Journal*, **3**, 272.

Baes, H. (1968) Photosensitivity caused by nalidixic acid. *Dermatologica*, **136**, 61–64.

Bendixen, G. & Søborg, M. (1963) Human lymphocyte migration as a parameter of hypersensitivity. *Acta medica scandinavica*, **181**, 247–256.

Birkett, D., Garrett, M. & Stevenson, C. (1969) Phototoxic bullous eruptions due to nalidixic acid. *British Journal of Dermatology*, **81**, 342–344.

Boger, W. P., Sherman, W. B., Schiller, I. W., Siegal, S. & Rose, B. (1953) Allergic reactions to penicillin. A panel discussion. *Journal of Allergy*, **24**, 383–404.

Brauner, G. (1975) Bullous photoreaction to nalidixic acid. *American Journal of Medicine*, **58**, 576.

Brehm, G. & Korting, G. (1972) Bullöse Hautreaktion auf Nalidixinsaure. *Medizinische Welt*, **21** (NF), 423–429.

Brigden, W. D., Amos, H. E. & Camps, M. (1976) *Lancet*. In press.

Brostoff, J. (1972) The leucocyte migration test in drug allergy. In *Mechanisms in Drug Allergy*, a Glaxo Symposium, ed. Dash, C. H. & Jones, H. E. H., pp. 177–178. Edinburgh and London: Churchill Livingstone.

Brown, B. C., Price, E. V. & Moore, M. B. (1964) Penicilloyl-polylysine as an intradermal test of penicillin sensitivity. *Journal of the American Medical Association*, **189**, 599–604.

Brown, P., Baddeley, H., Read, A. E., Davies, J. D. & McGarry, J. (1974) Sclerosing peritonitis, and unusual reaction to a adrenergic blocking drug (practolol). *Lancet*, **2**, 1477–1481.

Burge, K. M. & Winkelmann, R. K. (1970) Mercury pigmentation. An electron microscope study. *Archives of Dermatology*, **102**, 51.

Burrows, D., Bell, T. K. & Bridges, J. M. (1968) The influence of penicillin on platelet serotonin uptake and release in penicillin allergy. *British Journal of Dermatology*, **80**, 387–390.

Burry, J. N. (1969) Lipstick and lupus erythematosus. *New England Journal of Medicine*, **19**, 358.

Cameron, S. J. & Richmond, J. (1972) Ampicillin hypersensitivity lymphatic leukaemia. *Scottish Medical Journal*, **16**, 425–427.

Caron, G. A. & Sarkany, I. (1965) Lymphoblast transformation in sulphonamide sensitivity. *British Journal of Dermatology*, **77**, 556–559.

Caspary, E. A. & Comaish, J. S. (1967) Release of serotonin from human platelets in hypersensitivity states. *Nature (London)*, **214**, 286.

Chantler, S., Hansen, J., & Jacobson, J. (1973) Incidence of nuclear antibodies in patients and in related and unreleated groups from a community with a 'microepidemic' of systemic lupus erythematosus. *Clinical Immunology and Immunopathology*, **2**, 9–15.

Comaish, S. (1968) Platelet serotonin release in penicillin allergy. *British Journal of Dermatology*, **80**, 765–766.

Coombs, R. R. A. & Gell, P. G. H. (1968) Classification of allergic reactions responsible for clinical hypersensitivity and disease. In *Clinical Aspects of Immunology*, 2nd edn, Gell, P. G. H. & Coombs, R. R. A., pp. 575–596. Oxford and Edinburgh: Blackwell Scientific.

Copeman, P. W. M. (1972) Drug rashes. *British Journal of Hospital Medicine*, **7**, 339–358.

David, J. R., Askari, S. A., Lawrence, H. S. & Thomas, L. (1964) Delayed hypersensitivity in vitro. I. The specificity of inhibition of cell migration by antigens. *Journal of Immunology*, **93**, 264.

De Matteis, F. (1967) Disturbances of liver porphyrin metabolism caused by drugs. *Pharmacological Reviews*, **19**, 523.

De Weck, A. L. (1972) Immunochemical mechanisms in drug allergy. In *Mechanisms in Drug Allergy*, a Glaxo Symposium, ed. Dash, C. H. & Jones, H. E. H., pp. 2–17. Edinburgh and London: Churchill Livingstone.

De Weck, A. L. & Girard, J. P. (1972) Specific inhibition of allergic reactions to penicillin in man by a monovalent hapten. II. Clinical studies. *International Archives of Allergy*, **42**, 798–815.

De Weck, A. L. & Schneider, C. H. (1972) Specific inhibition of allergic reactions to penicillin in man by a monovalent hapten. I. Experimental immunological and toxicological studies. *International Archives of Allergy*, **42**, 782–797.

Dewdney, J. M., Smith, H. & Wheeler, A. W. (1971) The formation of antigenic polymers in aqueous solutions of beta-lactain antibiotics. *Immunology*, **21**, 517–525.

Dummett, C. O. (1965) Oral mucosa discolorations related to pharmacotherapeutics. *Journal of Oral Therapeutics and Pharmacology*, **1**, 106–110.

Evans, D. A. P., Manley, D. A. & McKusick, V. A. (1960) Genetic control of isoniazid metabolism in man. *British Medical Journal*, **2**, 485–491.

Evans, D. A. P., Davison, D. & Pratt, R. T. C. (1965) The influence of acetylator phenotype on the effects of treatment depression with phenelzine. *Clinical Pharmacology and Therapeutics*, **6**, 430–435.

Farr, M. J., Wingate, J. P. & Shaw, J. N. (1975) Practolol and the nephrotic syndrome, *British Medical Journal*, **2**, 68–69.

Felix, R. H., Ive, F. A. & Dahl, M. G. C. (1974) Cutaneous and ocular reactions to practolol. *British Medical Journal*, **4**, 321–324.

Fellner, M. J. (1968) An immunologic study of selected penicillin reactions involving the skin. *Archives of Dermatology*, **97**, 503–519.

Feltkamp, T. E. W., Dorhout, E. J. & Nieuwehnuis, G. (1970) Autoantibodies related to treatment with chlorthalidone and alpha-methyldopa. *Acta medica scandinavica*, **187**, 219–223.

Gaylande, D. M. & Sarkany, I. (1975) Side effects of practolol. *British Medical Journal*, **3**, 435.

Gell, P. & Coombs, R. (1963) *Clinical Aspects of Immunology*. Oxford: Blackwell Scientific.

Girard, J. P., Rose, N. R., Kunz, M. L., Kobayashi, S. & Arbesman, C. E. (1967) In vitro lymphocyte transformation in atopic patients: induced by antigens. *Journal of Allergy*, **39**, 65–81.

Green, G. R. & Rosenblum, A. (1971) *Report of the Penicillin Study Group—American Academy of Allergy and Clinical Immunology*, **48**, 331–343.

Hahn, B. H., Sharp, G. C., Irvin, W. S., Kantor, O. S., Gardner, C. A., Bagby, M. K., Perry, H. M. & Osterland, C. K. (1972) Immune responses to hydralazine and nuclear antigens in hydralazine-induced lupus erythematosus. *Annals of Internal Medicine*, **76**, 365–374.

Halpern, B., Ky, N. T. & Amache, N. (1967) Diagnosis of drug allergy in vitro with the lymphocyte transformation test. *Journal of Allergy*, **40**, 168–181.

Hansen, A., Rhemneo, P. E. R. & Oberius Kaptejin, J. (1975) Sclerosing peritonitis and practolol: and other letters. *Lancet*, **1**, 275–276.

Harpey, J. P. (1973) Drugs and disseminated lupus erythematosus. *Adverse Drug Reaction Bulletin* No. 43.

Haven, E. & Geerts, J. (1967) Lichtovergvoeligheid Veroorzaaktdoor nalidixinuur. *Archives Belges dermatologie et de syphiligraphie*, **23**, 421.

Hirschhorn, K., Bach, F., Kolodry, R. L., Firschein, L. L. & Hashem, N. (1963) Immune responses and mitosis of human peripheral blood lymphocytes in vitro. *Science*, **142**, 1185–1187.

Holland, P. & Mauer, A. M. (1964) Drug-induced in vitro stimulation of peripheral lymphocytes. *Lancet*, **1**, 1368–1369.

Hughes, G. R. V. (1971) Significance of anti-DNA antibodies in systemic lupus erythematosus. *Lancet*, **2**, 861–863.

Idsøe, O., Guthe, T., Willcox, R. R. & De Weck, A. L. (1968) Nature and extent of penicillin side reactions with particular reference to fatalities from anaphylactic shock. *Bulletin of the World Health Organisation*, **38**, 159–188.

Jaffe, L. A. (1968) Effects of penicillamine on the kidney and on taste. *Postgraduate Medical Journal*, **44**, Suppl. Penicillamine, 15–18.

Jeghers, H. (1944) Pigmentation of the skin. *New England Journal of Medicine*, **231**, 181.

Juhlin, L. & Wide, L. (1972) IgE antibodies and penicillin allergy. In *Mechanisms in Drug Allergy*, a Glaxo Symposium, ed. Dash, C. H. & Jones, H. E. H., pp. 139–147. Edinburgh and London: Churchill Livingstone.

Karna, T. & Chyrek-Borowska, S. (1975) Zastosowanie testu zahamowania migracji leucocyton (T. Z. M.) w diagnostyce alergii na antybiotyki. *Polski Tygodnik Lekarksi*, **30**, 185.

Klemola, E. (1970) Hypersensitivity reactions to amphicillin in cytomegalovirus mononucleosis. *Scandinavian Journal of Infectious Diseases*, **2**, 29.

Knudsen, E. T. (1969) Ampicillin and urticaria. *British Medical Journal*, **1**, 846–847.

Korotzer, J. & Haddad, Z. H. (1970) In vitro detection of human IgE-mediated immediate hypersensitivity reactions to pollens and penicillin (S) by a modified rat mast cell degranulation technique. *Journal of Allergy*, **45**, 126.

Lee, S. L. & Chase, P. H. (1975) Drug-induced systemic lupus erythematosus: a critical review. *Seminars in Arthritis and Rheumatism*, **V** (1), 83–103.

Lee Potter, J. P. (1972) Skin reactions to ampicillin. *British Medical Journal*, **1**, 749.

Levene, G. M. (1972) Hyposensitisation to drugs. In *Mechanisms in Drug Allergy*, a Glaxo Symposium, ed. Dash, C. H. & Jones, H. E. H., pp. 59–63. Edinburgh and London: Churchill Livingstone.

Levene, G. M. & Baker, H. (1968) Drug reactins. II. Lymphocyte transformation in vitro and drug hypersensitivity. *British Journal of Dermatology*, **80**, 415–418.

Levene, G. M. & Calnan, C. D. (1971) Platinum sensitivity: treatment by specific hyposensitisation. *Clinical Allergy*, **1**, 75.

Levene, G. M. & Withers, A. F. D. (1969) Anaphylaxis to streptomycin and hyposensitisation. *Transactions of the St John's Hospital Dermatological Society (London)*, **55**, 184.

Levine, B. B. (1966) Immunologic mechanisms of penicillin allergy. *New England Journal of Medicine*, **275**, 1115–1125.

Lichtenstein, L. M. & Osler, A. G. (1964) Studies on the mechanisms of hypersensitivity phenomena. I. Histamine release from human leucocytes by ragweed pollen antigen. *Journal of Experimental Medicine*, **120**, 507.

Locher, G. W., Schneider, C. H. & De Weck, A. L. (1969) Hemmung allergischer Reaktionen auf Penicillin durch Penicilloyl-ox Amide und chemisch Verwandten Substanzen. *Zeitschrift für Immuniätsforschung und experimentelle Therapie*, **138**, 299–323.

Lowell, F. C. (1965) Rationale of treatment with injected aqueous extracts of air-borne allergens. In *Immunological Diseases*, ed. Samter, M. & Alexander, H. L., p. 600. Boston: Little, Brown and Company.

Luscombe, H. (1970) Photosensitivity reaction to nalidixic acid. *Archives of Dermatology*, **101**, 122.

Nazareth, I. J. (1971) Ampicillin and mononucleosis. *British Medical Journal*, **2**, 48.

Novack, M. A. & Paine, R. (1975) Procainamide-induced lupus. *Journal of the American Medical Association*, **232**, 1269.

Parker, C. W. (1975a) Drug therapy: drug allergy (first of three parts). *New England Journal of Medicine*, **292**, 511–514.

Parker, C. W. (1975b) Drug therapy: drug allergy (second of three parts). *New England Journal of Medicine*, **292**, 732–736.

Parker, C. W. (1975c) Drug therapy: drug allergy (third of three parts). *New England Journal of Medicine*, **292**, 957–960.

Parker, C. W., Shapiro, J., Kern, M. & Eisen, H. N. (1962) Hypersensitivity to penicillanic acid derivatives in human beings with penicillin allergy. *Journal of Experimental Medicine*, **115**, 821–838.

Patel, B. M. (1967) Skin rash with infectious mononucleosis and ampicillin. *Pediatrics, Springfield*, **40**, 910.

Perelmutter, L., Liakopoulou, A. & Larose, C. (1970) Detection of human IgE-type reagins utilising rat mast cells, *Journal of Allergy*, **45**, 126.

Perrudet-Badoux, A. & Frei, P. C. (1971) The detection of antibodies on blood lymphocytes in drug hypersensitivities using a rosette technique. *International Archives of Allergy and Applied Immunology*, **41**, 149–156.

Perry, H. M., Jr, Sakamato, A. & Tan, E. M. (1967) Relationship of acetylating enzyme to hydralazine toxicity. *Journal of Laboratory and Clinical Medicine*, **70**, 1020–1021.

Perry, T. L., Culling, C. F. A., Berry, K. & Hansen, S. (1964) 7-Hydroxychlorpromazine: potential toxic drug metabolite in psychiatric patients. *Science*, **146**, 81.

Peters, J. H., Gordon, G. R., Gelber, R., Levy, L. & Glazko, A. J. (1970) Polymorphic acetylation of dapsone (4,4'-diaminodiphenyl sulphone—DDS) in man. *Federation Proceedings. Federation of American Societies for Experimental Biology*, **29**, 803.

Phills, J. A. & Perelmutter, L. (1974) IgE mediated and non-IgE mediated allergic reactions to aspirin. *Acta allergerlogica*, **29**, 474–490.

Pullen, H. (1969) Ampicillin and urticaria. *British Medical Journal*, **1**, 247.

Pullen, H., Wright, N. & Murdoch, J. McC. (1968a) Hypersensitivity reactions to antibacterial drugs in infectious moconucleosis. *Lancet*, **2**, 1176.

Pullen, H., Wright, N. & Murdoch, J. McC (1968b) Hypersensitivity to the penicillins. *Lancet*, **1**, 1090.

Raftery, E. B. & Denman, A. M. (1973) Systemic lupus erythematosus syndrome induced by practolol. *British Medical Journal*, **2**, 452–455.

Ramsay, C. A. (1973) Photosensitivity from nalidixic acid. *Proceedings of the Royal Society of Medicine*, **4**, 747.

Ramsay, C. A. & Obreshkova, E. (1974) Photosensitivity from nalidixic acid. *British Journal of Dermatology*, **91**, 523–528.

Redmond, A. P. & Levine, B. B. (1968) Delayed skin reactions to benzylpenicillin in man. *International Archives of Allergy and Applied Immunology*, **33**, 193–206.

Ripps, C. S. & Fellner, M. J. (1966) Lymphocytes and drug hypersensitivity. *Lancet*, **2**, 803.

Rose, B. (1953) In Boger, W. P., Sherman, W. B., Schiller, I. W., Siegal, S. & Rose, B. Allergic reactions to penicillin, a panel discussion. *Journal of Allergy*, **24**, 383–404.

Rytel, M. W., Klion, F. M., Arlander, T. R. & Miller, L. F. (1963) Detection of penicillin hypersensitivity with penicilloyl-*p* polylysine. *Journal of the American Medical Association*, **186**, 894–898.

Sarkany, I. (1967) Lymphocyte transformation in drug hypersensitivity. *Lancet*, **1**, 743–745.

Sarkany, I. (1968) Clinical and laboratory aspects of drug allergy. *Proceedings of the Royal Society of Medicine*, **61**, 891.

Schild, H. O., Hawkins, D. F., Mongar, J. L. & Herxheimer, H. (1951) Reactions of isolated human asthmatic lung and bronchial tissue to a specific antigen. *Lancet*, **2**, 376.

Schultz, K. H. (1964) Allergische Hautreaktionen und Arzneimittelgruppen. *Archiv für klinische und experimentelle Dermatologie*, **219**, 277.

Schultz, K. H. & Schmidt, P. (1967) Fixe Exantheme durch drei verschiedene Arzneimittel mit getrennter Lokalisation. *Beitrag zur Frage der Barbituratallergie, Zentrolblatt für Haut- u. Geschlechtskrankheiten; Zeitschrift für Haut- u. Geschlechtskrankheiten*, **42**, 561.

13§

Schwartz, J., Klopstoack, A., Zidert-Duverani, P. & Honig, S. (1965) Detection of hyper-sensitivity by indirect rat mast cells degranulation. *International Archives of Allergy*, **26**, 33.

Selroos, O. & Edgren, J. (1975) Lupus-like syndrome associated with pulmonary reaction to nitrofurantoin. *Acta medica scandinavica*, **197**, 125.

Shapiro, S. et al (1972) Boston collaborative drug surveillance program. Excess of ampicillin rashes associated with allopurinol or hyperuricemia. *New England Journal of Medicine*, **286**, 505.

Shelley, W. B. (1962) New serological tests for allergy in man. *Nature (London)*, **195**, 1181–1183.

Shelley, W. B. (1963) Indirect basophil degranulation test for allergy to penicillin and other drugs. *Journal of the American Medical Association*, **184**, 171–178.

Shelley, W. B. & Juhlin, L. (1961) A new test for detecting anaphylactic sensitivity: the basophil reaction. *Nature (London)*, **191**, 1056–1058.

Spark, R. P. (1971) Fatal anaphylaxis due to oral penicillin. *American Journal of Clinical Pathology*, **56**, 407.

Thiel, J. A., Mitchell, S. & Parker, C. W. (1964) The specificity of hemagglutination reactions in human and experimental penicillin hypersensitivity. *Journal of Allergy*, **35**, 399–424.

Thivolet, J., Perrot, H. & Pellerat, J. (1970) Toxidermie á l'acide nalidixique (Negram). *Bulletin de la Société française de dermatologie et de syphiligraphie*, **77**, 286–288.

Van Joost, Th., Crone, R. A. & Overdijk, A. D. (1976) Ocular cicatrical pemphigoid associated with practolol therapy. *British Journal of Dermatology* (in the press).

Vischer, T. L. (1966) Lymphocyte cultures in drug hypersensitivity. *Lancet*, **2**, 467–469.

Webster, A. W. & Thompson, R. A. (1974) The ampicillin rash: lymphocyte transformation by ampicillin polymer. *Clinical and Experimental Immunology*.

Wide, L., Bennich, H. & Johansson, S. G. O. (1967) Diagnosis of allergy by an in vitro test for allergen antibodies. *Lancet*, **2**, 1105–1107.

Winfield, J. B. & Davis, J. S. (1974) Anti-DNA antibody in procainamide-induced lupus erythematosus. *Arthritis and Rheumatism*, **17**, 325–326.

Windsor, W. O., Kurrein, F. & Dyer, N. H. (1975) Fibrinous peritonitis, a complication of practolol therapy. *British Medical Journal*, **2**, 68.

Wiseman, R. A. (1971) Practolol-accumulated data on unwanted side effects. *Postgraduate Medical Journal*, **47** Suppl. 68–71.

Wright, P. (1975) Untoward effects associated with practolol administration. Oculomucocu-taneous syndrome. *British Medical Journal*, **2**, 595–598.

INDEX

Note: Numbers in square brackets indicate the number of separate mentions on the page.

PRINTED BY ADLARD AND SON LTD, BARTHOLOMEW PRESS, DORKING